COMPREHENSIVE INTRA-AORTIC
BALLOON PUMPING

D0103133

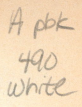
A pbk
490
White

COMPREHENSIVE INTRA-AORTIC BALLOON PUMPING

WITHDRAWN
Y 10 2

SUSAN J. QUAAL, R.N., C.V.S., M.S., CCRN

Cardiovascular Clinical Specialist,
Veterans Administration Medical Center,
and Clinical Instructor, College of Nursing,
University of Utah, Salt Lake City, Utah

with **359** illustrations

The C. V. Mosby Company

ST. LOUIS   TORONTO   1984

MOSBY

A TRADITION OF PUBLISHING EXCELLENCE

Editor: Barbara Ellen Norwitz
Assistant editor: Sally Gaines
Manuscript editor: Selena V. Bussen
Book design: Jeanne Bush
Cover design: Suzanne Oberholtzer
Production: Judy England, Judy Bamert

Copyright © 1984 by The C.V. Mosby Company

All rights reserved. No part of this publication may be reproduced, stored in a retrieval system, or transmitted, in any form or by any means, electronic, mechanical, photocopying, recording, or otherwise, without prior written permission from the publisher.

Printed in the United States of America

The C.V. Mosby Company
11830 Westline Industrial Drive, St. Louis, Missouri 63146

Library of Congress Cataloging in Publication Data

Quaal, Susan J.
   Comprehensive intra-aortic balloon pumping.

   Bibliography: p.
   Includes index.
   1. Intra-aortic balloon counterpulsation.
2. Heart failure—Treatment. 3. Heart failure—Nursing.
I. Title. [DNLM: 1. Assisted circulation. WG 168
Q103c]
RC684.I58Q3   1983   617'.413   83-897
ISBN 0-8016-4090-3

TS/VH/VH 9 8 7 6 5 4 3   02/B/269

RC
684
.I 58Q3
1984

Consulting board

DAVID BREGMAN, M.D.

Chairman, Department of Surgery, St. Joseph's Hospital and Medical Center,
Patterson, New Jersey

BERENICE LACKEY, R.N., CCRN

Regional Manager, Kontron Cardiovascular Inc.,
Chicago, Illinois

S.D. MOULOPOULOS, M.D.

Professor, University of Athens School of Medicine,
Athens, Greece

KEVIN D. MURRAY, M.D.

Surgical Research Fellow, Division of Artificial Organs, University of Utah,
Salt Lake City, Utah

MARJORIE SELF, R.N., CCRN

Clinical Education Manager, Datascope Corp.,
Paramus, New Jersey

EDMOND H. SONNENBLICK, M.D.

Professor of Medicine, Chief of Cardiology, Albert Einstein College of Medicine,
Bronx, New York

GEORGE VEASY, M.D.

Chief of Cardiology, Primary Children's Medical Center, Salt Lake City, Utah

WILLIAM F. MAAG LIBRARY
YOUNGSTOWN STATE UNIVERSITY

v

To
Mary
who believed in me

Preface

It was in the spring of 1971 on a Sunday afternoon that I was summoned to an in-service presentation on the intra-aortic balloon pump at St. Luke's Hospital in Fargo, North Dakota. Twenty-four hours later I was caring for a patient who was receiving balloon assist. This assignment was undertaken with a great deal of trepidation and with scarce literature available to help prepare me for this responsibility. Thanks to the comprehensive and steadfast instruction provided by Dr. Clif S. Hamilton, Jr., Mr. Howard McConnell, and Mr. Tony Harris, the patient and I both survived. Twelve years later I find that there is still a deficit in comprehensive teaching literature available on balloon pumping. Having had exposure to many nurses, perfusionists, and physicians who identified the need for a reference text on balloon pumping, I undertook the task of writing this book.

The individual who is introduced to balloon pumping for the first time may be overwhelmed by complicated technical data. Therefore the primary objective in writing this text is to provide a comprehensive yet practical approach to balloon pumping. An emphasis is placed on instruction of clinical concepts that are essential to the bedside care of the patient requiring balloon pumping. Ideally the text will serve as a beneficial resource for the novice balloon pump operator as well as for those who have already gained clinical experience in the care of the patient receiving balloon assistance. Most important, the concepts presented in this reference will prepare the nurse to care totally for the patient using the balloon pump by meeting his psychological as well as physiological needs.

Mechanical assistance for the failing heart now includes clinical use of the left ventricular assisting device and the Jarvik-7 artificial heart in humans. The reader is presented with factual information about these devices primarily based on animal research and limited human clinical trials.

Troubleshooting problems relevant to specific balloon consoles are deliberately omitted. All manufacturers provide supurb resource personnel and reference literature on the operation of their specific pumps. This volume makes no pretension of supplanting the training and information available from these manufacturers. The reader is therefore cautioned to obtain operating instructions relevant to the particular balloon console used in his or her institution before assuming the responsibility of caring for a patient requiring this assist modality.

Susan J. Quaal

Acknowledgments

It is with pleasure that I acknowledge my indebtedness to the following:

Willem J. Kolff, M.D., Robert K. Jarvik, M.D., Don Olsen, D.V.M., and the staff at the Division of Artificial Organs, University of Utah, for their kind assistance in the preparation of Chapter 33.

Reed Gardner, Ph.D., Chairman, Department of Biophysics, Latter Day Saints Hospital, Salt Lake City, Utah, for serving as an advisor to Chapter 21.

John Norman, M.D. (National Institutes of Health), **Robert Berger, M.D.,** Boston University, and **Jeffry Peters, M.D.,** University of Utah, for providing photographs of the left ventricular assist devices.

Berenice Lackey, R.N., CCRN, for improving my approach to timing, granting permission to reproduce tracings 8, 9, 12, 16, 18, and 19 in Chapter 15.

Bentley Laboratories, Datascope Corporation, American Edwards Laboratories, Kontron Cardiovascular, Inc., Hoek Loos, Sorenson Research, Sarns Inc., and SMEC Inc. for granting permission to quote and reproduce illustrations from their marketing literature.

Kathleen Stokes, R.N., M.S., and Elaine Kiess Daily, R.N., R.C.V.T., for their early reviews and constructive criticism.

Katie Mackin for her excellent illustrations, undertaken with great zeal, accuracy, and independent research.

Leo Schamroth, M.D., for teaching me the art of using simplistic illustrations.

Bobbi Maire and Renata von Glehn for their precision in the preparation of the manuscript.

Friends and colleagues who afforded constructive criticism, and most importantly to all my patients whose cases served as sources for my learning.

Contents

COMPREHENSIVE INTRA-AORTIC BALLOON PUMPING

CHAPTER 1 Introduction

Medical management of the patient with a catastrophic cardiac problem has traditionally centered around treatments that rested the failing heart while maintaining circulation. Options available in treatment modalities have changed drastically from the days of bed rest and the digitalis leaf. Today's available therapy includes sophisticated intensive care units equipped with nurses and physicians who are trained to render expert care to the patient. Preparation for this responsibility has included training in arrhythmia recognition, hemodynamic monitoring, and judicious use of therapeutic agents.

Despite the impressive array of treatment modalities available to the patient who is seriously ill from a cardiac problem, and regardless of the level of proficiency of intensive nursing care, infarction, which is complicated by cardiogenic shock, has remained the major cause of mortality from cardiac disease.[9] A reversal of the cardiogenic shock process has been demonstrated in humans with the use of mechanical circulatory assistance in the form of intra-aortic balloon pumping (IABP).[14] The profoundly depressed left ventricle, once capable of satisfactory ejection, has demonstrated dramatic recuperative powers if allowed to rest. Expanded use of the IABP now includes the following: (1) unstable angina refractory to medical therapy, (2) preoperative and intraoperative assist, (3) circulatory stabilization in patients with sudden development of ventricular septal defect and mitral regurgitation, and (4) postoperative interim organ support. Pediatric application of balloon pumping is an expanded development of the 1980s.[15] Patients with less than optimal cardiac performance have also benefited from balloon support while undergoing general surgical procedures.[12]

Mechanical support of the failing heart is therefore evolving into a discipline nearly unto itself. During the past three decades, considerable progress has been made in the development of devices that augment, supplement, and replace the heart. Numerous designs are currently marketed for the purpose of mechanical support of the failing heart, but their principles are uniformly simple. Circulatory assist centers on reducing or totally replacing the work effort of the heart as a pump and improving systemic and coronary circulation.

Circulatory support devices may be temporary, thus allowing corrective surgery to be performed on the heart (extracorporeal circulation) or assisting the recovery of the failing natural heart (IABP). The IABP essentially is an intravascular volume displacement device that augments the circulation by the displacement of aortic blood volume in diastole and reduces the work load of ventricular ejection in systole. Temporary mechanical assistance can also be achieved with a left ventricular assist device that allows the left ventricle to completely rest during systole. Finally the permanent design of mechanical assist, the artificial heart, is currently receiving the major emphasis on development.

It is fascinating to note the historical development of mechanical support. An early method of counterpulsation was developed from the research of Clauss and associates in 1961.[4] A pump actuator was used to withdraw a fixed volume of blood from bilateral femoral arterial catheters during systole, which reduced pressures in the aortic root. This volume of blood was reinfused during diastole. Each exchange was timed to the electrocardiogram. In the normotensive person, left ventricular work decreased, and coronary perfusion was increased; myocardial oxygen supply and demand were improved. This concept was initially received with great enthusiasm and was reported to have been used successfully. However, the extracorporeal handling of blood was a major problem clinically.[6]

Conception, design, assembly, and testing of the first intra-aortic balloon pump took place in Dr. Willem Kolff's laboratory at the Cleveland Clinic in 1961.[13] Stephen R. Topaz, a mechanical engineering graduate from Purdue and Dr. Spiro Moulopoulos, a cardiologist from Athens, tested their engineering genius on an intra-aortic balloon in a mock-circulatory loop. They combined the concepts of counterpulsation and diastolic augmentation with an approach of introducing a distensible balloon placed over a catheter into the aorta. When inflated with carbon dioxide, this balloon displaced a volume of blood in the aorta, corresponding to that removed by the actuator in the early design by Clauss. Intra-aortic compartmental blood displacement eliminated red blood cell traumatization by external instrumentation. Over a 6-month period, the balloon was modified and tested on animals. It was finally clinically tested in a resuscitation attempt following catheterization on a patient of Dr. Mason Sones.

The original IABP was used only a few times in terminal circumstances, and there were no survivors.[14] Further development and testing ensued over the next 5 years, sponsored by the artificial heart program of the National Heart and Lung Institute. Clinical application of intra-aortic balloon counterpulsation is credited to Kantrowitz in 1967.[7] A single-chambered helium-driven balloon was inserted in two patients with medically refractory left ventricular power failure. The circulatory status of both patients improved, and one individual was eventually discharged from the hospital.

Researchers at the AVCO Everett Research Laboratory and the surgical cardiovascular unit at Massachusetts General Hospital collaborated their efforts in perfecting balloon design. As studies progressed, the importance of the aortic diameter in relation to balloon size became obvious. Aortic diameter was known to decrease with hypotension, which severely altered the inflation pattern of a single-chambered balloon. In 1968 Kantrowitz[8] fabricated a polyurethane trisegmented balloon that inflated from the central segment and then toward the ends with reusable helium. Kantrowitz's balloon design brought impressive results in clinical trials with 27 patients. Feola[5] advanced the technique of balloon pumping by studying counterpulsation under fluoroscopy. He produced data that indicated that the timing of inflation and deflation was of critical importance.

Hemodynamic benefits of balloon pumping were seriously researched by Buckley,[3] initially in animal models and later in humans in 1970. Buckley documented that balloon inflation in diastole augmented perfusion, but equally important he dramatically illustrated how balloon deflation just before systole markedly reduced the resistance to left ventricular ejection and thereby reduced cardiac work and myocardial oxygen consumption.

In an attempt to develop a balloon that would more effectively improve cardiovascular dynamics, Bregman and Goetz[1] developed a dual-chambered balloon in 1972 that was designed with a large proximal balloon and a smaller distal balloon. The rationale behind this design was to produce a unidirectional blood flow proximally to the brain and coronary arteries by initial inflation of the distal, smaller balloon. This resulted in a blocking of the distal blood flow and an augmenting of proximal or forward flow.

In 1970 Mundth and his associates[14] introduced balloon pumping in the treatment of patients with cardiogenic shock, and they extended this application to those who required cardiac surgery following myocardial infarction. Aside from clinical pilot studies, the lag time from IABP conception (1961) to widespread clinical use was approximately 10 years.

By 1976, in the United States, more than 5000 patients with circulatory insufficiency following cardiotomy received balloon assistance. An equal number of patients received balloon support in other countries.[15] Today IABP is the most widely accepted and clinically used form of ventricular assist; the principle has not changed since the original inception in 1962. Pulsatile assist devices, percutaneous insertion technique, and modification of balloon pumping for pediatric usage have evolved within the last decade. Current research developments in the field of balloon pumping lie in improvements in console design and accompanying patient monitoring devices.

More recently, logical progression of mechanical assist in the form of intravascular volume displacement has extended to the use of extravascular volume capturing devices, such as true, implantable extracorporeal and intracorporeal blood pumps. These devices are sought when the IABP is insufficient to assist the failing heart. The left ventricular assist device has now been clinically used successfully in weaning patients from cardiopulmonary bypass, in cardiogenic shock following infarction, and as a bridge to cardiac transplantation during the interim period of searching for a suitable donor.

The principal emphasis on mechanical assist research today lies in the total artificial heart. Although the aforementioned techniques of counterpulsation reduce cardiac work, the pumping heart still maintains the circulation. In the event of circulatory collapse from cardiac pump failure, mechanical flow assistance is necessary. Transplant is more highly developed than permanent mechanical circulatory support, but the problems of limited donor availability and transplant rejection prevent cardiac allografting from becoming the leading treatment for patients with myopathies.

The Jarvik-7 total artificial heart, developed at the University of Utah, is the only artificial heart design that has received Food and Drug Administration approval for human implant. Animal experience with this device strongly suggests that it is within current technical grasp for an artificial heart to function for a long period in humans and for the recipient to maintain good health. On December 2, 1982, the Jarvik-7 artificial heart was implanted in a 61-year-old man at the University of Utah. The patient survived for 112 days.

Critical care team members are currently poised on an era in which care of the patient requiring the IABP is becoming commonplace. With that premise in mind, the reader is guided through this text with the purpose of more comprehensively understanding concepts of balloon pumping and other modes of ventricular assist.

Hemodynamic monitoring is included as an adjunct to balloon pumping. Balloon flotation catheterization of the central circulation clearly provides meaningful and vitally important data for the management of the patient who needs balloon pump assist. Essential to beneficial patient hemodynamic monitoring is an appreciation for the basic principles of bio-instrumentation and the significance of normal and abnormal physiological data retrieved. Such is the approach taken in the supportive chapters on hemodynamic monitoring.

REFERENCES

1. Bregman, D., and Goetz, R.H.: A new concept in circulatory assistance—the dual-chambered intra-aortic balloon, Mt. Sinai J. Med. N.Y. **39:**123, 1972.
2. Buckley, M.J., et al.: Hemodynamic evaluation of intra-aortic balloon pumping in man, Circulation **41**(suppl. 2):130, 1970.
3. Buckley, M.J., et al.: Intra-aortic balloon pump assist for cardiogenic shock after cardiopulmonary bypass, Circulation **48**(suppl. 3):90, 1973.
4. Clauss, R.H., et al.: Assisted circulation I. The arterial counterpulsator, J. Thorac. Cardiovasc. Surg. **41:**447, 1961.
5. Feola, M., et al.: Intraaortic balloon pumping in the experimental animal. Effects and problems, Am. J. Cardiol. **27:**129, 1971.
6. Jacoby, J.A., et al.: Clinical experience with counterpulsation in coronary artery disease, J. Thorac. Cardiovasc. Surg. **56:**848, 1968.
7. Kantrowitz, A., et al.: Initial clinical experiences with intra-aortic balloon pumping in cardiogenic shock, JAMA **203:**135, 1968.
8. Kantrowitz, A., et al.: Phase-shift balloon pumping in medically refractory cardiogenic shock. Results in 27 patients, Arch. Surg. **99:**739, 1969.
9. Mason, D.T., et al.: Diagnosis and management of myocardial infarction and shock. In Eliot, R.S., et al., editors: Cardiac emergencies, ed. 2, Mount Kisco, N.Y., 1982, Futura Publishing Co., Inc.
10. McGee, J.E.: Intra-aortic balloon pump: a perspective, J. Nat. Med. Assoc. **73:**885, 1981.
11. Michaels, R., et al.: Intra-aortic balloon pumping in myocardial infarction and unstable angina, European Heart J. **1:**31, 1980.
12. Miller, M., and Hall, S.V.: Intra-aortic balloon counterpulsation in a high-risk cardiac patient undergoing emergency gastrectomy, Anesthesiology **42:**103, 1975.
13. Moulopoulos, S.E., et al.: Diastolic balloon pumping (with carbon dioxide) in the aorta—a mechanical assistance to the failing circulation, Am. Heart J. **63:**669, 1962.
14. Mundth, E.D., et al.: Circulatory assistance in emergency direct coronary artery surgery for shock complicating acute myocardial infarction, N. Engl. J. Med. **283:**1382, 1970.
15. Norman, J.D.: Mechanical circulatory assistance and replacement: an evolving perspective, Bull. Texas Heart Institute **4:**445, 1980.
16. Veasy, L.G., et al.: Preclinical evaluation of intra-aortic balloon pumping for pediatric use, Trans. Am. Soc. Artif. Organs **27:**490, 1981.

CHAPTER 2 Physiological fundamentals relevant to balloon pumping

Essential to an understanding of the physiological benefits of balloon pumping is a foundation of normal cardiac physiology. Specifically, the series circuit arrangement of the right and left heart pumps and the intricate dynamics of left pump function must be appreciated. Working in a series circuit, these two pumps provide the force necessary to propel the venous blood into the pulmonic circulation and the oxygenated blood into the systemic circulation (Fig. 2-1). Intra-aortic balloon assist may be employed when the left ventricle fails to provide the pumping effort required.

The pulmonary circuit is a low-pressure system, offering little resistance to blood flow from the right ventricle. Conversely, the high-pressure systemic circulation presents considerably greater resistance to left ventricular blood flow. Therefore the work load of the right ventricle is much lighter than that of the left, and right ventricular wall thickness is

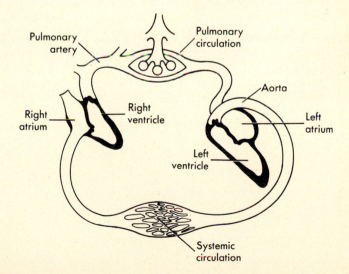

FIG. 2-1 Normal cardiopulmonary circulation. Right and left ventricles are in series circuit with pulmonary and systemic circulations.

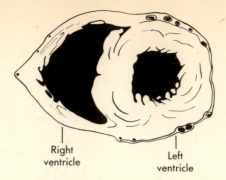

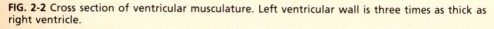

FIG. 2-2 Cross section of ventricular musculature. Left ventricular wall is three times as thick as right ventricle.

only one third that of the left ventricle (Fig. 2-2). A review of left ventricular function is necessary before proceeding to a discussion of the physiological action of balloon pumping because the principal goal of balloon assistance is to reduce the work load of the left ventricle. Normal left ventricular performance expectations must first be reviewed. Concepts of preload and afterload apply to both the right and left pumps, but the discussion that follows is restricted to a definition applicable to the left ventricle and balloon pumping. We begin with a rudimentary and brief review of the duties of each heart chamber and then concentrate on principles specific to left ventricular function.

The heart
Right atrium

The right atrium functions as a conduit to transport the systemic blood returned through the vena cava and the coronary sinus to the right ventricle (Fig. 2-3, *A*). Right atrial venous return flows passively through the tricuspid valve into the right ventricle. An additional 20% of ventricular filling occurs during atrial contraction; this added contribution to the cardiac output is termed the *atrial kick*.

Right ventricle

Work required of the right ventricle is modest compared to demands placed on the left ventricle. Normally the pulmonary bed offers little resistance to right ventricular contraction (Fig. 2-3, *B*). Resistance may drastically increase in the presence of a pulmonary embolism, which could cause massive right ventricular failure. The most common cause of right ventricular failure, however, is left ventricular failure. A look at the series circuit arrangement lends appreciation for the influence left-sided failure exerts on the right side.

Left atrium

The left atrium passively empties the oxygenated blood received from the lungs via four pulmonary veins, through the mitral valve, and into the left ventricle (Fig. 2-3, *C*).[6] Since no true valves separate the pulmonary veins from the left atrium, elevation of left atrial pressure is readily reflected retrogradely into the pulmonary vasculature.

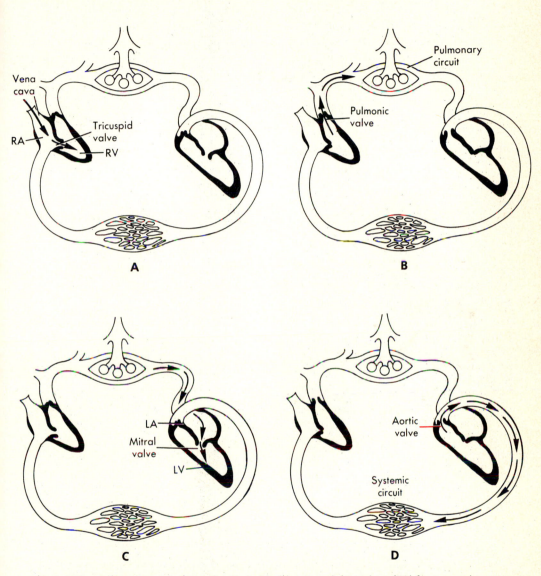

FIG. 2-3 Blood flow through series circuit. **A,** Blood enters right atrium *(RA)* from superior vena cava, inferior vena cava, and coronary sinus and flows passively to right ventricle *(RV)* through tricuspid valve. **B,** Blood volume is propelled from RV through pulmonic valve and out into lungs. **C,** Oxygenated blood flows from lungs via four pulmonary veins to left atrium *(LA),* through mitral valve, and into left ventricle *(LV).* **D,** High pressure generation by LV finally propels blood through aortic valve and out into aorta and systemic circulation during ventricular systole.

WILLIAM F. MAAG LIBRARY
YOUNGSTOWN STATE UNIVERSITY

Left ventricle

High pressure generation is a requirement of left ventricular function to overcome the resistance of the systemic circulation and to deliver the blood through the aortic valve to the peripheral arterial tree (Fig. 2-3, *D*). Contributing to the development of high pressure during left ventricular contraction is the circular shape and thick musculature of this chamber (see intramyocardial wall tension, p. 17). The intraventricular septum also contributes to the powerful compression sustained during contraction.[9]

Conduction system

Synchronized contraction and relaxation of the previously mentioned chambers follow an inherent rhythmicity of the cardiac muscle. Fig. 2-4 illustrates the conduction network. The highest level of automaticity lies in the sinoatrial (SA) node located in the posterior wall of the right atrium, immediately beneath the point of entry of the superior vena cava. Once the impulse is discharged from the SA node, it travels first to the atria, causing them to depolarize and contract, and then it propagates to the atrioventricular (AV) node, where it is delayed a few hundredths of a second before it is released to pass through the bundle of His, the bundle branches, and the Purkinje network. This delay of the impulse in the AV node allows blood to flow from atria to ventricles before ventricular contraction.[12,21]

Depolarization and repolarization: action potential

Electrochemical activity precedes the mechanical contraction of the heart muscle. Intracellular and extracellular fluids are electrolyte solutions composed of negative and positive ions. Ion fluxes across the cell membrane shift the electrical charges, which causes depolarization and repolarization. Depolarization of the myocardial cell occurs when the inside of the cell becomes less negative. Repolarization is the process by which the cell returns to its resting state. These changes in electrical potential across the cell membrane constitute what is referred to as the *cardiac action potential*. Insertion of a

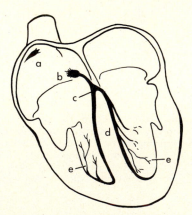

FIG. 2-4 Conduction system of heart. *a,* SA node; *b,* AV node, *c,* Bundle of His; *d,* Bundle branches; *e,* Purkinje fibers.

microelectrode into the cell allows the recording of this action potential (Fig. 2-5).

Five phases are characteristic of a myocardial cell action potential. Briefly, when the microelectrode is introduced into the myocardial muscle cell (nonpacemaker cell), the graph reading plunges to about -90 millivolts. Phase 0 represents rapid cellular depolarization. Phases 1 through 3 represent the three stages of repolarization, and phase 4 is the period of electrical diastole. Phase 4 of the myocardial fiber differs from a pacemaker cell in that the myocardial fiber requires some sort of stimulus to jar the cell membrane to cause an ion flux—hence depolarization. A pacemaker cell is therefore self-perpetuating and continuously generating new action potentials during phase 4.[14]

Ventricular systole and diastole

Understanding the systolic and diastolic phases of the cardiac cycle is important in later chapters in which the physiological outcome of intra-aortic balloon inflation and deflation and the timing of this inflation-deflation sequence in proper synchronization with the cardiac cycle are discussed. Physiologically, systole is considered to begin approximately with closure of the AV valves and to end approximately with their opening.[10] The breakdown of ventricular systole and diastole has been approached in several ways. More important is an understanding of the events that occur during contraction and relaxation of the ventricles. Both systole and diastole are described in terms of early and late phases (Fig. 2-6). In early diastole the mitral and tricuspid valves are open, and blood entering the atria through venous channels flows passively and rapidly into the ventricles through the open AV valves. Finally the atria contract, contributing an additional 20% to ventricular volume. At this point, the ventricular filling phase reaches a plateau. Such an interval of unchanging ventricular volume is termed the *period of diastasis*. In early systole the papillary muscles are excited and begin to contract. The shortening papillary muscles exert traction on the chordae tendinae, drawing the AV valves into apposition. Since all four valves are closed, the contracting muscles elevate the pressure in the ventricle but do not change the volume contained in the ventricle. Thus the interval during which ventricular

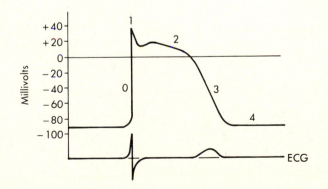

FIG. 2-5 Myocardial cell action potential. Phase 0, rapid influx of sodium (depolarization); phases 1 to 3, stages of repolarization; phase 4, electrical diastole.

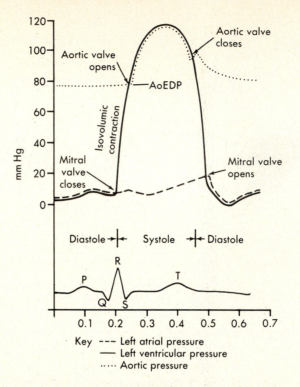

FIG. 2-6 Electrical and mechanical cycles of left heart. P wave is noted (atrial depolarization) to immediately precede the atrial pressure wave generated by atrial contraction. QRS complex represents ventricular depolarization, which is followed by left ventricular contraction and rise of left ventricular pressure to 120 mm Hg during peak systole. Systole begins with QRS complex and ends with T wave. Diastole begins with T wave and ends with onset of QRS complex. Aortic pressure curve is represented as 120 mm Hg in systole and 80 mm Hg in diastole. *(AoEDP, Aortic end-diastolic pressure.)*

pressure rises to a level sufficient to open the semilunar valves by overcoming the aortic end-diastolic pressure is termed *isovolumic contraction*. This is an extremely important phase of the cardiac cycle to understand in relation to balloon pumping, and it is discussed later in greater detail. As soon as the ventricular pressure exceeds the aortic end-diastolic pressure, the aortic valve opens, and ventricular ejection into the systemic circulation occurs.[2,3,20]

Blood flow

Ventricular systole causes a propulsion of blood from the left ventricle to the systemic circuit. During ventricular relaxation, or diastole, this driving force is absent, but blood flow to the peripheral tissues continues. The elastic proximal aorta and large arteries stretch to accommodate cardiac stroke volume in systole.[1] This permits much of the force imparted to the blood by ventricular contraction to be stored as potential energy in the elastic arterial wall. When the heart relaxes and the intravascular pressure falls, these stretched fibers in aorta recoil, maintaining a pressure head (Fig. 2-7). Runoff into the peripheral tissues continues in diastole under the pressure head created by the stored elastic

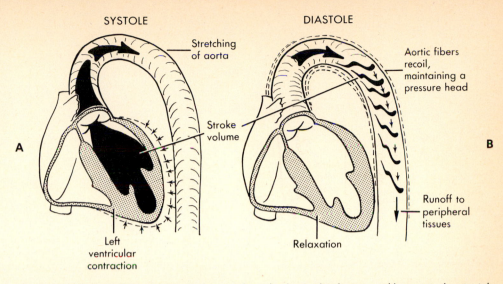

SYSTOLE   DIASTOLE

Stretching of aorta

Aortic fibers recoil, maintaining a pressure head

Stroke volume

A   B

Runoff to peripheral tissues

Left ventricular contraction   Relaxation

FIG. 2-7 Windkessel effect. **A,** Ventricular systole—elastic proximal aorta and large arteries stretch to accommodate cardiac stroke volume. Force imparted to blood by ventricular contraction is stored as potential energy in elastic arterial wall. **B,** Ventricular diastole—fibers in aorta, which were stretched in systole, now recoil, maintaining a pressure head. Runoff into peripheral tissues continues in diastole under this pressure head created by stored elastic energy in the aorta.

energy in the aorta. The temporary storage of much of the stroke volume during the ejection period is termed the *Windkessel effect*. This effect serves to smooth out the flow of blood in the circulation so that flow continues during diastole. Without the Windkessel effect, the blood would reach the tissues in spurts.[3,18]

Determinants of cardiac output

Cardiac output is the product of heart rate and stroke volume. Stroke volume, the volume of blood pumped by the ventricle per beat, averages 70 ml in the adult. Thus at a heart rate of 70 beats per minute, the cardiac output would equal 4900 ml per minute. Stroke volume, which represents myocardial performance, is dependent on the following four distinct but interrelated variables: preload, afterload, contractility or inotropic state of the heart, and heart rate (Fig. 2-8).[6,25]

Preload: Frank-Starling law of the heart. In 1884 Howell and Donaldson[8] presented their findings that the heart possesses an intrinsic mechanism by which its output is adjusted to the venous input. This concept, known as *preload*, establishes that the length of the ventricular fiber before contraction (fiber stretch caused by end-diastolic volume) determines the strength of the contraction. The capacity of the intact ventricle to vary its force of contraction on a beat-to-beat basis as a function of end-diastolic fiber length constitutes the *Frank-Starling law of the heart*.[5,22] When cardiac muscle fibers are stretched before contraction because of increased end-diastolic volume, a greater contractile effort ensues[2] (Fig. 2-9). Simplistically this concept can be presented by examining the effect on the water pressure generated with release of the balloon (Fig. 2-10) from varying volumes of water in a balloon before its release. Increasing the water volume before release of the

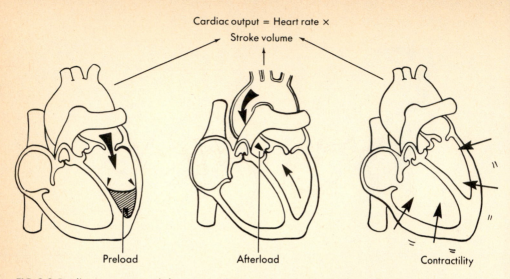

FIG. 2-8 Cardiac output equals heart rate times stroke volume. Factors influencing stroke volume are preload, afterload, and contractility (see text for discussion).

balloon nets a greater force of pressure generated when the balloon is released.

The gain falls off when myocardial fibers are stretched beyond "physiological limits"; further stretching fails to produce a positive effect on the force of ventricular contraction (Fig. 2-11). Because end-diastolic fiber length and intraventricular pressure are normally related to each other, it is common in clinical practice to monitor the left ventricular end-diastolic pressure or pulmonary artery wedge pressure as representative of left ventricular fiber length. In this normal Starling curve very slight changes in fiber length, produced by small changes in left ventricular end-diastolic pressure, are associated with significant increases in stroke volume. In many cases a patient's myocardial muscle appears to operate chronically at the maximal projection length. Therefore he is unable to significantly respond to increased filling or stretch with a greater force of contraction.[1,2,11,13,15]

Afterload. The resistance to left ventricular ejection is termed the *afterload* component of cardiac work. For the left ventricle the major contributors of afterload are the aortic impedance and the peripheral vascular resistance. The aortic end-diastolic pressure represents the pressure resistance the left ventricle must overcome to push open the aortic valve during the phase of isovolumic contraction (Fig. 2-12).[13,20] Aortic end-diastolic pressure is an extremely important landmark in balloon pumping; the net outcome is to produce a lowering of this aortic end-diastolic pressure. Approximately 90% of myocardial oxygen consumption occurs during this isovolumic phase as the heart works against the afterload. Anticipated physiological improvement to the patient with balloon assistance would be to reduce the afterload and myocardial oxygen consumption during isovolumic contraction.

Contractility. Contractility refers to the changes in the force of myocardial contraction

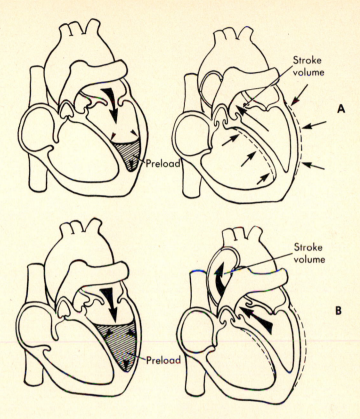

FIG. 2-9 A, Increased preload (end-diastolic volume) stretches contractile fibers just before systole, enabling left ventricle to contract with greater vigor. **B,** Additional preload results in even greater stroke volume ejected during systole.

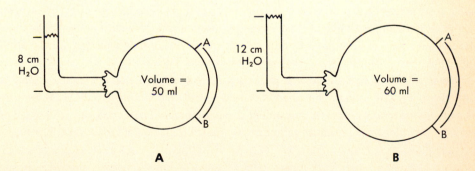

FIG. 2-10 Effect of preload on ensuing ventricular systole, using analogy of balloon filled with water and attached to manometer **(A)**. Balloon is filled with 50 ml of water. On release, 8 cm of water pressure is generated **(B)**. Balloon is now filled with 60 ml of water. Added stretch is placed on balloon wall (tangent A to B). On release of balloon, 12 cm of water pressure is generated.

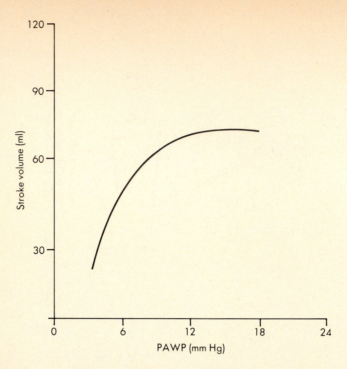

FIG. 2-11 Starling's curve of the heart. Increasing preload (pulmonary artery wedge pressure, *PAWP*) results in greater force of contraction in systole, but only to a certain physiological point. Thereafter, increasing end-diastolic volume does not facilitate greater force of contraction, and eventually with continued added stretch on fibers, the ventricle may fail.

and is a function of the interaction between the contractile elements (actomyosin cross-bridges, Chapter 3) at the cellular level. By definition contractility refers to the alterations in the force of contraction that occur independently of myocardial fiber length. Contractility may be increased by sympathetic stimulation that may occur with endogenous production of catecholamines or with those exogenously administered in the form of epinephrine, norepinephrine, isoproterenol, dopamine, or calcium. These drugs effect an increase in inotropic (increased force of contraction) performance of the heart muscle. Myocardial contractility may be decreased by hypoxemia and by the following drugs: propranolol, quinidine, procainamide, lidocaine, and barbiturates.[2,6,19]

Heart rate. Acceleration of the frequency of contraction increases stroke volume at any given level of filling. This phenomenon is termed the *staircase* or *Bowditch effect*. However, the reduction in the duration of diastole at rapid heart rates can interfere with ventricular filling time, ultimately limiting the rise in cardiac output associated with tachycardia.[7,16]

Factors influencing vascular resistance

Braunwald[2] identifies the major stimuli that are responsible for alterations in vessel caliber and therefore vascular resistance as the following: (1) metabolic, hormonal, or

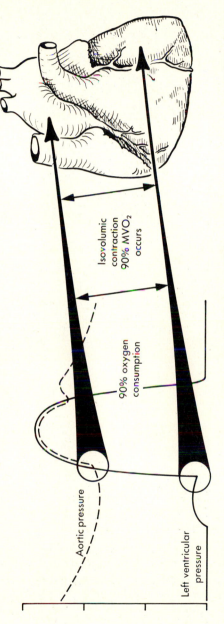

FIG. 2-12 Isovolumic contraction—early systolic phase of cardiac cycle. All four heart valves are closed, and left ventricle is required to generate enough pressure to overcome aortic end-diastolic pressure to push open aortic valve. Systolic ejection then follows. Approximately 90% of myocardial oxygen consumption (MVO$_2$) occurs during isovolumic contraction.

Isovolumic
contraction
90% MVO$_2$
occurs

90% oxygen
consumption

Aortic pressure

Left ventricular
pressure

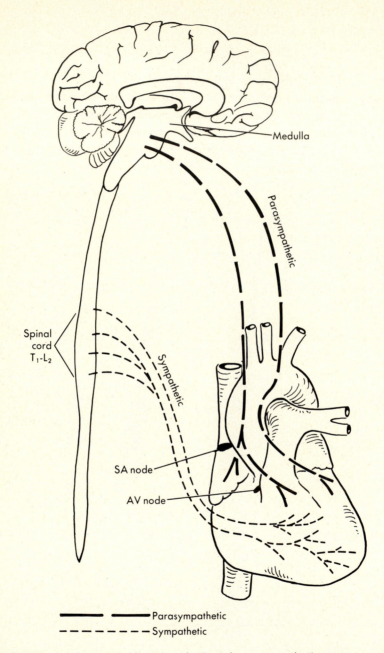

Medulla

Parasympathetic

Spinal
cord
T_1-L_2

Sympathetic

SA node

AV node

————— Parasympathetic
– – – – – – Sympathetic

FIG. 2-13 Heart is innervated by sympathetic and parasympathetic nervous systems.

chemical substances that are carried in the blood or released locally and (2) the autonomic nervous system.

Metabolic, hormonal, or chemical substances. A decrease of oxygen, an increase in potassium, or an increase in osmolality produces vasodilation. Conversely, systemic release of norepinephrine and epinephrine by the adrenal medulla, as occurs in stressful situations, can initiate potent vasoconstriction (Chapter 7).

Autonomic nervous control of the heart. Intrinsic pacemaker systems enable the heart to operate without any nervous influences. However, the efficacy of the heart action can be changed by the tonic influence of the autonomic nervous system. The heart interconnects with the autonomic nervous system via the parasympathetic (vagi) and sympathetic nerves (Fig. 2-13). Sympathetic fibers originate in the spinal cord (T1-L2) and articulate with the heart via the cervical sympathetic ganglia. Sympathetic nervous fibers supply both the atria and the ventricles. Norepinephrine is the mediator, and its effect on the heart is to increase the force of contraction and the heart rate by its stimulation of the sinus node. Sympathetic system–induced tachycardia decreases the period of diastole and coronary artery filling time.

Parasympathetic fibers originate in the medulla and reach the heart via the vagus nerve. Stimulation of the vagi causes the hormone acetylcholine to be released, causing the rate of impulse discharge from the sinus node and conduction of the impulses through the AV node to slow.[3,9,10,12]

Myocardial oxygen use: supply and demand

If the heart is deprived of oxygen for only a few minutes, mechanical activity ceases; the metabolic processes of contraction are almost totally aerobic; the heart extracts 75% to 80% of the arterial oxygen content of coronary blood. Thus the balance between oxygen supply and demand is so intricate that the demands of accelerated myocardial work can only be provided by augmenting coronary blood flow through vasodilation, since extrapolation is already extraordinarily high[17] (Fig. 2-14).

Myocardial oxygen consumption

Determinants of myocardial oxygen consumption are expressed in Fig. 2-15. Afterload, preload, contractility, and heart rate have been previously discussed. Intramyocardial wall tension is determined by the following: (1) pressure generated by the contracting ventricle in systole and (2) size of the ventricular cavity. During isovolumic contraction, ventricular radius decreases, which builds tension that contributes to the left ventricle overcoming the aortic end-diastolic pressure (afterload). An expansion of the chamber radius (cardiac dilation) nets an increased *intramyocardial wall tension*. Therefore a dilated heart requires more oxygen than a normal heart.[2,6]

Coronary circulation

Fig. 2-16 depicts a cutaway view of the left ventricle and aorta, representing anatomical locations of the coronary arteries. Orifices of the right and left coronary arteries are located within the sinuses of Valsalva in the aorta, immediately above the aortic valve.

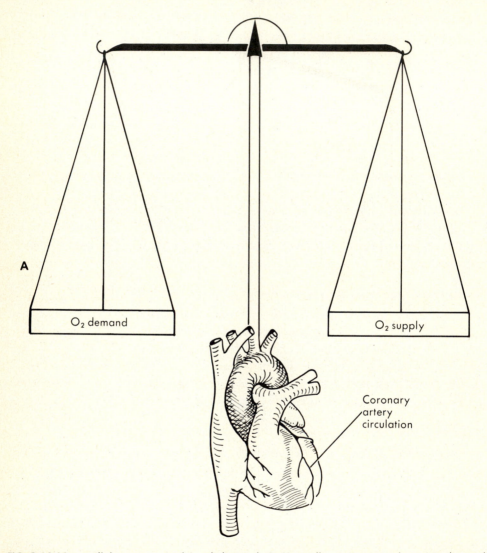

FIG. 2-14 Myocardial oxygen supply and demand. **A,** Normally, oxygen supply meets demand required with myocardial work performance.

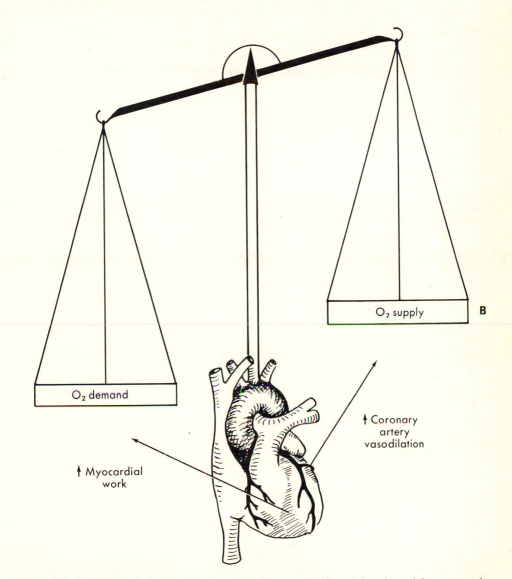

O₂ supply

O₂ demand

↑ Coronary
artery
vasodilation

↑ Myocardial
work

FIG. 2-14, cont'd B, Increased myocardial work (as may occur with peripheral arterial vasoconstriction) adds to demand for oxygen. Coronary artery vasodilation may occur as compensatory mechanism to increase perfusion and oxygen delivery to myocardium.

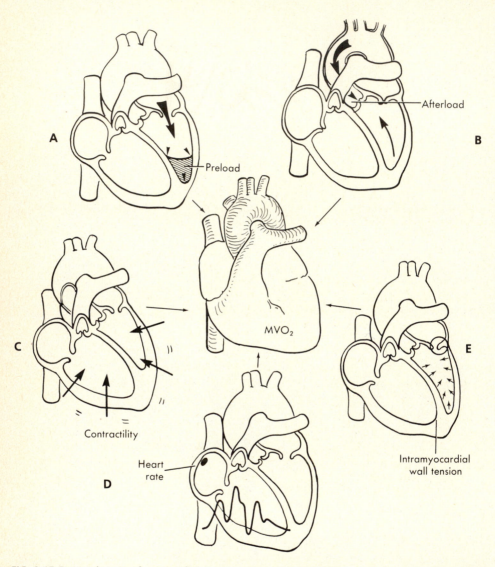

FIG. 2-15 Determinants of myocardial oxygen consumption (MVO$_2$). **A**, Preload. **B**, Afterload. **C**, Contractility. **D**, Heart rate. **E**, Intramyocardial wall tension (determined by pressure generated by contracting ventricle in systole and radius of ventricular cavity).

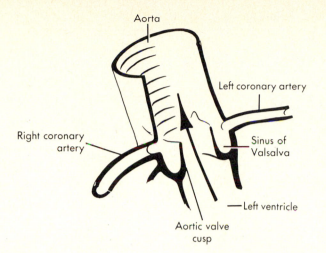

FIG. 2-16 Cutaway view of left ventricle and aorta, representing anatomical location of coronary arteries. Orifices of right and left coronary arteries are located within sinuses of Valsalva, which arise from aortic walls, immediately above aortic valve.

TABLE 2-1 Right coronary artery subdivisions

Anterior branches	Area supplied
Conus	Outflow tract of right ventricle (infundibulum)
Marginal	Anterior and posterior right ventricle
Posterior branches; transverses high across the posterior heart along the intraventricular groove that separates the two ventricles	Crux of the heart (juncture of the AV and intraventricular grooves)
Posterior descending	Posterior interventricular septum; supplies adjacent areas of the right and left ventricles
Obstruction to blood flow of the right coronary artery =	Inferior myocardial infarction

These sinuses of Valsalva appear as pockets just above the aortic valve cusps. During diastole, blood flows into and distends the sinuses and then flows out into the right and left coronary arteries. The right and left main coronary arteries and their subdividing branches are illustrated in Fig. 2-17. Arising from the anterior surface of the aorta, the right coronary artery passes diagonally toward the right side of the heart and descends in the groove between the right atrium and ventricle (the AV groove). Table 2-1 lists the subdivisions of the right coronary artery. In about 80% of the population the right coronary artery provides the posterior descending coronary vessel. The right coronary is then said to be *dominant*. In the remaining 20%, the posterior descending vessel arises from the terminal portion of the left coronary artery, which is then termed a *predominant left coronary system*.[6,7,12]

TABLE 2-2 Left coronary artery subdivisions

Branch		Area supplied
LEFT ANTERIOR DESCENDING BRANCHES		
Septal		Anterior part of interventricular septum
Anterior branches		Anterior surface of left ventricle
Diagonal branch		Supplies lateral margin of left ventricle
Obstruction to blood flow of anterior descending branch		Anterior, anterior-septal, or anterior-lateral myocardial infarction
CIRCUMFLEX BRANCHES		
Marginal		Posterior surface of left ventricle
Obstruction to circumflex branch	=	Posterior myocardial infarction

Data compiled from Hurst, J.W., et al., (editors): The heart, ed. 5, New York, 1982, McGraw-Hill Book Co.

Arising from the posterior surface of the aorta and left of the sinus of Valsalva is the left coronary artery. The short stub of a main left vessel soon divides into the following two major vessels: the anterior descending branch and the circumflex branch. The subdivisions and areas of the heart supplied by these tributary vessels are listed in Table 2-2.

Venous coronary circulation (Fig. 2-17). Once blood has circulated through the rich network of coronary capillaries, about 90% returns to the right atrium through the coronary sinus; the remainder returns through the thebesian vessels that empty directly into the right atrium.

Phasic coronary blood flow. Blood flows from the main coronary artery vessels through branches over the outer surface of the heart and then into smaller arteries in the cardiac muscle.[17] The outer, epicardial layer of the heart is supplied with blood from coronary branches that arise at acute angles from the main coronary branches (Fig. 2-18). Smaller vessels also branch at right angles from the right and left coronary arteries, which penetrate into the myocardium and endocardium (intramural arteries). The heart muscle is supplied with an unusually rich network of capillaries, but blood flow through this rich network is phasic with systolic and diastolic cycles of myocardial contraction. In contrast to blood flow in the other portions of the circulation, perfusion through the coronary arteries is generally greater in diastole than in systole. Fig. 2-19 illustrates coronary capillary circulation in systole and in diastole. Strong compression of the cardiac muscle around the deeply embedded coronary capillaries creates a marked rise in coronary vascular resistance and a phasic reduction in blood flow. During diastole, the cardiac muscle relaxes completely and no longer obstructs blood flow.

Recently Chilian and Marcus[4] at the University of Iowa studied phasic coronary circulation. During controlled conditions, the percentage of total coronary blood flow veloc-

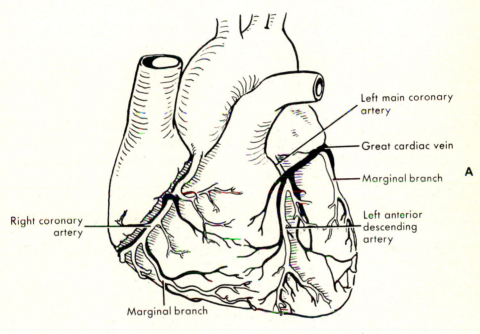

FIG. 2-17 Coronary arteries and veins. **A,** Anterior view.
Continued.

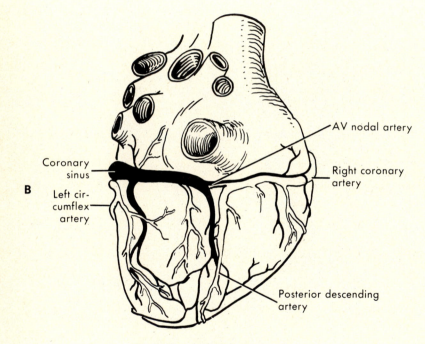

FIG. 2-17, cont'd B, Posterior view.

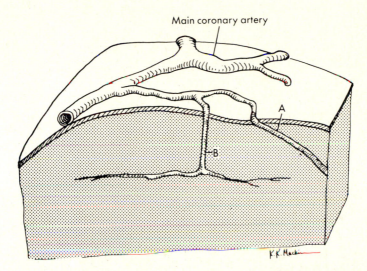

FIG. 2-18 Intramyocardial distribution of coronary arteries (A). Epicardial arteries arise at acute angles from main coronary vessels to supply epicardial surface of heart (B). Smaller vessels branch at oblique angles from main coronary vessels that penetrate deeper into myocardium and endocardium (intramural arteries).

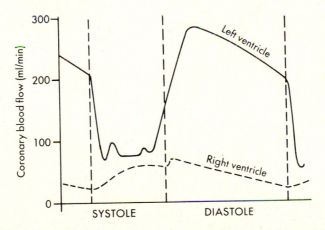

FIG. 2-19 Phasic flow of blood through coronary arteries of right and left ventricle. (From Guyton, A.: Textbook of medical physiology, ed. 5, Philadelphia, 1976, W.B. Saunders, Co. By permission.)

ity occurring during diastole per cardiac cycle was significantly greater ($p \leqq 0.05$) in the intramural artery (septal—92%) than in the epicardial artery (left anterior descending—75%). The phasic blood velocity pattern in penetrating coronary arteries was found to be different from large epicardial arteries. Blood flow velocity during mid-systole was retrograde in the intramural vessel and antegrade in the epicardial vessel. During vasodilation, following nitroglycerin, the mid-systolic retrograde flow component of the intramural artery persisted, despite large increases (300% to 400%) in the mid-systolic antegrade flow of the epicardial artery.

The right ventricular coronary capillary circulation also undergoes phasic changes in perfusion. However, the force of right ventricular contraction is significantly less than the left ventricle. Therefore the phasic reduction in coronary flow is relatively mild compared to the left ventricle.

Autoregulation of coronary blood flow. Coronary blood flow is controlled by the process of autoregulation within the coronary bed. Autoregulation is an intrinsic mechanism, maintaining a balance between local myocardial oxygen supply and demand. Myocardial tissue hypoxia is the most potent stimulus for increasing coronary blood flow and oxygen supply through vasodilation. Conversely, a reduction in oxygen demand produces a decrease in coronary blood flow through vasoconstriction.[1,11]

Collateral circulation. When a gradual narrowing of a coronary artery occurs, intercoronary communications (collateral flow) are established (Fig. 2-20). The major areas of

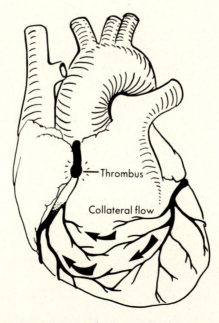

FIG. 2-20 Collateral coronary circulation. A thrombus or atherosclerotic lesion can obstruct blood flow through major coronary vessel. Intertributary communication allows flow to be reestablished distal to area of occlusion via blood flow through collateral vessels.

anastomotic connections are at the posterior surface, where the terminal portions of the right coronary artery and the left circumflex branch unite and at the apex of the heart, where the terminal portion of the anterior and posterior descending and marginal branches of the right coronary artery all converge. Collateral flow, communication in blood flow to the narrowed vessel from an alternative branch, is then established.

REFERENCES

1. Alpert, N.R., et al.: Heart muscle mechanics, Annu. Rev. Physiol. **41**:521, 1979.
2. Braunwald, E., et al.: The contraction of the normal heart. In Braunwald, E.: Heart disease: a textbook of cardiovascular medicine, Philadelphia, 1980, W.B. Saunders Co.
3. Burton, A.C.: Physiology and biophysics of the circulation, ed. 2, Chicago, 1972, Year Book Medical Publishers, Inc.
4. Chilian, W.M., and Marcus, M.L.: Phasic coronary blood flow velocity in intramural and epicardial coronary arteries, Circ. Res. **50**:775, 1982.
5. Frank, O.: On the dynamics of cardiac muscle, Am. Heart J. **58**:282, 1959. (Translated by Chapman, C.B., and Wasserman, E.)
6. Guyton, A.C.: Textbook of medical physiology, ed. 6, Philadelphia, 1982, W.B. Saunders Co.
7. Hirsch, E.F.: The innervation of human heart. IV. (1) The fiber connections of the nerves with the perimysial plexus (Gerlach-Hofmann); (2) The role of nerve tissues in the repair of infarcts, Arch. Pathol. **75**:378, 1963.
8. Howell, W.H., and Donaldson, F., Jr.: Experiments upon the heart of the dog with reference to maximum volume of blood sent out by the left ventricle in a single beat, Philos. Trans. R. Soc. Lond. (Biol.) **175**:139, 1884.
9. James, T.L., et al.: Anatomy of the heart. In Hurst, J.W., et al., editors: The heart, ed. 5, New York, 1982, McGraw-Hill Book Co.
10. Katz, A.M.P.: Physiology of the heart, New York, 1977, Raven Press.
11. Little, R.C.: Physiology of the heart and circulation, Chicago, 1977, Year Book Medical Publishers, Inc.
12. Little, R.C., editor: Physiology of atrial pacemakers and conductive tissue, Mount Kisco, N.Y., 1980, Futura Publishing Co., Inc.
13. Mahler, F., et al.: Effects of changes in preload, afterload, and inotropic state on ejection and isovolumic phase measures of contractility in the conscious dog, Am. J. Cardiol. **36**:626, 1975.
14. Marriott, H.J.L., and Conover, M.: Advanced concepts in arrhythmias, St. Louis, 1983, The C.V. Mosby Co.
15. Mirsky, I., et al.: Cardiac mechanics: physiological, clinical and mathematical considerations, New York, 1974, John Wiley & Sons, Inc.
16. Mitchell, J.H., et al.: Intrinsic effects of heart rate on left ventricular performance, Am. J. Physiol, **205**:411, 1963.
17. Pasyk, S., et al.: Systemic and coronary effects of coronary artery occlusion in the unanesthetized dog, Am. J. Physiol, **220**:646, 1971.
18. Rushmer, R.F.: Cardiovascular dynamics, ed. 4, Philadelphia, 1976, W.B. Saunders Co.
19. Sarnoff, S.J.: Myocardial contractility as described by ventricular function curves: observations on Starling's law of the heart, Physiol. Rev. **35**:107, 1955.
20. Schlant, R.C., and Sonnenblick, E.B.: Pathophysiology of heart failure. In Hurst, J.W., et al., editors: The heart, ed. 5, New York, 1982, McGraw-Hill Book Co.
21. Sommers, J.R., and Johnson, E.A.: A comparative study of purkinje fibers and ventricular fibers, J. Cell Biol. **36**:497, 1968.
22. Starling, E.H.: The Linacre lecture on the law of the heart, London, 1918, Longmans, Green and Co., Ltd.
23. Wiggers, C.J.: Determinants of cardiac prformance, Circulation **4**:485, 1951.

CHAPTER 3 Cardiac muscle ultrastructure and function

Understanding the fundamental mechanisms of contraction of the normal and failing heart is essential to a textbook on IABP. Impaired contractile function, resulting in cardiac failure, is a precipitating factor that may necessitate IABP. Contraction of the myocardium is a result of the integrated function of its individual contractile elements. This chapter initially defines the ultrastructure of the myocardium and correlates the described organelles with their functional activities during the contraction process.

Myocardial ultrastructure

Myocardial ultrastructure, as described by Fawcett and McNutt[6] is illustrated in Fig. 3-1. The myocardium is composed of longitudinal series of bundles of myocardial cells that interdigitate with each other to form a fiber, the myofibril. Most of these fibers are arrayed parallel to one another with the mitochondria, the energy source for contraction, sandwiched between the myofibrils.

Within the cell the myocardial ultrastructure consists of the following organelles: the cell membrane or sarcolemma, the intercalated disk, sarcomeres, myofibrils, actin, myosin, tropomyosin and troponin proteins, the sarcotubular system, and the mitochondria.[7]

Sarcolemma (cell membrane)

The sarcolemma separates intracellular constituents from the extracellular fluid. Numerous vesicles are found immediately external to and within the membrane as well as within the cytoplasm of the cell. These vesicles are termed *pinocytotic,* capable of absorbing liquids by phagocytosis, and are presumably involved in cellular metabolism. The functions ascribed to the sarcolemma are (1) separation of intracellular and extracellular environments, (2) membrane transport activity as necessary for cellular metabolism, (3) active maintenance of the ionic composition of the cell, and (4) transmembrane movement of ions, producing electrical currents that are manifested in the electrocardiogram.[4,15]

Intercalated disk

Electron microscopic examination reveals that each cell is separated by an intercalated disk. Therefore the cells of the working myocardium are not an anatomical *syncytium* (a

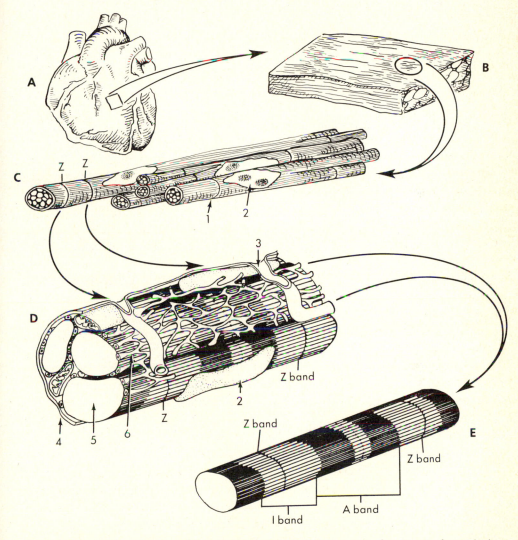

FIG. 3-1 Microscopic structures of heart muscle. **A** to **B,** Enlargement of segment of ventricular myocardium. **C,** Myofibril *(1),* intercalated disk *(2),* and mitochondria. **D,** Microscopic ultrastructure *(3),* T tubule, *(4)* sarcolemma, *(5)* myofibril, and *(6)* sarcoplasmic reticulum. **E,** Enlargement of myofibril. (See text for discussion.)

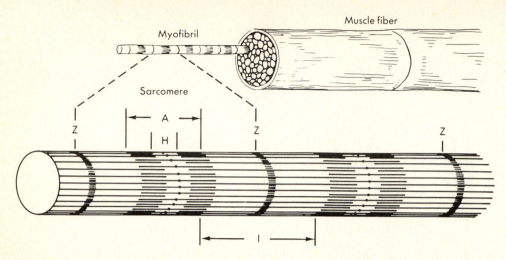

FIG. 3-2 Ultrastructure of working myocardial cell, illustrating Z band (separates each contractile unit or sarcomere), I band (actin filaments), A band (overlapping of myosin filaments from actin filaments), and H zone (region occupied only by myosin filaments).

group of cells in which the protoplasm of one cell is continuous with that of adjoining cells). However, these boundaries offer little electrical resistance so that the myocardium is considered a functional syncytium. In working myocardial cells the myofibrils insert into the region of the intercalated disk. The disk must therefore possess great strength to support the forces generated by repeated contraction of the myofibrils.[4,10,11]

Myofibrils

Each cardiac muscle fiber contains a group of branching longitudinal, striated strands approximately 1 μm in diameter, termed *myofibrils*. The myofibrils exhibit a characteristic pattern of light and dark transverse bands and are subdivided into a series of repeating contractile units, the sarcomeres, by a dark, transverse line, the *Z band* (Fig. 3-2). The sarcomere functions as the contractile unit of the cell and is ideally suited to the structural aspects of contraction as a result of its elongated shape.[9,12]

Sarcomeres exhibit a band appearance because they are composed of an ordered array of two different overlapping protein filaments, *actin* (thin) and *myosin* (thick). Actin filaments extend in both directions from the Z band that produces a light area, the *I band* (Fig. 3-2), so called because it rotates polarized light under the electron microscope. Myosin fibrils overlap onto the actin filaments, which gives rise to a darker, transverse band, the *A band*. The central light area *(H zone)* of the A band represents the regions occupied only by the myosin filaments.[8,16]

Myosin filaments

The myosin (thick) filaments extend throughout the A band, from one A-I band boundary to the next (Fig. 3-3). Myosin is a rod-shaped molecule with a globular enlargement at one end. Localized in this globular head are two important biological properties.

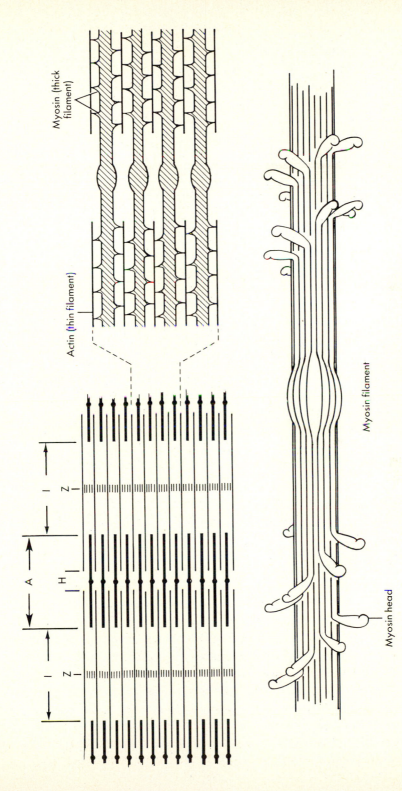

Myosin (thick filament)

Actin (thin filament)

Myosin filament

Myosin head

FIG. 3-3 Organization of thick myosin filaments of sarcomere.

1. Myosin has the ability to hydrolyze the polyphosphate chain on adenosine triphosphate (ATP), thereby releasing chemical energy.

2. Myosin heads come together with the actin filaments to form cross-bridges in a sliding mechanism that results in contraction[8,20] (Chapter 4).

Actin, tropomyosin, troponin proteins

Thin filaments are composed of the following three proteins: actin, tropomyosin, and troponin. The actin protein is much smaller than myosin. Unlike myosin, which is a highly asymmetrical structure, actin forms a slightly ovoid shape. The thin actin filaments are helically arranged like a double string of beads twisted together (Fig. 3-4). Tropomyosin has no biological properties. Similar to the tail of the myosin molecule, tropomyosin was found to be a coiled tail.[1] Troponin is the receptor for calcium and acts to modulate the interaction between actin and myosin through alterations in tropomyosin.[2,10]

The troponin complex is now recognized to be made up of three proteins. Troponin-I, like tropomyosin, has the ability to inhibit the interaction of actin and myosin. Troponin-T serves to bind the troponin complex to tropomyosin, and troponin-C contains the binding site for calcium.[2,19] Therefore the major effect of the troponin-tropomyosin complex is to inhibit the ability of actin to interact with myosin. The contribution of calcium to the contraction process is further discussed in Chapter 4.

Sarcotubular system

Membrane-limited microtubules, the *sarcotubular system,* fill the interfibrillar spaces of cardiac muscle. The network is composed of the following two elements: a transverse component called the *T system* and a longitudinal component, the *sarcoplasmic reticulum (SR)* (Fig. 3-1).

The T-tubule system originates from invaginations along the surface of the sarcolemma. This transverse tubular system provides an extension of the sarcolemma into the cell; hence the tubular content is continuous with the extracellular fluid, possibly has a similar ionic content, and may be involved in the movement of substrates into the cell and the removal of metabolic end products from the cell.[17,18]

The SR is an entirely intracellular system of tubules that forms a membrane-limited network around each myofibril. A single T tubule passes between two myofibrils, each of which is encircled by an SR system. This point of close association of the two systems is called a *triadic junction,*[11] although direct membrane continuity has not been observed.

The sarcotubular system plays an important role in electrochemical coupling involved in the initiation and regulation of contraction and relaxation. Calcium is thought to be bound within the sarcotubular system, specifically in a portion of the SR called the *terminal cisterrae.*[1,3,21] When an action potential courses over the surface of a cardiac muscle fiber, a wave of depolarization spreads passively along the membranes of the sarcotubular system, which leads to a release of bound calcium. The calcium then diffuses within the SR toward the A-band region of the sarcomere, where it is involved in the activation of cardiac contraction.[19]

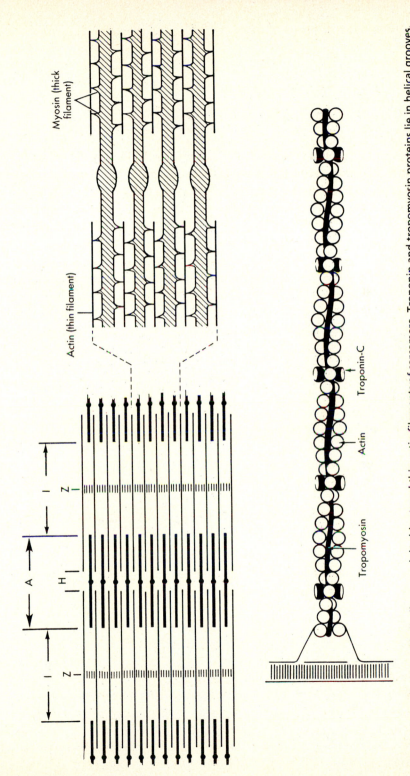

Myosin (thick filament)

Actin (thin filament)

A

H

Z

I

Z

I

Z

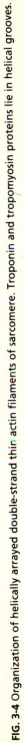

Troponin-C

Actin

Tropomyosin

FIG. 3-4 Organization of helically arrayed double-strand thin actin filaments of sarcomere. Troponin and tropomyosin proteins lie in helical grooves.

Mitochondria

Between 25% and 50% of the entire myocardial mass is composed of *mitochondria*. These cylindrical bodies are found arranged systematically between and in close approximation to the parallel rows of sarcomeres (Fig. 3-1). Oxidative phosphorylation, the process by which ATP is produced with the energy contained in carbohydrates, lipids, and proteins, occurs within the mitochondria. The exact mechanism for transfer of ATP from the mitochondrion to the myofibril is not known. The great number of mitochondria in the myocardium is commensurate with the massive demand for energy by the continuously contracting heart muscle, in contrast to the conduction tissue, where only 10% of its volume is occupied by mitochondria.[5,7,14,21]

REFERENCES

1. Bond, E.: Physiology of the heart. In Underhill, S., et al.: Cardiac nursing, Philadelphia, 1982, J.B. Lippincott Co.
2. Ebashi, S.: Regulatory mechanism of muscle contraction with special reference to the Ca-troponin-tropomyosin system. In Campbell, P.N., and Dickens, F., editors: Essays in biochemistry, vol. 10, London, 1974, Academic Press, Inc.
3. Ebashi, S., and Lipmann, F.: Adenosine triphosphate linked concentrations of cations in a particular fraction of rabbit muscle, J. Cell Biol. **14:**389, 1962.
4. Fawcett, D.W.: Physiologically significant specializations of the cell surface, Circulation **26:**1105, 1962.
5. Fawcett, D.W.: Mitochondria. In Briller, S.A., and Conn, J., editors: The myocardial cell: structure, function and modification by cardiac drugs, Philadelphia, 1966, University of Pennsylvania Press.
6. Fawcett, D.W., and McNutt, N.S.: The ultrastructure of the cat myocardium; capillary muscle, J. Cell Biol. **43:**1, 1969.
7. Hurst, J.W.: The heart, ed. 5, New York, 1982, McGraw-Hill Book Co.
8. Huxley, H.E.: The double-array of filaments in cross-striated muscle, J. Biophys. Biochem. Cytol. **3:**63, 1957.
9. Johnson, E.A., and Sommer, J.R.: A strand of cardiac muscle: its ultrastructure and the electrophysiological implications of its geometry, J. Cell Biol. **33:**103, 1967.
10. Katz, A.M.: Contractile proteins of the heart, Physiol. Rev. **50:**63, 1970.
11. Kawamura, K., and James, T.N.: Comparative ultrastructure of cellular junctions in working myocardium and the conduction system under normal and pathologic conditions, J. Mol. Cell. Cardiol. **3:**31, 1971.
12. Moore, D.H., and Rustu, H.: Electron microscopic study of mammalian cardiac muscle cell, J. Biophys. Biochem. Cytol. **3:**261, 1957.
13. Peachy, L.D.: The sarcoplasmic reticulum and trans-tubules of the frog's sartorius, J. Cell Biol. **25:**209, 1965.
14. Rendi, R., and Valter, A.E.: Possible location of phospholipids and structural protein in mitochondrial membranes, Protoplasma **63:**200, 1967.
15. Robertson, J.D.: The molecular structure and contact relationships of cell membranes, Prog. Biophys. Mol. Biol. **10:**343, 1960.
16. Rushmer, R.F.: Cardiovascular dynamics, Philadelphia, 1976, W.B. Saunders Co.
17. Simpson, F.O.: The transverse tubular system in mammalian myocardial cells, Am. J. Anat. **117:**1, 1965.
18. Simpson, F.O., and Dertelis, S.J.: The fine structure of sheep myocardial cells; subsarcolemmal invaginations and transverse tubular system, J. Cell Biol. **12:**91, 1962.
19. Sonnenblick, E.H., and Stam, A.C., Jr.: Heart excitation, conduction and contraction, Annu. Rev. Physiol. **31:**647, 1968.
20. Spiro, D., and Sonnenblick, E.H.: The structural basis of the contractile process in heart muscle under physiological and pathological conditions, Prog. Cardiovasc. Dis. **7:**295, 1965.
21. Weeks, L.: Cardiovascular physiology. In Kinney, M.R., et al.: AACN's clinical reference for critical care nursing, New York, 1981, McGraw-Hill Book Co.

CHAPTER 4 Myocardial excitation and contraction

Properties of myocardial muscle
Excitation and contraction

Katz[6] described the properties of myocardial muscle contraction observed during the interaction of the myosin heads with the actin to form cross-bridges. These properties include the following: (1) adenosine triphosphate (ATP) hydrolysis and liberation of energy, (2) physiochemical changes in which the chemical energy derived from ATP hydrolysis is converted to mechanical work, and (3) regulation of contraction by the regulatory proteins, tropomyosin and troponin (dependent on the cellular levels of calcium).

Depolarization and release of calcium

Calcium triggers the contractile process by reversing the inhibitory effect of the regulatory protein, troponin-C. Following ventricular or individual myocardial cell membrane depolarization, the electrical impulse propagates through the transverse tubules to the inside of the cell (Fig. 4-1). Depolarization causes calcium to be released from its stores in the T-tubule system and sarcoplasmic reticulum.* Calcium then migrates to the thin actin filaments and binds with the troponin-C protein. Calcium therefore removes the inhibition that is present, and a cross-bridge is formed.[3,10,11]

Formation of actin and myosin cross-bridges

Theories of myocardial muscle contraction have been simplified by the introduction of the Huxley sliding filament hypothesis of contraction.[5] Calcium binds to troponin-C and causes tropomyosin to shift out of the way, allowing the physical interactions to develop between the myosin heads and the active sights of the actin filaments. The myosin heads then hydrolyze ATP and form cross-bridges. Attachment of the cross-bridges at each end of the myosin filament to a binding site on the appropriate actin filament draws the actin filaments into the A band in a sliding mechanism and reduces the length of the sarcomere, which is the process of contraction (Fig. 4-2). The cross-bridges systematically detach

---

*The mitochondria contain ample stores of calcium. Its release, however, is too slow to be effectively used to trigger contraction.

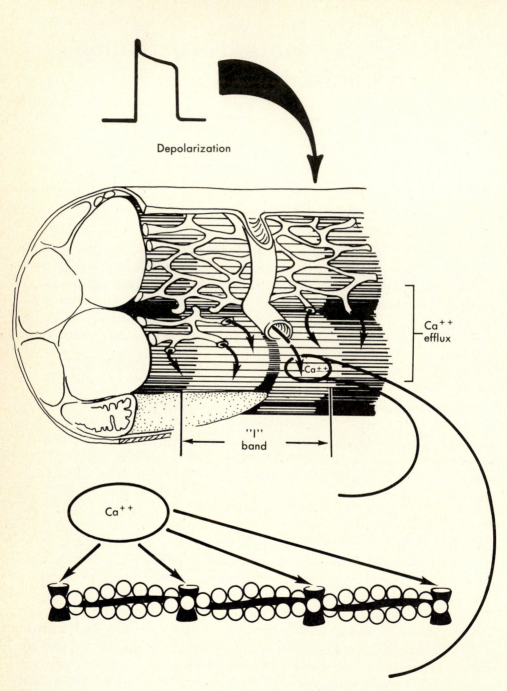

FIG. 4-1 Depolarization of myocardial cell and release of Ca^{++} from sarcoplasmic reticulum and T tubules.

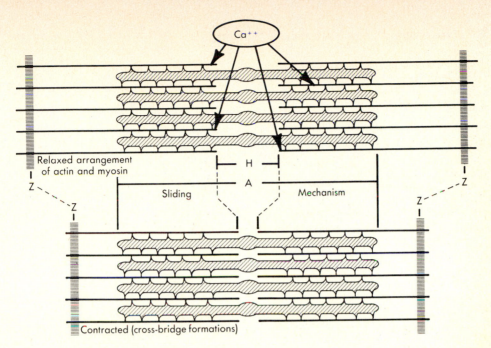

FIG. 4-2 Actin filaments drawn into A band (sliding over myosin filaments) to form cross-bridges.

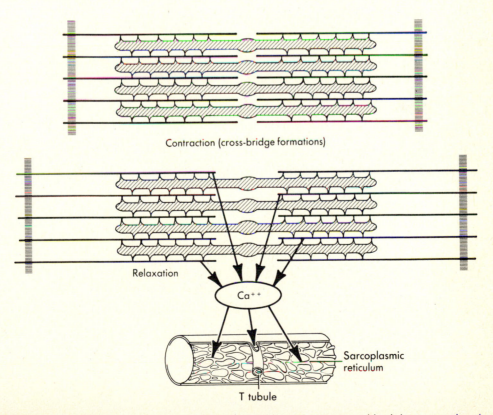

FIG. 4-3 Relaxation of actin and myosin cross-bridges (Ca^{++} sequestered back into sarcoplasmic reticulum and T tubules).

from the reactive sites, return to their original configuration, and reattach to new reactive sites on the actin filaments, beginning a new cycle of ATP splitting. Repeated attachments of the cross-bridges to the actin filaments are believed to occur.[12] The cross-bridges are thought to attach to the actin filaments, swivel to a new position, release, reattach to a new site, and repeat the process in rapid succession.[1,2,7,13]

Relaxation

Repolarization of the cell membrane is associated with relaxation of the myocardial muscle. Relaxation is initiated by an unknown stimulus that produces sequestration of calcium back into the sarcoplasmic reticulum. Recapture of calcium by the sarcoplasmic reticulum requires use of energy from the splitting of ATP. This removal of calcium from the troponin-binding sites results in inhibition of the hydrolysis of ATP, breaking of the cross-bridge attachments, and finally relaxation of the muscle (Fig. 4-3).[4,8]

REFERENCES

1. Barany, M.: ATPase activity of myosin correlated with speed of muscle shortening, J. Gen. Physiol. **50**:6, 1962.
2. Braunwald, E., Ross, J., Jr., and Sonnenblick, E.H.: Mechanism of contraction of the normal and failing heart, ed. 1, Boston, 1968, Little, Brown & Co.
3. Gergely, J.: Some aspects of the role of the sarcoplasmic reticulum and the tropomyosin-troponin system in the control of muscle contraction by the calcium ions. Circ. Res. **35** (suppl. 3):74, 1974.
4. Huxley, H.E.: The mechanism of muscular contraction, Science, **164**:1356, 1969.
5. Huxley, H.E., and Hanson, J.: Changes in the cross striation of muscle during contraction and stretch and their structural interpretation, Nature **173**:973, 1964.
6. Katz, A.M.: Physiology of the heart, New York, 1977, Raven Press.
7. Katz, A.M., and Brady, A.Y.: Mechanical and biochemical correlates of cardiac contraction, Mod. Concepts Cardiovasc. Dis. **40**:39, 1971.
8. Langer, G.A.: Heart: excitation-contraction coupling, Annu. Rev. Physiol. **35**:55, 1973.
9. Noble, D.: Application of Hodgkin-Huxley equation to excitable tissue, Physiol. Rev. **46**:1, 1966.
10. Peachy, L.D.: The role of transverse tubules in excitation contraction coupling in striated muscles, Ann. N.Y. Acad. Sci. **137**:1025, 1966.
11. Reuter, H., and Beeter, G.W.: Calcium current and activation of contraction in ventricular myocardial fibers, Science **163**:399, 1969.
12. Rushmer, R.I.: Cardiovascular dynamics, Philadelphia, 1976, W.B. Saunders Co.
13. Weeks, L.: Cardiovascular physiology. In Kinney, M.R., et al.: AACN'S clinical reference for critical care nursing, New York, 1981, McGraw-Hill Book Co.

CHAPTER 5 Myocardial energetics

Cardiac metabolism

The heart normally functions as an aerobic organ, converting metabolic energy to intracardiac pressure that is necessary to produce ventricular ejection; the net result is perfusion of blood to the tissues and vital organs. Myocardial energetics encompass metabolism of nutrients provided to the myocardial muscle and turn it into a usable energy source to accomplish the work of systole.

With an adequate supply of oxygen provided to the myocardium, free fatty acids and glucose, among other substrates, are extracted from the blood by the myocardial cell and are oxidized to pyruvate, which is catabolized in the Krebs' cycle. Adenosine triphosphate (ATP) is generated via the Krebs' cycle, which provides the necessary energy source for myocardial contraction (Fig. 5-1).[3,4]

Activation of the contractile elements in early systole produces a longitudinally oriented tension within the muscle fibers that causes the myofibrils to press on the blood in the same manner that a stretched rubber band placed around a tube occludes the lumen. Tension increases, and muscle length remains constant. This early systolic phase is termed *isometric contraction*. Shortening of the ventricular myocardium occurs later as the aortic and pulmonic valves open, and blood is ejected (i.e., *isotonic contraction*).[1,5] Tension that develops during this transfer of metabolic energy to ventricular pressure is affected by ventricular volume. Displacement of this volume during systole constitutes what is termed *cardiac work*.

Cardiac work

Physics terminology describes work as energy transfer that occurs when a mass is moved or a volume is displaced. External and internal work are involved in myocardial transfer of energy from its metabolic substrate to the pressure developed in contraction.

External work. Relating ventricular volume and pressure to the cardiac cycle graphically illustrates the principle of left ventricular external work (Fig. 5-2). During the isovolumic phase of ventricular contraction (A to B), pressure increases, but volume remains unchanged. Ventricular volume decreases rapidly during ventricular ejection (B to C), whereas the pressure continues to rise. Ventricular pressure falls rapidly after the aortic valve closes during isovolumic relaxation (C to D). Finally ventricular volume rises with only a small increase in pressure (D to A). The area bounded by the loop ABCDA represents the pressure-volume work, (i.e., the external work of the left ventricle).[2]

Static and dynamic external work. Static work refers to the development and mainte-

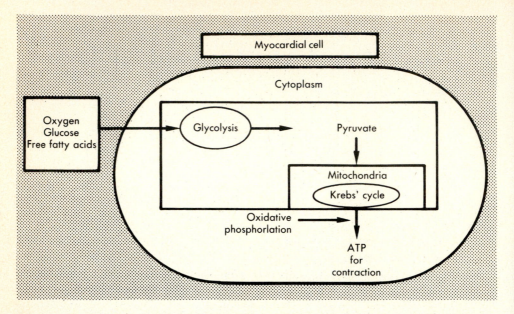

FIG. 5-1 Myocardial metabolism in presence of adequate oxygen. Among other substances, glucose and fatty acids are extracted from blood by myocardial cell and oxidized to pyruvate. Oxygen than enables oxidation of pyruvate to adenosine triphosphate (ATP) during Krebs' metabolic cycle, which occurs in mitochondria of cell.

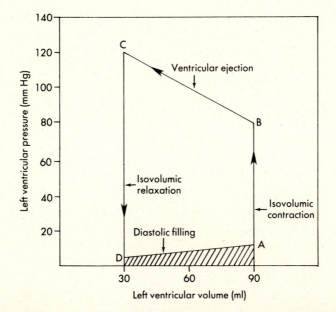

FIG. 5-2 Schematic representation of relationship between left ventricular pressure and volume during complete cardiac cycle. (See text for discussion.)

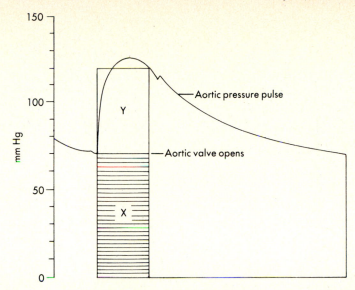

FIG. 5-3 Schematic representation of static *(X)* and dynamic work *(Y)* involved with ventricular ejection. Static work is isometric effort that occurs as left ventricle generates and sustains pressure necessary to push open aortic valve. Dynamic work occurs during ejection itself. (From Little, R.C.: Physiology of the heart and circulation, ed. 2, Chicago, Year Book Medical Publishers, Inc., Copyright 1981. By permission. [Modified from Wiggers, C.J.: Circulatory dynamics, New York, 1952, Grune & Stratton, Inc.])

nance of ventricular pressure before the opening of the aortic valve. Dynamic work occurs during the process of ventricular ejection. Little[5] beautifully describes the division of external cardiac work into static and dynamic by making an analogy to the forces involved in pouring a pail of water over a fence. Static effort is constituted by lifting the pail of water to a height equal to or slightly above the top of the fence. Additional energy (dynamic) must be used to tip the pail so that the water pours out over the fence.

Static and dynamic work can be graphically illustrated by drawing a horizontal line at the level of the diastolic pressure of an aortic pressure pulse (Fig. 5-3). Static work encompasses the effort involved in raising the ventricular pressure to a level sufficient to open the aortic valve and then holding that pressure for the duration of systole. Therefore static work is an isometric effort that requires a large amount of energy. Dynamic work involves systolic ejection.

Internal work. Energy dissipated in the form of heat or used to open and close valve cusps and to carry out the normal basal tissue activity is termed *internal cardiac work.*[5]

REFERENCES

1. Bond, E.F.: Physiology of the heart. In Underhill, S., et al.: Cardiac nursing, Philadelphia, 1982, J.B. Lippincott Co.
2. Burton, A.C.: Physiology and biophysics of the circulation, ed. 2, Chicago, 1972, Year Book Medical Publishers, Inc.
3. Huxley, H.E.: The contraction of muscle, Sci. Am. **199**:66, 1958.
4. Katz, A.M.: Physiology of the heart, New York, 1977, Raven Press.
5. Little, R.C.: Physiology of the heart and circulation, ed. 2, Chicago, 1981, Year Book Medical Publishers, Inc.

CHAPTER 6 Pump failure

Problem of heart failure

Heart failure defines the pathophysiological state in which the cardiovascular system fails to provide nutrients (blood) to the tissues at a rate commensurate with metabolic needs and to adequately remove metabolic products from the cells.[3] Myocardial failure (i.e., defaulting myocardial contraction) is a common cause for heart failure and may require balloon pumping as a treatment modality. However, heart failure may be present as a clinical syndrome without detectable myocardial malfunction. The implication is that a healthy heart could be made to fail if extreme demands of performance were placed on it.

The accumulation of salt and water as a result of excess blood or fluid administration, salt-retaining steroids, or acute glomerulonephritis may cause a circulatory overload and thereafter heart failure without primary myocardial contractile dysfunction. Secondary failure may ensue as a result of increased venous return as noted with an arteriovenous fistula or acute aortic regurgitation. Constrictive pericarditis, which hampers cardiac filling, can produce heart failure without contractile pumping dysfunction.[31] Finally hypovolemia, severe anemia, beriberi, and hyperthyroidism can induce circulatory failure without pump failure. Myocardial pump failure always produces circulatory failure, but the reverse is not necessarily true.

The following discussion focuses on basically illustrating how impairments in the normal mechanical action of the heart affect the patient. The physiological gains from balloon counterpulsation as an intervention to treat mechanical pump failure can then perhaps be better understood. Experimental data gathered from studies of isolated cardiac muscle provide a basis for our understanding of the pathophysiology of heart failure.

Normal circulation: a series circuit

A simplified circuit depicting the right and left ventricles arranged in a series within the circulation is illustrated in Fig. 6-1. As the blood circulates continuously in this series circuit, the outputs of the two ventricles are approximately equal (5 to 6 L/minute). In a healthy circulatory circuit the systemic veins empty into the atrium; thereafter the blood profuses into the right ventricle and through the pulmonary artery to the low resistance pulmonary capillary bed. Oxygenated blood returns via the pulmonary veins to the left atrium, goes to the left ventricle, and is pumped out the aorta to the systemic circulation. Normal pressures within these chambers are defined in Fig. 6-2.

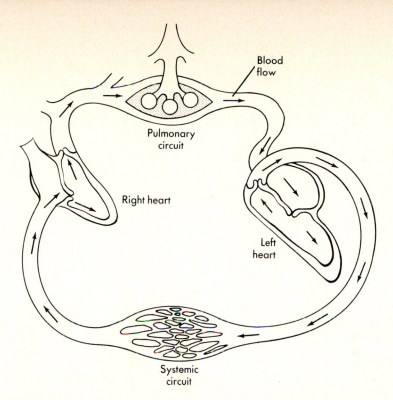

FIG. 6-1 Simplified series circuit, depicting right and left ventricles arranged in series within circulation. Pulmonary and systemic circuits are included as part of series circuit. Failure in one component of circuit affects other components as well.

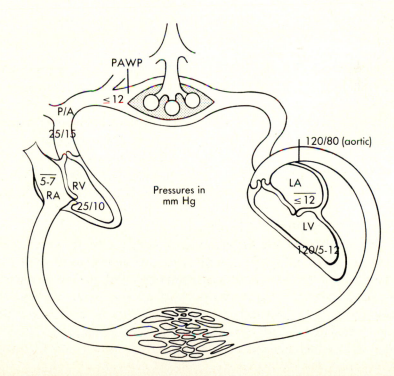

FIG. 6-2 Normal pressures within series circuit. *RA*, Right atrium. *RV*, Right ventricle. *P/A*, Pulmonary artery. *PAWP*, Pulmonary artery wedge pressure. *LA*, Left atrium. *LV*, Left ventricle.

Left and right ventricular failure

Left and *right ventricular failure* are terms used to label the ventricle with the primary impairment. Because of this series arrangement of the ventricles, neither left nor right ventricular failure occurs in a "pure" form. Pumping impairment, which may initially be unilateral, does not exist as a totally isolated condition for any length of time because the muscle bundles within the ventricles are continuous. To affirm the biventricular effects, even if the initial impairment was unilateral, Chandler, and others[9] observed an alteration in the activation of actomyosin adenosine triphosphatase (ATPase), the enzyme necessary for actin-myosin interaction, in both ventricles of animals in which the hemodynamic failure was induced in only one ventricle.

Left-sided failure

Etiology underlying left-sided failure may be atherosclerotic heart disease, hypertensive heart disease, myocardial infarction, myocarditis, pericarditis, and aortic and mitral valve disease. The left heart fails without initial concomitant failure of the right side; blood continues to be pumped to the lungs with vigorous right ventricular contraction, but the left ventricle fails to pump this volume out to the systemic circulation. As a result, the pulmonary filling pressure rises with a fall in the systemic filling pressure because of the large volume of blood shifted from the systemic to the pulmonary circulation.

As the volume of blood shifted to the pulmonary circulation increases, the pulmonary vessels enlarge (Fig. 6-3). If the pulmonary capillary wedge pressure rises above 28 mm Hg (above the colloid osmotic pressure of the plasma), fluid transudates out of the capillaries into the interstitial spaces and alveoli, resulting in pulmonary edema.[10,11]

Right-sided failure

The most common cause of right-sided failure is left-sided failure. Right ventricular failure may, however, result secondarily to chronic lung disease (i.e., emphysema). With unilateral right ventricular failure, the right ventricle fails to deliver its contained volume to the lungs; consequently, the volume backs up in the systemic venous circulation, and pressure builds up in the pulmonary arteries. The right ventricle fails because of the increased resistance encountered when pumping against high pulmonary pressures (Fig. 6-4). When right ventricular failure is secondary to lung disease, the situation is termed *cor pulmonale*.[3]

Forward versus backward failure

In oversimplified terms *forward* and *backward failure* have been used to describe clinical manifestations of heart failure that arise as a consequence of either inadequate cardiac output, forward failure, or damming up of blood behind one or both ventricles, backward failure.[28]

Forward theory. Mackenzie[22] proposed the forward theory, relating clinical manifestation of heart failure to inadequate cardiac output delivery. Mental confusion is associated with diminished cerebral perfusion, hypoperfusion to skeletal muscles is identified with

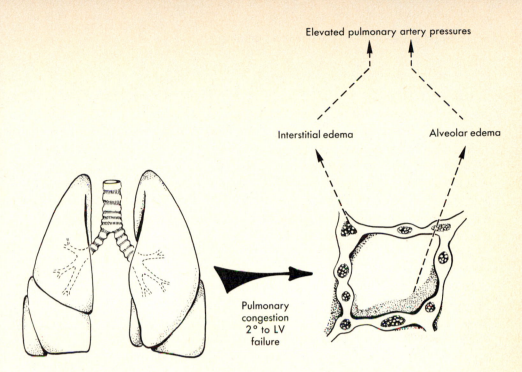

FIG. 6-3 Pathophysiology of pulmonary edema. When left ventricle fails to empty its volume, blood backs up into pulmonary circulation, and pulmonary vessels enlarge. If pulmonary capillary wedge pressure rises above 28 mm Hg (colloid osmotic pressure of plasma), fluid filters out of capillaries into interstitial spaces and alveoli, resulting in pulmonary edema.

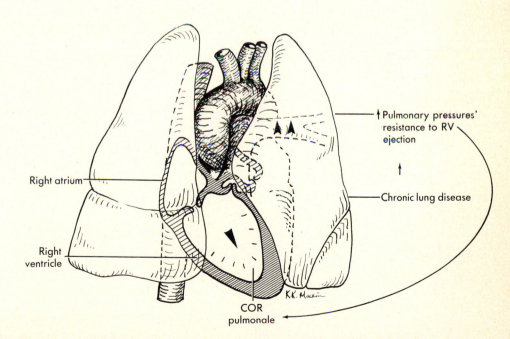

FIG. 6-4 Cor pulmonale. Right ventricular failure occurs secondary to chronic lung disease. Right ventricle cannot continue to pump adequately against increased pulmonary resistance.

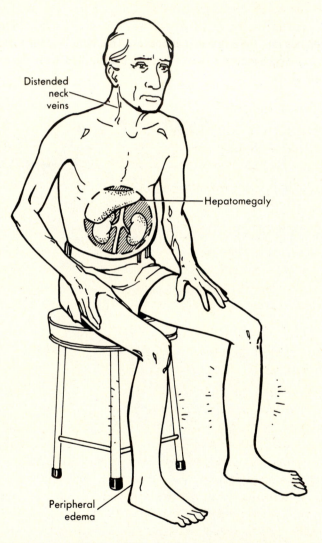

Distended
neck
veins

Hepatomegaly

Peripheral
edema

FIG. 6-5 Clinical picture of congestive heart failure. Venous congestion in systemic circulation may be visible as peripheral edema, hepatomegaly, and increased neck veins.

weakness, and inadequate blood supply to the kidneys leads to sodium and water retention through a series of complex mechanisms.

Backward theory. The backward theory of failure, first proposed by James Hope,[19] describes the situation in which the ventricle cannot discharge its volume adequately, causing increased volume and pressure in the pulmonic and systemic venous systems. If the heart cannot adequately discharge its volume, it cannot handle an additional returning venous supply. The rise in venous pressure may lead to an efflux of fluid across the capillary membranes into the extracellular spaces. This fluid is manifested as the clinical picture of edema. The backward theory has been identified with the congestive heart failure syndrome.

Congestive heart failure

When heart failure produces abnormal circulatory congestion because the heart is no longer able to transfer the blood satisfactorily from one circulation to the other, congestive heart failure is said to exist.[24] Transudation of fluid occurs from the capillaries to the interstitial spaces. If the rate of transudation exceeds the rate of lymphatic drainage in the pulmonary system, pulmonary edema becomes apparent from a chest x-ray examination and later from audible ausculatory rales. Congestive failure usually develops chronically with associated sodium and water retention. Venous congestion in the systemic circulation may be visible as peripheral edema, hepatomegaly, and increased neck veins (Fig. 6-5). Congestive failure usually manifests as a chronic state, but acute congestive failure may occur secondarily to massive myocardial infarction or following rupture of papillary muscle that culminates in an acute shift of blood from the systemic to the pulmonic circulation.[34]

Right- and left-sided failure as reflected on pressures in the series circuit

Movement of blood in the series circuit decreases the reality of a separation between forward and backward failure. Effects of the failing chamber are manifested in front of and behind this chamber, within the series circuit. Fig. 6-6 depicts the series circuit with primary right ventricular failure as could occur with cor pulmonale secondary to chronic lung disease. The pressures on the left side of the heart are normal. Pulmonary artery, right ventricular, and right atrial pressures are elevated. Forward effects of right ventricular failure manifest as decreased cardiac output, since initially there is a decreased volume delivered from the right ventricle to the lungs. This volume is appreciable in the left ventricle, depleting cardiac output available for delivery to the systemic circulation (Fig. 6-7).

Fig. 6-8 represents the pressure changes within the series circuit as a consequence of left ventricular failure. Pressures increase as volume dams up behind the left ventricle. Left atrial, pulmonary artery wedge, pulmonary artery, and finally right-sided pressures become elevated. The most common cause of right failure is left ventricular failure. Backward and forward effects of left ventricular failure are outlined in Fig. 6-9.

Text continued on p. 52.

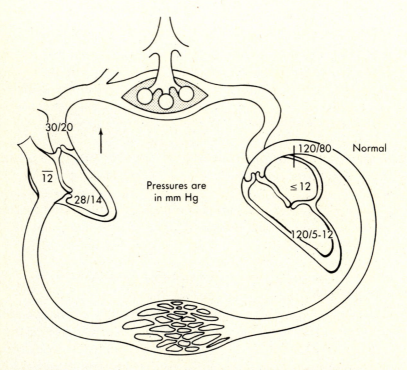

FIG. 6-6 Series circuit, outlining pressure changes observed in right ventricular failure, secondary to chronic lung disease. Pulmonary artery, right ventricular and right atrial pressures are elevated. Left-sided pressures are normal.

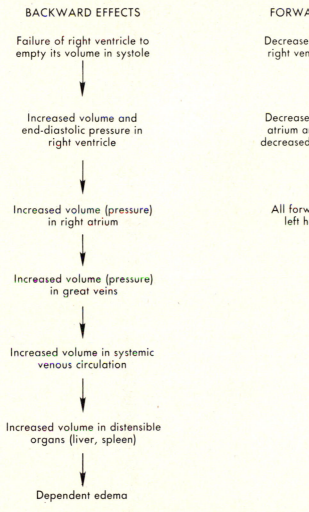

BACKWARD EFFECTS

Failure of right ventricle to
empty its volume in systole

↓

Increased volume and
end-diastolic pressure in
right ventricle

↓

Increased volume (pressure)
in right atrium

↓

Increased volume (pressure)
in great veins

↓

Increased volume in systemic
venous circulation

↓

Increased volume in distensible
organs (liver, spleen)

↓

Dependent edema

FORWARD EFFECTS

Decreased volume from
right ventricle to lungs

↓

Decreased return to left
atrium and subsequent
decreased cardiac output

↓

All forward effects of
left heart failure

FIG. 6-7 Right heart failure.

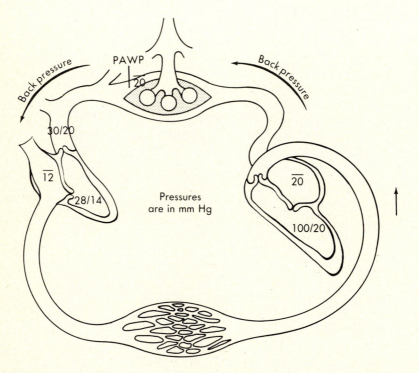

FIG. 6-8 Series circuit, outlining pressure changes observed in left ventricular failure. Left ventricular, end-diastolic, left atrial, pulmonary artery wedge, pulmonary artery, and finally right-sided pressures become elevated.

BACKWARD EFFECTS

Failure of left ventricle
to empty its stroke volume
in systole

↓

Increased volume and pressure
in left ventricle (end-diastolic
pressure rises)

↓

Increased volume (pressure)
in left atrium

↓

Increased volume (pressure) in
pulmonary veins

↓

Increased volume (pressure) in
pulmonary capillary bed

↓

Transudation of fluid from
capillaries to alveoli

↓

Pulmonary edema

↓

Right ventricle may fail
secondarily to elevated
pulmonary pressures

FORWARD EFFECTS

Decreased cardiac output

↓

Decreased perfusion of
body tissues

↓

Decreased blood flow to
body organs

↓

Increased reabsorption of
sodium and water via stimulation of renin-angiotensin
aldosterone mechanism

↓

Increased extracellular fluid
volume and blood volume

FIG. 6-9 Left heart failure.

Ultrastructural changes observed in the failing heart

The evaluation of pathological tissue of the failing heart is complicated by the rapid deterioration of pathological tissues, which alters penetration of fixatives. Thus a degree of critical objectivity must remain in attributing cause and effect to ultrastructure tissue alteration observed in the failing heart.[32]

Normally the ventricle operates on a sharply rising Frank-Starling curve, where small changes in filling pressure or left ventricular end-diastolic pressure (LVEDP) yield appreciable changes in stroke volume (Fig. 6-10). Starling[33] concluded that cardiac responsiveness was primarily related to presystolic fiber length. His enunciation of this famous Starling theory has been validated by other investigators.[30] When ventricular failure occurs, ventricular function is characterized by a shift of the curve to the right and downward, relating stroke volume to LVEDP. Thus an initial compensatory increased preload (left ventricular end-diastolic volume) on the ventricle, up to about 12 mm Hg, places a stretch on the sarcomere unit, which strengthens the velocity of contraction and augments stroke volume.[2,26]

The ideal sarcomere length for maximum effective contraction is 2.3 to 2.4 μm. The failing ventricle nets a chronic residual left ventricular end-diastolic volume that further

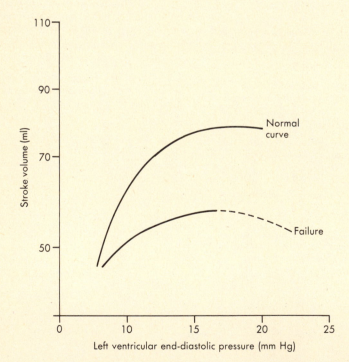

FIG. 6-10 Frank-Starling curve. Normally left ventricle operates on sharply rising Frank-Starling curve, where small changes in filling pressure (left ventricular end-diastolic pressure [LVEDP]) yield appreciable changes in stroke volume. Increasing filling pressure (LVEDP or preload) beyond about 12 mm Hg yields no additional increases in stroke volume, and failure may ensue with added stretch on myocardial fibers before contraction.

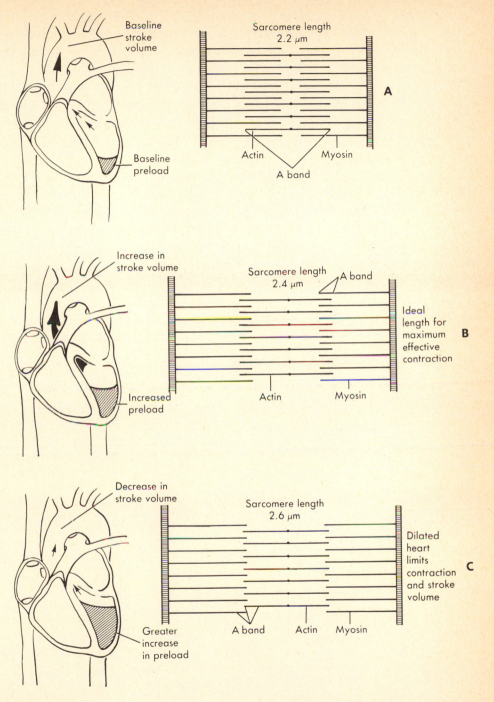

FIG. 6-11 Net effect of lengthened sarcomeres on cardiac output. **A,** Baseline preload, producing stretch on sarcomeres, which lengthens them to 2.2 μm. **B,** Ideal sarcomere length for maximum effective contraction. **C,** Further stretch on sarcomeres beyond 2.4 μm produces ineffective actin-myosin coupling. These elongated sarcomeres reflect withdrawal of actin filaments from A band and a decrease in myosin overlap. Force of contraction and resultant stroke volume are reduced.

stretches the sarcomere unit, limiting the contractile ability; the heart is then said to be *dilated*.[5] Fig. 6-11 illustrates the net effect of lengthened sarcomeres on the stroke volume. A small amount of stretch on the contractile units actually increases the force of the contraction and the resultant stroke volume. Further stretch on the myocardial sarcomeres (beyond 2.3 to 2.4 μm) produces an ineffective actin-myosin coupling, thereby reducing the force of contraction and stroke volume.[27] These elongated sarcomere lengths actually reflect a withdrawal of the thin actin filaments from the center of the A band and a decrease in myosin overlap. Destruction of the thin filaments, beginning at the I band, has been described.[29,32]

At first thought ventricular dilation may seem advantageous. With an increased end-diastolic volume and resultant increased sarcomere length, each sarcomere would seem to have to shorten less to eject a given volume of blood. The hemodynamic consequence of

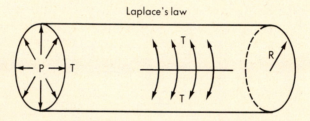

FIG. 6-12 Laplace's law. *T*, Tension. *P*, Pressures. *R*, Radius. Tension on wall of chamber is product of pressure in chamber times radius.

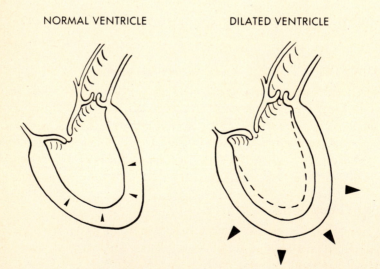

FIG. 6-13 Effect of ventricular size on afterload. Dilated ventricle on right must generate more tension than normal ventricle on left during systole to achieve a systolic pressure of 120 mm Hg. In the normal ventricle, radius decreases appreciably during systole, which contributes to generation of tension. Radius of dilated ventricle decreases less in systole. Therefore ventricular dilation creates added afterload, as more tension must be generated to achieve same pressure.

ventricular dilation is the need for the dilated myocardial wall fibers to develop greater tension to produce a given pressure in the ventricle, which is explained by Laplace's law (Fig. 6-12).[6,7] The equation states that the tension in the wall is the product of pressure and radius. In a normal ventricle the radius decreases appreciably during ejection. The effect of a rapidly decreasing ventricular wall radius on generating wall tension is greater than the opposing effect of pressure rising in the ventricle during systole. As a result, the myocardial fiber tension actually decreases soon after the beginning of ejection in a normal ventricle. Therefore the tension is less at the moment of peak systolic ejection than at the beginning of ejection.[6,16,34]

Laplace's law expresses the disadvantage of the dilated ventricle as failure of the ventricular radius to appreciably decrease during systole, which may consequently result in a rise in tension from the beginning of ejection to the point of peak systole. Schlant explains that this tension is, in a sense, an additional type of afterload encountered in ventricles that are significantly dilated by an increased preload (Fig. 6-13).

Because of the increase in myocardial systolic wall tension resulting from the Laplace relationship, the oxygen consumption of the myocardium may be significantly increased in patients with heart failure. This may result in a greater amount of oxygen extracted from coronary blood flow and a widening of the arteriovenous oxygen difference. In one study of a group of patients with left ventricular failure, the left ventricular oxygen consumption averaged 16% of the total oxygen consumed by the body compared to 5% in normal subjects.[21]

Mitochondria and the failing heart

The mitochondria of failing hearts have been observed to be slightly larger and differ in aspects of their internal structure with a significant decrease in the ratio of mitochondria to myofibrils.[10,36] The importance of this observation in relation to impaired contractions is unclear.

Calcium and heart failure

Studies of in vitro systems suggest that there is impairment of the delivery of calcium for activation of the contractile process in heart failure. The uptake of calcium by the sarcoplasmic reticulum is dependent on the activity of the enzyme ATPase. Reduction in the activities of the myofibrillar ATPase has been identified in patients who died of heart failure.[1,13,15] Therefore a disturbance in the uptake of calcium by the sarcoplasmic reticulum could interfere with cardiac performance.[13]

Clinical manifestations of heart failure

The signs of heart failure (i.e., objective manifestations) are usually caused by the elevated systemic venous pressure that is secondary to right ventricular failure. Symptoms or abnormalities perceived by the patient correlate with increased pulmonary pressure and a fall in cardiac output. The patient usually complains of weakness, fatigue, and shortness of breath. Paroxysmal nocturnal dyspnea (PND) may occur when the patient is asleep. Classically the patient awakens, coughing with a feeling of choking and suffocation.

Transudation of fluid across the pulmonary capillary membrane occurs when the left

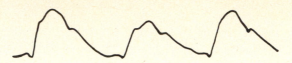

FIG. 6-14 Arterial pulse, demonstrating "pulsus alternans." Alternating strong and weak pulsations are noted.

ventricle cannot handle its pumping load; the pulmonary capillaries and alveoli become engorged (i.e., pulmonary edema). There may be ruptures of the small capillaries, and the patient may expectorate frothy pink mucus. Symptoms include sudden dyspnea, wheezing, orthopnea, peripheral cyanosis, apprehension, and a weak, rapid pulse. Chest examination findings include an enlarged heart, and bubbling rales may be heard on auscultation. An enlarged liver and fluid in the abdominal cavity (ascites) as well as edema in the dependent parts of the body may be noted.[34]

Characteristically, *pulsus alternans,* an alteration in the peripheral arterial pulse despite a regular rhythm (Fig. 6-14), is observed in patients suffering from myocardial dysfunction.[11] Alternate strong and weak contractions are detected by palpating the peripheral pulse. This change in pulse magnitude is best appreciated in a large distal artery, such as the brachial, which has a slightly wider pulse pressure than the carotid artery. The mechanism of this finding is controversial. Some clinicians believe that it is a manifestation of a variation in left ventricular end-diastolic volume, which causes an alteration in the force of contraction.[25] Another theory proposes that there is a failure of electromechanical coupling on alternate beats in certain damaged regions of the heart, which results in an alternation in the number of muscle cells participating in contraction.[17] Both mechanisms may be operant in patients with myocardial infarction.

Decreased cardiac output and compensatory adjustments

A decrease in established cardiac output prompts the body to make certain compensatory adjustments. Sympathetic stimulation causes vasoconstriction in an attempt to elevate the blood pressure and assure perfusion of the brain, kidneys, and heart muscle. The coronary arteries respond to sympathetic stimulation by vasodilation. Another acute adjustment is an increase in heart rate that assists in attempting to maintain the needed cardiac output.

Kidneys respond to hypoperfusion by an increased reabsorption of sodium and water. There is an increase in release of the adrenocortical hormone aldosterone and in the formation of the antidiuretic hormone. An understanding of the renin-angiotensin mechanism is presented to clarify the process of tubular reabsorption of sodium and water.[8]

Renal adjustments in heart failure

Studies in the 1940s indicated that alteration in renal function does occur in patients with heart failure.[12] Blood flow to the kidneys proportionally diminishes with the decline in cardiac function. Consequently, vasoconstriction of the renal arterioles occurs, and the capacity to excrete sodium, chloride, and water is reduced.

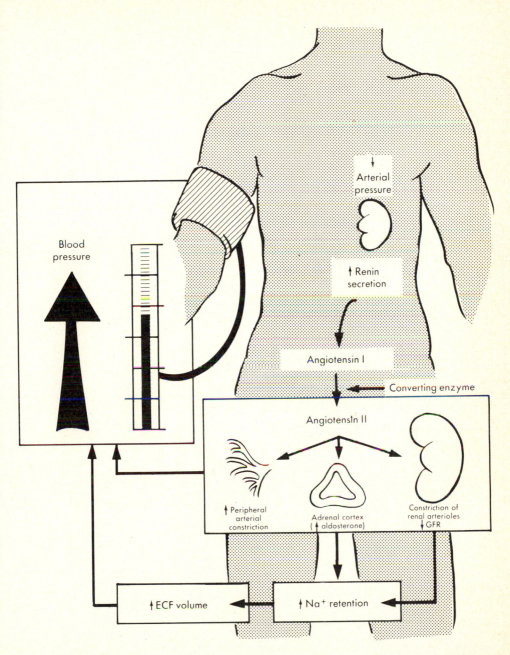

FIG. 6-15 Renin-angiotensin mechanism in heart failure. As systemic pressure drops, blood flow to the kidney decreases proportionately with resultant renal vasoconstriction. Renin is secreted by kidney in defense of hypotension, which acts to release angiotensin I from blood, and that is converted to angiotensin II (potent vasoconstrictor). Angiotensin II prompts release of aldosterone from adrenals. *ECF,* Extracellular fluid. *GFR,* Glomerular filtration rate.

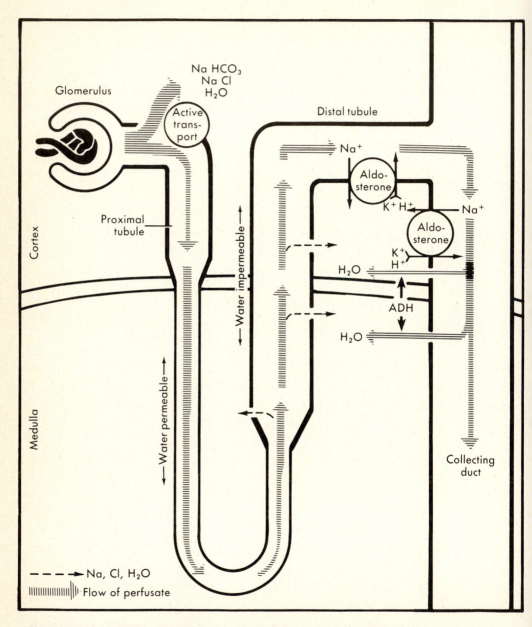

FIG. 6-16 Aldosterone acts on distal tubules and collecting ducts of kidney to increase tubular reabsorption of sodium, chloride, and water in exchange for potassium and hydrogen ions.

Homeostatic adaptations occur within the renal system in defense of the falling arterial blood pressure associated with heart failure. The most important hormonal system involved is the renin-angiotensin-aldosterone system. Increased secretion of the protein renin occurs in the kidney in response to hypoperfusion and possibly to the increased distention of the ventricles, atria, and large veins.[18]

Renin acts on a substrate in the blood to release the peptide angiotensin I, which is converted to angiotensin II by the action of a converting enzyme, primarily found in the lungs but also in a lesser amount in the blood vessels and kidneys. Angiotensin II produces vasoconstriction of arteriolar smooth muscle; it is the most potent pressor substance released by the body—10 times more potent than norepinephrine[7] (Fig. 6-15).

Angiotensin II is one of the most important stimuli to the adrenal secretion of aldosterone. Aldosterone acts on the distal tubules and collecting ducts of the kidney to increase tubular reabsorption of sodium, chloride, and water in exchange for potassium and hydrogen ions (Fig. 6-16).[35]

In mild heart failure the retained fluid increases blood volume and venous return to the heart; cardiac output is increased, and arterial blood pressure and tissue perfusion are maintained. The resultant elevation of arterial pressure deactivates renin secretion once the kidney is no longer ischemic.

Advanced heart failure does not lend itself to restoration of arterial pressure despite the sodium and water retention catalyzed by the renin-angiotensin-aldosterone mechanism. Since the blood pressure is not restored to normal in the ventricles, the atria and the great veins remain distended, and stimuli to the secretion of renin and aldosterone persist.

Aldosterone is metabolized by the liver. Degradation may decrease in heart failure if hepatic blood flow is reduced, thereby increasing the circulating concentration. The kidneys, therefore play an extremely important role in the pathogenesis of heart failure.

The aforementioned body adaptations related to heart failure are usually associated with a slow to moderate rate of degeneration of myocardial function. The cardiac output can fall extremely low immediately following a severe myocardial infarction. This leads to a greatly diminished blood flow through the body and can culminate in a state of cardiogenic shock.

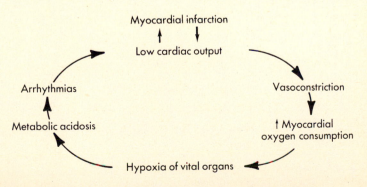

FIG. 6-17 Self-perpetuating cycle of cardiogenic shock.

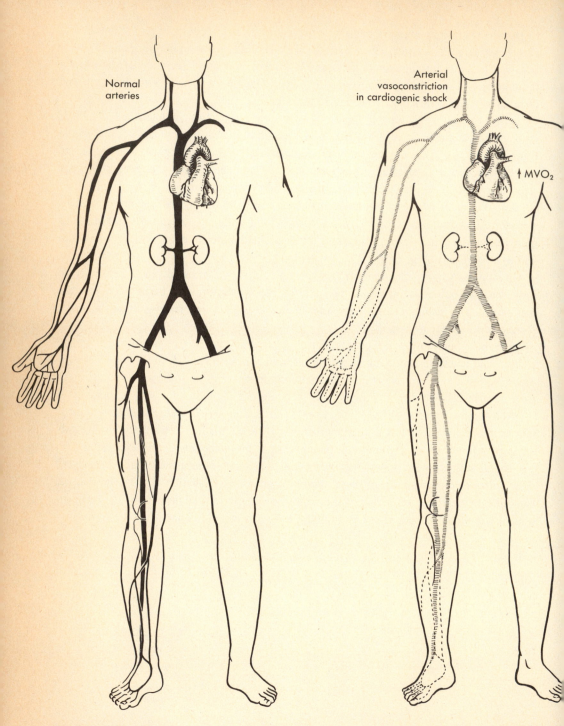

FIG. 6-18 Reflex vasoconstriction in cardiogenic shock. Increased resistance imposed by arterial constriction increases afterload of left ventricle. Blood is ejected by left ventricle at higher outflow impedance. Increased myocardial oxygen consumption (MVO_2) ensues.

Severe cardiac failure: cardiogenic shock

Cardiogenic shock, or severe heart failure, develops in about 15% of patients with acute myocardial infarction.[23] As a result of the failure of the left ventricle to maintain an adequate cardiac output for perfusion of the body, tissues deteriorate rapidly, and death ensues. The mortality from left ventricular pump failure, following an acute myocardial infarction, approximates 85% to 90%.[2]

A self-perpetuating cycle of progressive left ventricular dysfunction characterizes the cardiogenic shock syndrome (Fig. 6-17). Extensive myocardial damage impairs contractility to the degree of reducing cardiac output and arterial pressure dramatically. Hypotension decreases coronary artery perfusion with resultant myocardial and systemic hypoperfusion, hypoxia, and acidosis. Coronary flow to the potentially viable ischemic myocardium is compromised, extending the size of the infarction and increasing the degree of ventricular dysfunction. To compensate for this hypoperfusion, the resultant hypotension activates the baroreceptors of the carotid sinus and aorta, calling for massive vasoconstriction to maintain arterial pressure.[3]

Although reflex vasoconstriction does support arterial perfusion pressure and coronary blood flow, this increased vascular resistance imposes an increased work load on the injured left ventricle that must consequently eject blood at a higher outflow impedance. Unfortunately then, these compensatory mechanisms increase the work of the injured myocardium and increase oxygen consumption of the already hypoxic heart (Fig. 6-18).

REFERENCES

1. Alpert, N.R., and Gordon, M.S.: Myofibrillar adenosine triphosphate activity in congestive failure, Am. J. Physiol. **202**:940, 1962.
2. Beutsaert, D.L., and Sonnenblick, E.H.: Cardiac muscle mechanics in the evaluation of myocardial contractility and pump function: problems, concepts, and directions, Prog. Cardiovasc. Dis. **16**:337, 1973.
3. Braunwald, E.: Heart disease—a textbook of cardiovascular medicine, Philadelphia, 1980, W.B. Saunders Co.
4. Braunwald, E., et al.: Mechanisms of contraction of the normal and failing heart, ed. 2, Boston, 1976, Little, Brown & Co.
5. Burch, G.E.: Theoretic considerations of the time courses of pressure developed and volume ejected by the normal and dilated left ventricle during systole, Am. Heart J. **50**:352, 1955.
6. Burton, A.C.: The importance of the shape and size of the heart, Am. Heart J. **54**:801, 1957.
7. Burton, A.C.: Physiology and biophysics of the circulation, ed. 2, Chicago, 1972, Year Book Medical Publishers, Inc.
8. Cannon, P.J.: The kidney in heart failure, N. Engl. J. Med. **296**:26, 1977.
9. Chandler, B.M., et al.: Association of depressed myofibrillar adenosine triphosphatase and reduced contractility in experimental heart failure, Circ. Res. **21**:717, 1967.
10. Chidsey, C.A., et al.: Biochemical studies of energy metabolism in the failing human heart, J. Clin. Invest. **45**:40, 1966.
11. Crawford, M.H., and O'Rourke, R.A.: The bedside diagnosis of the complications of myocardial infarction. In Eliot, P.S., et al.: Cardiac emergencies, ed. 2, Mount Kisco, N.Y., 1982, Futura Publishing Co., Inc.
12. Davis, J.L.: The physiology of congestive heart failure. In Hamilton, W.F., and Dow, P., editors: Handbook of physiology, III. Washington, D.C., 1965, American Physiological Society.
13. Endo, M.: Calcium research from sarcoplasmic reticulum, Physiol. Rev. **57**:71, 1977.

14. Gleason, W.L., and Braunwald, E.: Studies on Starling's law of the heart. VI. Relationships between left ventricular end-diastolic volume and stroke volume in man with observations on the mechanism of pulsus alternans, Circulation **25:**841, 1962.
15. Gordon, M.S., and Brown, A.L.: Myofibrillar adenosine triphosphate activity of human heart tissue and congestive failure: effects of ouabain and calcium, Circ. Res. **19:**534, 1966.
16. Grossman, W., and Braunwald, E.: Contractile state of the left ventricle in man as evaluated from end-systolic pressure-volume relations, Circulation **56:**845, 1977.
17. Guntheroth, W.G., et al.: Alternate deletion and potentiation as the cause of pulsus alternans, Am. Heart J. **78:**669, 1969.
18. Haber, E.: The race of renin in normal and pathological cardiovascular homeostasis, Circulation **54:**849, 1976.
19. Hope, J.A.: Treatise on the diseases of the heart and great vessels, London, 1832, Williams-Kidd.
20. Karb, G., and Totovic, G.: Electron microscopic studies on experimental ischemic lesions of the heart, Ann. N.Y. Acad. Sci. **165:**48, 1969.
21. Levine, H.J., and Wagman, R.J.: Energetics of the human heart, Am. J. Cardiol. **9:**372, 1968.
22. Mackenzie, J.: Diseases of the heart, ed. 3, London, 1913, Oxford University Press.
23. Mason, D.T., et al.: Diagnosis and management of myocardial infarction shock. In Eliot, R.S., et al.: Cardiac emergencies, ed. 2, Mount Kisco, N.Y., 1982, Futura Publishing Co., Inc.
24. McKee, P.A., et al.: The natural history of congestive heart failure. The Framingham study, N. Engl. J. Med. **285:**1441, 1971.
25. Mitchell, J.N., et al.: The dynamics of pulsus alternans: alternating end-diastolic fiber length as a causative factor, J. Clin. Invest. **42:**55, 1963.
26. Ross, J., Jr., et al.: Architecture of the heart in systole and diastole: technique of rapid fixation and analysis of left ventricular geometry, Circ. Res. **21:**409, 1967.
27. Ross, J., Jr., et al.: Diastolic geometry and sarcomere lengths in the chronically dilated left ventricle, Circ. Res. **28:**49, 1971.
28. Rushmer, R.F.: Cardiovascular dynamics, ed. 4, Philadelphia, 1976, W.B. Saunders Co.
29. Sarnoff, S.J.: Myocardial contractility as described by ventricular function curves: observations on Starling's law of the heart, Physiol. Rev. **35:**107, 1955.
30. Sarnoff, S.J., and Bergland, E.: Ventricular functions. In Starling's law of the heart studies by means of simultaneous right and left ventricular function curves in the dog, Circulation **9:**706, 1954.
31. Schlant, R.C., and Sonnenblick, E.B.: Pathophysiology of heart failure. In Hurst, J.W., et al., editors: The heart, ed. 5, New York, 1982, McGraw-Hill Book Co.
32. Sonnenblick, E.H., et al.: Ultrastructure of the heart in systole and diastole: changes in sarcomere length, Circ. Res. **21:**423, 1967.
33. Starling, E.H.: The lineac lecture on the law of the heart, London, 1918, Longmans, Green & Co., Ltd.
34. Waters, D., and Forrester, J.: Diagnosis and management of congestive heart failure and pulmonary edema. In Eliot, R.S., et al.: Cardiac emergencies, ed. 2, Mount Kisco, N.Y., 1982, Futura Publishing Co., Inc.
35. Watkins, J., Jr., et al.: The renin-angiotensin-aldosterone system in congestive failure in conscious dogs, J. Clin. Invest. **57:**1606, 1976.
36. Wollenberger, A., et al.: Some metabolic characteristics of mitochondria from chronically overloaded hypertrophied hearts, Exp. Mol. Pathol. **2:**251, 1963.

CHAPTER 7 **Traditional pharmacological management of pump failure**

Left ventricular dysfunction, which may evolve following an acute myocardial infarction, is characterized by severe impairment of circulatory function. The expanded picture may include an elevated left ventricular filling pressure and decreased stroke work index. Systemic vascular resistance rises as the arterial system constricts in a compensatory effort to conserve blood flow to the major organs.[13] Clinical improvement in these hemodynamic regressions may be achieved by administering pharmacological agents that increase myocardial force of contraction *(inotropic)* or augment cardiac output by increasing the heart rate *(chronotropic)*. Other drugs may act directly on the peripheral arterioles to dilate them, thereby easing the work of contraction of the failing left ventricle (afterload reduction).

Each of the drugs traditionally used for treatment of pump failure has distinct effects on the heart itself as well as on the peripheral vascular system. Careful consideration must be given when prescribing a drug; trade-offs must be made. For example, a specific drug may improve cardiac output by increasing heart rate; however, this effect may in turn increase myocardial oxygen consumption (MVO_2). When the clinician achieves an understanding of the attempts made to improve pump failure by pharmacological endeavors and considers their limitations, an appreciation for the balloon pump's effect on a failing heart is more easily and comprehensively grasped.

Treatment of pump failure is undertaken with the following four main goals in mind:[19]

1. To increase cardiac output.
2. To decrease work of the heart.
3. To decrease the oxygen requirements of the heart.
4. To reduce myocardial ischemia and limit infarct size.

Alpha and beta receptors

Alquist[1] first demonstrated the existence of tissue receptor sites, responding to catecholamine-mediated stimuli—the *adrenergic receptors*. These receptors were classified by Alquist as alpha (α) or beta (β), according to their response to adrenergic drugs.

Adrenergic simply defines the response of the sympathetic nerve fiber when stimulated (i.e., release of sympathin, a neurohumoral substance). Acceptance of Alquist's classification with full realization of the potential impact on cardiac physiology resulted in a revolutionary change in the pharamacological therapy of cardiac diseases. Subsequently, beta-adrenergic receptor sites were subdivided into beta$_1$ and beta$_2$ subtypes.[14]

The functional classification of the beta-adrenergic receptor sites is listed in Table 7-1. Stimulation of alpha receptors causes sphincter constriction, glycogenolysis, and sweat gland acitivty. Beta-receptor stimulation increases impulse generation and conduction in the sinoatrial (SA) and atrioventricular (AV) nodes, enhances myocardial contractility,

TABLE 7-1 Functional classification of the adrenergic receptor sites

Heart	β_1
Arterioles	
Coronary	$\alpha\beta_2$
Skin	α
Skeletal muscles	$\alpha\beta_2$
Pulmonary	$\alpha\beta_2$
Abdomen	$\alpha\beta_2$
Veins	$\alpha\beta_2$
Bronchi	β_2
Kidney	$\beta_{(? 1 or 2)}$
Sex organs (male)	α
Liver	β_2
Pancreas	
Acini	α
Islets (B cells)	β_2
Fat	β_1

From Goodman, L.S., and Gilman, A., editors: The pharmacological basis of therapeutics, ed. 6, New York, 1980, Macmillan Publishing Co., Inc. By permission.

TABLE 7-2 Specific adrenergic receptor activity of sympathomimetic amines

	Alpha peripheral	Beta$_1$ cardiac	Beta$_2$ peripheral
Isoproterenol	0	+ + + +	+ + + +
Dobutamine	+	+ + + +	+ +
Norepinephrine	+ + + +	+ + + +	0
Methoxamine	+ + + +	0	0
Epinephrine	+ + + +	+ + + +	+ +
Dopamine*	+ + + +	+ + + +	+ +

From Sonnenblick, E.H., et al.: Dobutamine: a new synthetic cardioactive sympathetic amine, N. Engl. J. Med. **300:**18, 1979. By permission.
*Selectively dilates renal and mesenteric vascular beds by stimulating dopaminergic receptors.

dilates arteriolar and bronchial smooth muscles, promotes insulin and renin secretion, and stimulates lipolysis and lactate production. Use of alpha and beta adrenergic drugs in the treatment of pump failure is specifically directed to the effects of the drugs on the beta$_1$ receptors in the myocardium, the beta$_2$ receptors located in the arterioles and lungs, and the alpha receptors' response to stimulation in the peripheral arterioles. Functional clas-sification of the beta-adrenergic receptor sites is listed in Fig. 7-1.

Tissue receptor responses to various *sympathomimetic amine drugs* (agents that produce effects resembling those manifested from stimulation of the sympathetic nervous system) are listed in Table 7-2. The net action of any of these amines depends on their dominant receptor activity.

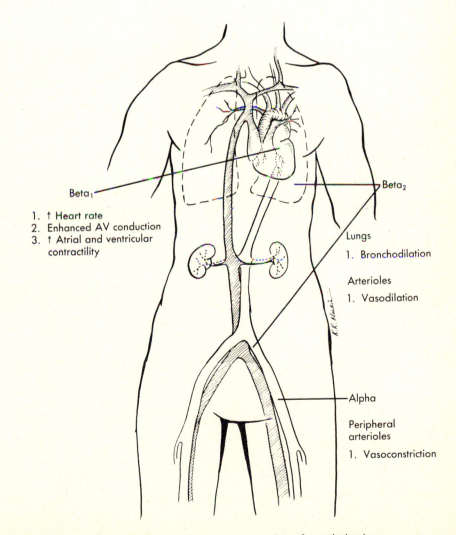

Beta$_1$
1. ↑ Heart rate
2. Enhanced AV conduction
3. ↑ Atrial and ventricular contractility

Beta$_2$

Lungs
1. Bronchodilation

Arterioles
1. Vasodilation

Alpha

Peripheral arterioles
1. Vasoconstriction

FIG. 7-1 Alpha- and beta-receptor action of catecholamines.

Brief drug monograph[5, 7, 12]

1. **Beta adrenergics**
   a. Isoproterenol (Isuprel)

Reconstituting solution	5% dextrose in water (D_5W), normal saline (NS)
IV onset	Immediate
Duration	Low dose—8 minutes
	High dose—50 minutes
Actions	Increased heart rate
	Increased cardiac output
	Increased MVO_2
	Increased pacemaker automaticity
	Dilated smooth muscles in bronchioles, skeletal muscle, and kidney
Dosage	2 to 20 µg per minute
Adverse effects	Tachycardia, headache, flushing, decreased renal perfusion as a result of shunting of blood to skeletal muscle, ventricular arrhythmias
Incompatibilities	Alkalies (HCO_3, lidocaine aminophylline, barbiturates)
	Isoproterenol may actually extend ischemic areas of the myocardium

   b. Dobutamine (Dobutrex)

Reconstituting solution	D_5W
IV onset	1 to 2 minutes
Action	Inotropic effect with increase in cardiac output; may decrease pulmonary artery wedge pressure minimally and increase heart rate slightly
Dosage	2.5 to 20 µg per kilogram per minute
Adverse effect	Palpitations, dyspnea, nervousness, restlessness, atrial and ventricular arrhythmias
Incompatibilities	Alkalies

2. **Alpha > beta adrenergics**
   a. Levarterenol (Levophed) (Norepinephrine)

Reconstituting solution	NS, D_5W less stable
IV onset	Rapid
Duration	1 to 2 minutes

Action	Increased systemic vascular resistance, increased systolic and diastolic pressure, decreased cardiac output, decreased renal perfusion
Dosage	2 to 15 μg per minute
Adverse effects	Increased angina pain, reflex bradycardia, altered mental status, arrhythmias
Incompatibilities	Alkalies

b. Metaraminol (Aramine)

Reconstituting solution	D_5W, NS
IV onset	1 to 2 minutes
Duration	20 minutes
Action	Similar to levarterenol; longer duration of action
Dosage	1 to 5 mg per minute, IV infusion
Adverse effects	Increased myocardial oxygen consumption, precipitating angina, arrhythmias, reflex bradycardia, decreased peripheral perfusion, extravasation (not as extensive as with levarterenol)
Incompatibilities	Sulfonamides, barbiturates, increased decomposition of penicillin, nafcillin, erythromycin, methicillin, Ringer's lactate, bicarbonate

3. **Pure alpha adrenergic**

a. Methoxamine (Vasoxyl)

Reconstituting solution	D_5W, NS
IV onset	2 minutes
Duration	60 minutes
Action	Increased systolic and diastolic blood pressures, vascular bed constriction, coolness of skin and tingling of extremities, increased systemic vascular resistance
Dosage	0.1 to 0.5 mg, IV bolus
	10 to 50 μg per minute, IV infusion
Adverse effects	Vomiting, reflex decrease in heart rate, paresthesias, increased desire to micturate
Interactions	Guanethidine, reserpine, tricyclic antidepressants cause enhanced effect
Incompatibilities	Alkalies

Pure alpha
adrenergics

4. Alpha = Beta adrenergics

a. Epinephrine (Adrenalin)

Reconstituting solution	NS, D_5W less stable
IV onset	Rapid
Action	At lower dosages the beta effect predominates; at normal dosages, alpha > beta but with shorter duration[5]
Adverse effect	Cardiostimulation and ventricular arrhythmias
Dosage	For asystole[5] 0.5 mg of 1:10,000 (5ml) solution in 5-minute intervals may be instilled tracheobronchially if no IV is available
Incompatibilities	Alkali and oxidizing agents—brown color signifies oxidation and should not be used; should not be given simultaneously with isoproterenol

5. Alpha = Beta adrenergics

(effects less dramatic than with epinephrine)

a. Dopamine (Intropin)[7,12,15,23,32]

Reconstituting solution	D_5W, NS
IV onset	2 to 4 minutes
Duration	10 minutes
Action	Increased systolic and diastolic pressure, increased systemic vascular resistance, increased cardiac output, increased heart rate, selectively dialates renal and coronary arteries at low rates (dopaminergic effect)
Dosage	1 to 2 μg per kilogram per minute = dopaminergic effect
	2 to 10 μg per kilogram per minute = predominately beta effect
	10 μg per kilogram per minute = predominately alpha effect
	15 μg per kilogram per minute = same effects as norepinephrine
Incompatibilities	Alkalies and oxidizing agents decompose drug (HCO_3 and aminophylline), ampicillin

Dopamine and dobutamine. Dopamine, the immediate precursor of norepinephrine, stimulates myocardial contractility by acting directly on beta$_1$-adrenergic receptors in the myocardium and indirectly by releasing norepinephrine from sympathetic nerve fibers.

Vasodilation mediated by dopamine is secondary to activation of specific dopaminergic receptors.[11] Dopamine-induced vasodilation is not related to activation of $beta_2$ receptors; vasodilation occurs in the renal, mesenteric, coronary, and cerebral vascular beds but not in the denervated skeletal muscle vascular bed. Dopamine-induced diuresis is observed in patients with heart failure secondary to the inotropic and renal vasodilator effects of this catecholamine drug[10] (Fig. 7-2, A).

The dosage at which the dopaminergic dilation effect is reversed is titratable for each patient. Generally, dosages beyond 15 to 20 µg per kilogram per minute cause constriction of arteries and veins in all vascular beds. Coronary vasodilation through action on dopaminergic receptors increases coronary flow. Larger dosages may increase coronary vascular resistance through stimulation of the coronary alpha receptors. Thus in low dosages, dopamine exerts beneficial hemodynamic and renal effects. Negative effects of tachycardia, vascular constriction, and increased MVO_2 may ensue with higher rates of infusion; the dopaminergic effects are then outweighed by the alpha effects[16] (Fig. 7-2, B).

Dobutamine exerts a weaker $beta_2$-adrenergic action than does isoproterenol and a weaker alpha-adrenergic action than does norepinephrine or dopamine. Slight vasoconstriction occurs at low dosages, and a biphasic vasoconstrictor-vasodilator response occurs at higher dosages.[11] Ventricular arrhythmias have been observed with both drugs.[28]

Comparisons between dopamine and dobutamine have been made in a crossover study[15] in patients with pump failure. Infusion rates were between 2.5 to 10.0 µg per kilogram per minute. Dobutamine produced a progressive rise in cardiac output by increasing stroke volume while simultaneously decreasing both systemic and pulmonary capillary wedge pressure. Heart rate did not increase nor did premature ventricular contractions arise at this level. With dopamine, pulmonary artery wedge pressure rose as arterial pressure increased. At a dosage greater than 6 µg per kilogram per minute, dopamine augmented heart rate. During a 24-hour infusion of each drug, only dobutamine produced a sustained increase of stroke volume, cardiac output, urine flow, urine sodium concentration, creatinine clearance, and peripheral blood flow.

Although dopamine can improve renal and mesenteric perfusion by selective vasodilation, a property not unique to dobutamine, this beneficial effect is reversed when dopamine is infused in larger dosages (10 to 15 µg per kilogram per minute).[7,32] Dosage-related vasoconstriction is titratable from patient to patient. Therefore when larger dosages of dopamine are necessary to sustain patients in frank hypotension, a careful ongoing assessment of urine output is essential.

Vasodilator therapy (pharmacological afterload reduction). When the left ventricular outflow is impeded because of peripheral vasoconstriction, vasodilation therapy may augment cardiac output by lowering this outflow resistance. Vasodilator therapy was first employed clinically by Majid and others.[18] They infused the alpha-adrenergic blocking agent phentolamine into normotensive patients with left ventricular dysfunction, following myocardial infarction. Vasodilation produced a fall in systemic vascular resistance accompanied by elevation of cardiac output and reduction of pulmonary artery pressure. The use of vasodilator therapy in pump failure has since been well documented.[29,30]

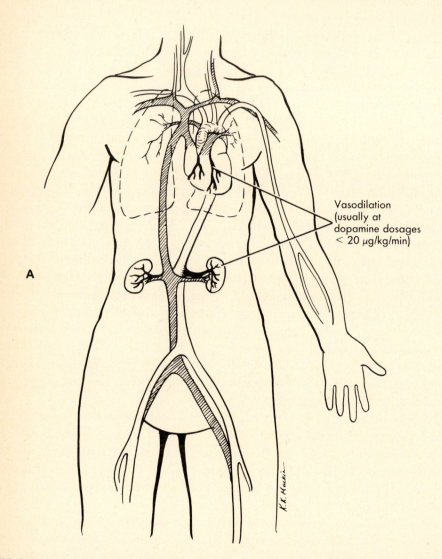

Vasodilation
(usually at
dopamine dosages
< 20 µg/kg/min)

A

FIG. 7-2 Dopamine's dosage-mediated effects on receptor sites. **A,** Dopaminergic response.

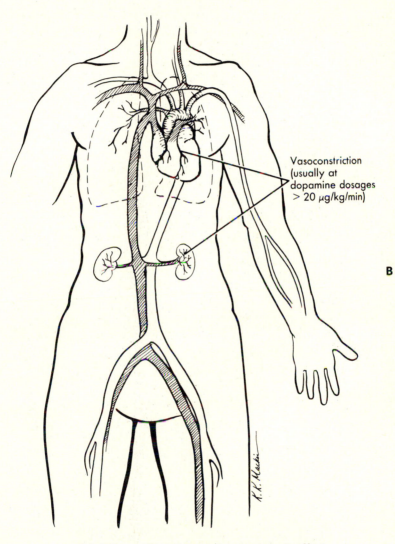

Vasoconstriction
(usually at
dopamine dosages
> 20 μg/kg/min)

B

FIG. 7-2, cont'd **B,** Reversed dopaminergic effect.

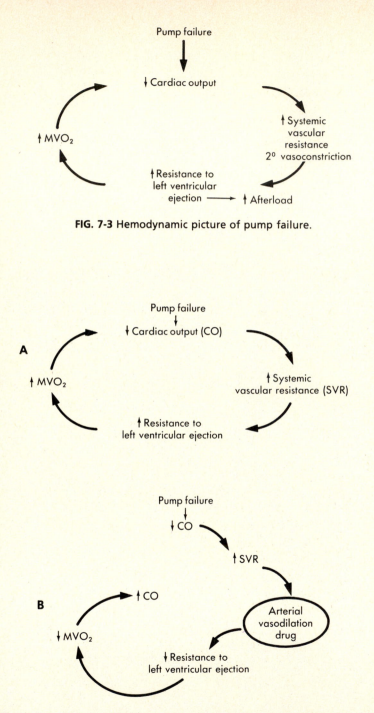

FIG. 7-3 Hemodynamic picture of pump failure.

FIG. 7-4 Effects of arteriolar vasodilation on vascular smooth muscles and resulting improvement in pump function. **A,** Hemodynamic status before arterial vasodilation. **B,** Hemodynamic status after arterial vasodilation.

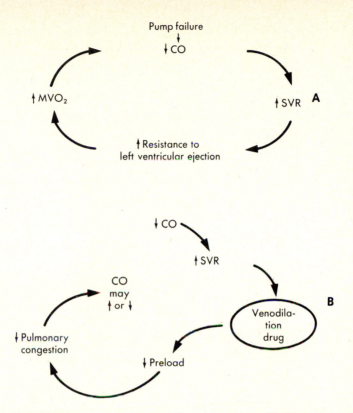

FIG. 7-5 Effects of venodilation on vascular smooth muscle and resulting improvement in pump function. **A,** Hemodynamic status before venodilation. **B,** Hemodynamic status after venodilation.

Fig. 7-3 illustrates the hemodynamic status of a patient who can perhaps be treated with a vasodilator agent. Compensatory vasoconstriction, secondary to myocardial ischemia, leads to a potentially vicious circle—increased resistance to left ventricular ejection increases the work load of the heart and increases oxygen consumption, which further increase myocardial ischemia.

Arteriolar and venodilators. Smith and Braunwald[27] delineated the mechanisms of arteriolar and venodilators. Arteriolar dilation intercepts the vicious circle triggered by peripheral vasoconstriction by dilating the arterioles and reducing afterload (Fig. 7-4). Pure vasodilators may produce a hemodynamic effect similar to a diuretic by redistributing blood volume. Venodilation produces a reduction in preload, contributes to a lower ventricular filling pressure, and may diminish symptoms of pulmonary congestion (Fig. 7-5). Reduction of pulmonary capillary pressure may occur at the expense of some reduction in cardiac output.

Intimate interactions exist in the vasodilator agents' effect on preload and afterload. A venodilator that reduces preload also lowers afterload by reducing ventricular volume (although systemic vascular resistance is not reduced). Conversely, an arterial vasodilator that diminishes arterial pressure, thereby enhancing ventricular emptying, indirectly lowers preload. Both arteriolar and venodilators effectively reduce MVO_2 and usually improve cardiac output.

Specific vasodilator agents

Sodium nitroprusside (Nipride). Sodium nitroprusside was introduced as a vasodilator agent for use in the treatment of left ventricular pump dysfunction as early as 1972.[9] A "balanced" vasodilator, nitroprusside acts directly to relax both vascular arterioles and veins.[24] Preload and afterload are decreased with a resultant improvement in left ventricular performance. The initial infusion rate in adults is usually 10 μg per minute, increased in amounts of 5 to 10 μg per minute every 5 minutes until the desired hemodynamic improvement is achieved, up to a maximum dosage of 400 to 500 μg per minute.[27]

Hypotension is a hazardous side effect that is usually reversed within 10 minutes after discontinuation of the drug. Normal metabolism produces cyanide molecules that are converted to thiocyanate by a hepatic enzyme and excreted by the kidneys.[30] In the presence of renal insufficiency, infusion of nitroprusside in dosages greater than 5 μg per kilogram per minute may result in thiocyanate toxicity. Manifestations include convulsions, psychosis, abdominal pain, muscle twitching, and dizziness. Cyanide toxicity interferes with tissue oxygen use, and anaerobic metabolism ensues. Hemoglobin may be reduced to methamoglobin, which interferes with normal oxygen transport. Serum thiocyanate levels should never exceed 6 mg per 100 ml. Nitroprusside loses its potency with exposure to light;[7] the manufacturer should be consulted for proper handling of the medication bottle to protect it from light and for the length of duration that the medication will remain stable in the reconstituted IV.

Nitrates

IV NITROGLYCERIN. Tridil (Arnar-Stone)[4] is an IV administrable form of nitroglycerin. Although venous effects predominate, nitroglycerin produces dilation of both arterial and venous beds. Therefore preload and afterload are reduced. Elevated central venous and pulmonary capillary wedge pressures and pulmonary and systemic vascular resistances should be reduced by intravenous nitroglycerin therapy. Heart rate is usually increased, presumably a reflex response to the fall in blood pressure. Coronary blood flow is usually improved more than with nitroprusside.

There is no fixed optimum dosage. The drug must be titrated to the responsiveness of the individual patient and the desired level of hemodynamic function. Nitroglycerin (50 mg, IV) is usually reconstituted in a 500 ml solution. Initial infusion should begin at 5 μg per minute delivered through an infusion pump. Initial titration should be at 5 μg per minute with increases made every 3 to 5 minutes. If no response is noted at an infusion rate of 20 μg per minute, increments of 10 and 20 μg per minute can be used. Once a partial reduction in blood pressure is observed, the dosage increase should be reduced and the interval between increases lengthened.[3]

Nitroglycerin readily migrates into many plastics. Polyvinyl chloride (PVC) tubing absorbs 40% to 80% of IV nitroglycerin. The higher rates of absorption occur when flow rates are low and nitroglycerin concentrations are high. A non-PVC administration set is provided with the medication to minimize diffusion of the drug.[4]

There are no infusion pumps that are totally acceptable for controlling infusion of IV nitroglycerin with the non-PVC administration set. Non-PVC tubing is less compliant than conventional PVC tubing. Infusion pumps tested with this administration set have been faulted in their inability to exert sufficient force to fully occlude the non-PVC tubing. This condition could result in excessive flow at low infusion rate settings or allow gravity flow after the pump has been turned off.[20] Therefore close monitoring of the infusion through a pump is essential. The roller clamp should be closed whenever the infusion is stopped.

Nitroglycerin ointment may be used for a more prolonged vasodilation action. A 0.5- to 4.0-inch strip is applied to the skin every 4 to 6 hours. An advantage with this form of administration is that it can be readily removed in case of adverse effects.

PHENTOLAMINE. Phentolamine, first used as a vasodilator in patients with heart failure,[18] has three actions: (1) it blocks alpha-adrenergic receptors of both arterioles and veins; (2) it is a direct relaxant of vascular smooth muscle; (3) it releases cardiac norepinephrine stores and thereby exerts positive chronotropic and inotropic effects.[30]

Phentolamine has a short-acting duration. The initial dosage is 0.1 mg per minute, which may be increased by a rate of 0.1 mg per minute every 5 minutes to a maximum of 2.0 mg per minute. Tachycardia and the high cost of this medication make it less desirable than nitroprusside as a vasodilator agent.

PRAZOSIN. Prazosin exerts direct relaxing effects on vascular smooth muscles. The circulatory effects mimic nitroprusside, since prazosin is a balanced vasodilator. It is orally effective; an oral dose displays maximum effectiveness in 45 minutes, persisting for 6 hours. The initial oral dosage is 1 mg that is adjusted upward but not to exceed 10 mg twice a day. The most common side effect is the so-called *first dose phenomenon*. Transient faintness, palpitations, and occasionally syncope may occur.[17]

HYDRALAZINE. Another orally effective vasodilator is found in hydralazine, which acts directly on arteriolar smooth muscle. The usual dosage is 25 to 100 mg three to four times daily. Onset of action is within 30 minutes and persists for about 6 hours. Because of hydralazine's predominant action on the arterial bed, afterload reduction and resultant improvement in cardiac output usually occur without preload reduction.[21]

Combined use of vasopressors and vasodilator drugs. Combined use of a vasodilator drug with an inotropic agent affords pharmacological support to minimize resistance to ejection and to optimize ventricular contraction.[25] The inotropic agent, such as dopamine or dobutamine, is infused at a dosage of 5 to 15 µg per kilogram per minute, whereas the vasodilator, such as IV nitroglycerin, is titrated based on the pulmonary artery wedge pressure, peripheral perfusion, and arterial pressure. Combined therapy produces greater improvement in left ventricular performance than either agent can when used alone.

Digitalization in pump failure. Digitalis preparations increase myocardial contractility by blocking a membrane-bound enzyme system called *sodium-potassium adenosin triphosphatase (ATPase),* which increases the availability of intracellular calcium to the contractile elements. Peripheral vascular resistance increases with administration of the digitalis preparations because of their acute vasoconstricting effects. Electrophysiological effects of digitalis result from a net increase in the refractory period, a decrease in conduction velocity in specialized conduction tissues, and a shortening of the refractory period in atrial and ventricular myocardium.

For patients with acute heart failure who are in sinus rhythm, digitalis probably adds little benefit.[33] Diminished contractile actions have been observed with ischemic myocardium following digitalis administration.[3] Therefore potentially deleterious effects can ensue when digitalis is administered to a patient with an acute condition of pump failure because of the vasodilating effects and diminished contractile action on ischemic myocardium.

REFERENCES

1. Alquist, R.P.: A study of the adrenergic receptors, Am. J. Physiol. **153**:586, 1948.
2. American Heart Association: Advanced life support standards, Dallas 1982, The Association.
3. Amsterdam, E.A., et al.: Myocardial infarction shock: mechanisms and management. In Maston, D.T., editor: Congestive heart failure, New York, 1976, Yorke Medical Publishers.
4. Arnar-Stone del Caribe Inc.: Tridil (nitroglycerin), package insert, McGaw Park, Ill., Sept. 1981.
5. Avery, G.S.: Drug treatment principles and practice of clinical pharmacology and therapeutics, ed. 2, New York, 1980, ADIS Press.
6. Chatterjee, K., et al.: Hemodynamic and metabolic responses of vasodilator therapy in acute myocardial infarction, Circulation **48**:1183, 1973.
7. Cohn, J.N.: Current therapy, Philadelphia, 1982, W.B. Saunders Co.
8. Cohn, J.N., and Franciosa, J.A.: Vasodilator therapy of cardiac failure, N. Engl. J. Med. **297**:27, 1977.
9. Franciosa, J.A., et al.: Improved left ventricular function during nitroprusside infusion in acute myocardial infarction, Lancet **1**:650, 1972.
10. Goldberg, L.I., et al.: Cardiovascular and renal actions of dopamine: potential clinical applications, Pharmacol. Rev. **24**:1, 1972.
11. Goldberg, L.I., et al.: Newer catecholamines for treatment of heart failure and shock: an update on dopamine and a first look at dobutamine, Prog. Cardiovasc. Dis. **19**:327, 1977.
12. Goodman, L.S., and Gilman, A., editors: The pharmacological basis of therapeutics, ed. 6, New York, 1980, Macmillan Publishing Co., Inc.
13. Hanosh, P., and Cohn, J.N.: Left ventricular function in acute infarction, J. Clin. Invest. **50**:523, 1971.
14. Lands, A.M., et al.: Differentiation of receptor systems activated by sympathomimetic amines, Nature **214**:597, 1967.
15. Leier, C.V., et al.: Comparative systematic and regional hemodynamic effects of dopamine and dobutamine in patients with cardiomyopathic heart failure, Circulation **58**:466, 1978.
16. Loch, A.S., et al.: Hemodynamic effects of dobutamine in man, Circ. Shock **2**:29, 1975.
17. Lowenstein, J., and Steele, J., Jr.: Prazosin, Am. Heart J. **95**:262, 1978.
18. Majid, P.A., et al.: Phentolamine for vasodilator treatment of severe heart-failure, Lancet **2**:719, 1971.
19. Mason, D., et al.: Diagnosis and management of myocardial infarction and shock. In Eliot, R.S., et al., editors: Cardiac emergencies, ed. 2, Mount Kisco, N.Y., 1982, Futura Publishing Co., Inc.
20. Nitroglycerin overinfusion with infusion devices through Tridil set IV administration sets, Health Devices Sourcebook, 1981-82 reference, Nov. 1981.
21. Packer, M., et al.: Dose requirements of hydralazine in patients with severe chronic congestive heart failure, Am. J. Cardiol. **45**(3):655, March 1980.
22. Parmley, W.W., and Chatterjee, K.: Vasodilator therapy, Curr. Probl. Cardiol. **2**:1, 1978.
23. Robie, N.W., and Goldberg, L.I.: Comparative systemic and regional hemodynamic effects of dopamine and dobutamine, Am. Heart J. **90**(3):340, 1975.
24. Shah, P.K.: Ventricular unloading in the management of heart disease: role of vasodilators. Part I, Am. Heart J. **93**(2):256, 1977.
25. Shearer, J.K., and Caldwell, M.: Use of sodium nitroprusside and dopamine hydrochloride in the postoperative cardiac patient, Heart Lung **8**:302, 1979.
26. Smith, T.W.: Drug therapy. Digitalis glycosides, N. Engl. J. Med. **288**:719, 1973.
27. Smith, T.W., and Braunwald, E.: The management of heart failure. In Braunwald, E., editor: Heart disease, a textbook of cardiovascular medicine, Philadelphia, 1980, W.B. Saunders Co.
28. Sonnenblick, E.H., et al.: Dobutamine: a new synthetic cardioactive sympathetic amine, N. Engl. J. Med. **300**:18, 1979.

29. Stemple, D.R., et al.: Combined nitroprusside-dopamine therapy in severe chronic congestive heart failure, Am. J. Cardiol. **42:**267, 1978.
30. Stern, M.A., et al.: Hemodynamic effects of intravenous phentolamine in low output cardiac failure. Dose-response relationships, Circulation **58:**157, 1978.
31. Tinker, J.H.: Dobutamine for inotropic support during emergence from cardiopulmonary bypass, Anesthesiology **44:**281, 1976.
32. Tuttle, R.R., and Mills, J.: Dopamine: development of a new catecholamine to selectively increase cardiac contractility, Circ. Res. **36:**185, 1975.
33. Waters, D., and Forrester, J.: Diagnosis and management of congestive heart failure and pulmonary edema. In Eliot, R.S., et al., editors: Cardiac emergencies, ed. 2, Mount Kisco, N.Y., 1982, Futura Publishing Co., Inc.

CHAPTER 8 Physiology of intra-aortic balloon pump counterpulsation

Intra-aortic balloon pump counterpulsation involves the placement of a distensible polyurethane, nonthrombogenic balloon in the descending thoracic aorta, just distal to the left subclavian artery, which is usually introduced through the femoral artery (Fig. 8-1). (Insertion techniques in Chapter 13). A Dacron graft sutured to the femoral artery facilitates insertion and avoids interruption of blood flow to the extremity.[3] The intra-aortic balloon is mounted on a vascular catheter that has multiple communications with the lumen of the balloon (Fig. 8-2), allowing transfer of helium or carbon dioxide gas in and out of the balloon, which alternately inflates and deflates it.[4] The balloon catheter extends outside the femoral arteriotomy and is attached to the balloon pump console (Fig. 8-3). The console is equipped with R-wave detector triggering circuitry and driving gas to phasically pulse the balloon in synchrony with the cardiac cycle.

Principles of counterpulsation

Raising of the intra-aortic pressure in diastole by inflation and deflation of the balloon with rapid withdrawal of the gas just before the next systole is termed *counterpulsation* (Fig. 8-4).[5] Therefore counterpulsation alters the normal physiological cycle of systolic and diastolic pressure. Mechanically, the intra-aortic balloon pump is a "volume-displacement device"; it actively synchronizes displacement of aortic blood. Blood volume within the aorta (see Windkessel effect, Chapter 2) is actually displaced proximally and distally at the time of balloon inflation in diastole. Elevation of the intra-aortic pressure during diastole is termed *diastolic augmentation*.

Two counterpulsation cycles are diagrammed in Fig. 8-5. The balloon rapidly inflates just after the aortic valve closes, represented by the dicrotic notch on the arterial waveform. Rapid deflation occurs just before the next systolic ejection, signaled by the R wave of the electrocardiogram (ECG).

To ensure proper coordination between the pump and cardiac cycle, complex logic systems are necessary within the console. Phasic volume changes of the balloon are effected by this external control mechanism that is synchronized with the ECG. Timing logic describes the method of synchronizing the system's mechanical function with an input ECG signal. The R wave of the standard ECG serves as an easily recognizable and reliable input signal for referencing the cardiac cycle.[4]

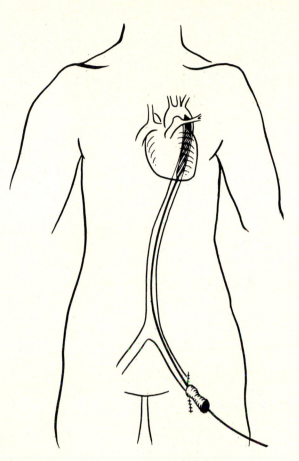

FIG. 8-1 Intra-aortic balloon may be introduced through femoral artery via Dacron graft. (Note percutaneous insertion technique in Chapter 13.)

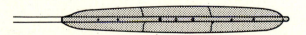

FIG. 8-2 Intra-aortic balloon is mounted on vascular catheter that has multiple communications with lumen of balloon.

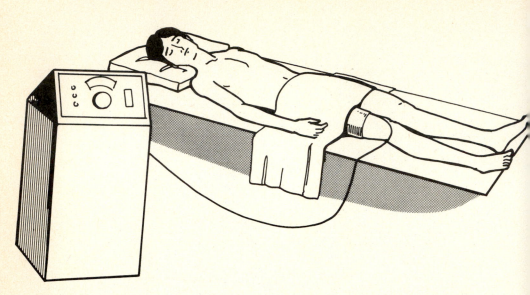

FIG. 8-3 Balloon catheter extends outside femoral arteriotomy and is attached to balloon pump console that is equipped with triggering circuitry and driving gas to phasically pulse balloon in synchrony with electrocardiogram.

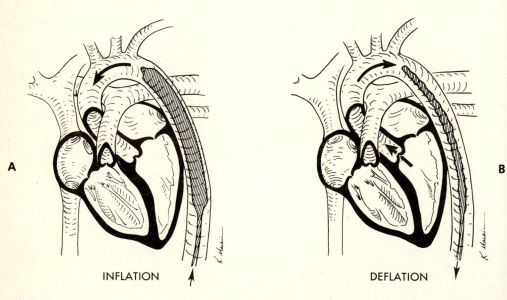

A

INFLATION

DEFLATION

B

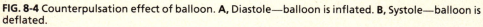

FIG. 8-4 Counterpulsation effect of balloon. **A,** Diastole—balloon is inflated. **B,** Systole—balloon is deflated.

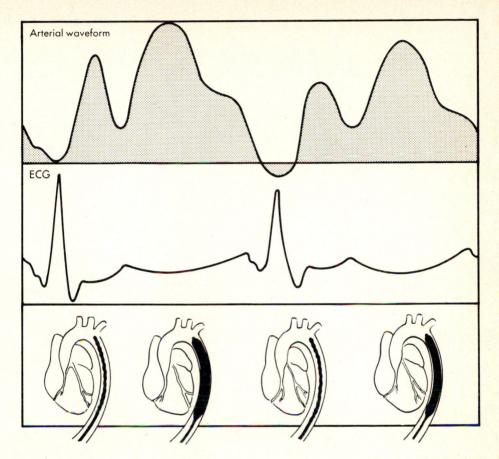

FIG. 8-5 Two counterpulsation cycles. Balloon is rapidly inflated at beginning of diastole just after aortic valve closes. Rapid deflation occurs just before next systole.

Machine controls for inflation-deflation allow the operator to manually adjust the inflation-deflation logic within defined safety limits to achieve ideal hemodynamic benefits from the counterpulsation sequence. *Though the ECG is used in triggering the pump, it is the arterial waveform that must be examined and continuously monitored to establish and evaluate the counterpulsation effect of balloon augmentation on the hemodynamic performance of the left ventricle (see Timing, Chapter 15).*

Balloon's action in diastole

The ventricles are relaxed in diastole. Immediately after the aortic valve closes, the gas in propelled into the balloon, which increases the intra-aortic volume and pressure (displacement principle); hence the term *augmentation of diastolic pressure.* Conceptually, balloon inflation can be visualized as "compartmentalizing" the aorta[2] (Fig. 8-6). The proximal compartment includes the aortic root and the coronary arteries. The distal com-

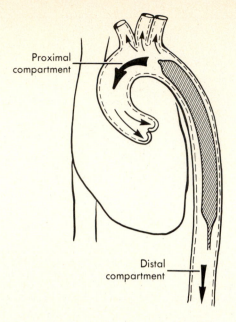

FIG. 8-6 Balloon inflation in diastole can be visualized as "compartmentalizing" aorta. *Proximal compartment* includes aortic root and coronary arteries. *Distal compartment* is composed of remainder of aorta, distal to balloon and systemic circulation.

partment includes the remainder of the aorta, distal to the balloon and the systemic circulation.

Effects of balloon inflation on the proximal compartment[2,4]

1. Total or regional coronary blood flow is increased by raising the perfusion pressure at the coronary ostia.
2. Collateral coronary circulation may be opened because of the principle just described.
3. Diastolic pressure is raised or augmented in the aorta, which increases perfusion to the vessels of the aortic arch.

Effects of balloon inflation on the distal compartment[2,4]

Systemic perfusion is increased because balloon inflation facilitates peripheral runoff, although the exact physiological mechanisms involved have not been conclusively clarified. The currently accepted theory is that the volume displaced by the balloon imparts momentum to the column of blood in the aorta (Windkessel effect, Chapter 2). This action boosts cardiac ejection.

Balloon's action in systole[4,5]

The ventricles are contracted in systole. Balloon deflation occurs just prior to systole before the aortic valve opens (Fig. 8-7). The gas is rapidly removed from the balloon,

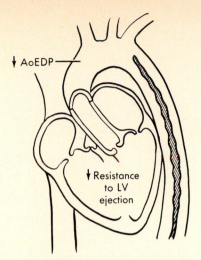

FIG. 8-7 Balloon deflation just before systole, which briefly decreases aortic end-diastolic pressure, thereby reducing resistance to left ventricular ejection (afterload).

which reduces the intra-aortic volume and pressure. Intra-aortic pressure (aortic end-diastolic or AoEDP) reduction is timed to occur just before systole, which reduces the afterload or resistance to left ventricular ejection. This is perhaps the most critical effect of the balloon because if afterload is reduced, the left ventricle empties more easily and completely. In summary, the net gains of balloon deflation just before systole are the following:

1. The rapid reduction of aortic pressure enables the left ventricle to eject against a lower pressure (afterload reduction).
2. Maximum tension developed by the left ventricle is reduced.

Counterpulsation and afterload reduction

Deflation is timed to occur just before the aortic valve opens, causing a sudden reduction in intra-aortic pressure (Fig. 8-8). Isovolumic contraction occurs as the early component of systole when the left ventricle generates tension by decreasing the chamber radius and elevating intracavity pressure (without a change in volume). The rising left ventricular pressure finally exceeds the AoEDP that pushes open the aortic valve, and systolic ejection occurs. Approximately 90% of myocardial oxygen consumption (MVO_2) occurs during isovolumic contraction.

Rapid balloon deflation during isovolumic contraction reduces the AoEDP (i.e., the afterload component of cardiac work or the resistance to left ventricular ejection).[5]

The balloon's effect on afterload reduction can be more easily understood if an analogy is made to a man trying to move a 1000-pound load. Fig. 8-9, *A*, illustrates a man trying to move the load by lifting, but he is unsuccessful. Again he attempts to move the load a

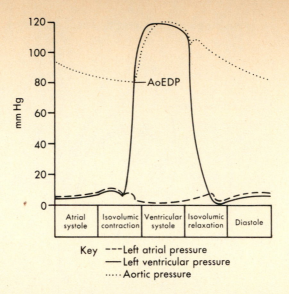

FIG. 8-8 Left aortic and ventricular pressure diagram. Isovolumic contraction occurs as early phase of systole when left ventricle generates tension by decreasing chamber radius and elevating intracavity pressure until enough force is generated to open aortic valve; ejection follows. Ninety percent of myocardial oxygen consumption occurs during isovolumic contraction.

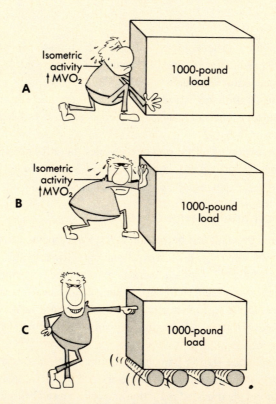

FIG. 8-9 **A,** Unsuccessful attempt is made to move 1000-pound load (resistance) by lifting. **B,** Another attempt is made to move load by pushing. During this isometric exercise, oxygen consumption is increasing. **C,** Rollers are placed under 1000-pound load, and it can be moved with little effort. Balloon's deflation also effects lowering of AoEDP, which makes left ventricle ejection less effort (rollers placed under left ventricle).

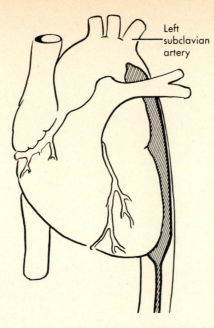

Left subclavian artery

FIG. 8-10 Balloon is positioned in descending thoracic aorta, just distal to left subclavian artery. Positioning in aortic arch would compromise flow to arch vessels.

distance by pushing it in Fig. 8-9, *B*, but to no avail. MVO_2 is increased during these isometric exercises. In Fig. 8-9, *C*, rollers are placed under the 1000-pound load. Now the man can easily move the load with one finger. MVO_2 is reduced as the afterload or impedance to moving the load is reduced by placing rollers under the load. That is precisely the effect of the IABP. It places rollers under the left ventricle by reducing AoEDP in the process of rapid balloon deflation just before left ventricular systole.

The enhanced aortic capacitance caused by peripheral runoff, the drop in AoEDP, and the balloon-affected augmentation of blood flow combine to reduce afterload, decrease cardiac work, and lower oxygen consumption.[6]

Positioning of the balloon

Risk of cerebrovascular insult, which could occur with positioning of the balloon in the carotid artery, dictates that the balloon be positioned in the descending aorta, just distal to the takeoff of the left subclavian artery (Fig. 8-10). Placement of the balloon in this position expands the proximal compartment to include the subclavian and carotid arterial systems. The remoteness of the balloon from the aortic valve imposes a time delay between actual balloon inflation and its physiological effect at the aortic root, which is considered when timing the balloon. Finally to minimize hemolysis and to prevent aortic wall damage, the balloon is inflated to occlude no more than 90% of the aorta.

REFERENCES

1. Alpert, J., et al.: Vascular complications of intra-aortic balloon pumping, Arch. Surg. **111:**1190, 1976.
2. Hollinger, W.A.: The intra-aortic balloon pump and other mechanical cardiac assist devices, CVP, **9:**19, 1981.
3. Kantrowitz, A., et al.: Clinical experience with cardiac assistance by means of intra-aortic phase-shift balloon pumping, Trans. Am. Soc. Artif. Intern. Organs **14:**344, 1968.
4. Mason, D.T., et al.: Diagnosis and management of myocardial infarction shock. In Eliot, R.S., et al., editors: Cardiac emergencies, ed. 2, Mount Kisco, N.Y., 1982, Futura Publishing Co., Inc.
5. Michels, R., et al.: Intra-aortic balloon pumping in coronary artery disease, Herz **4:**397, 1979.
6. Nichols, A.B., et al.: Left ventricular function during intra-aortic balloon pumping assessed by mutigated cardiac blood pool imagery, Circulation **58**(suppl. 1):entire issue, 1978.

CHAPTER 9 Balloon's effect on a failing heart

No currently available pharmacological therapy can as effectively combine the two physiological treatment goals of pump failure (reduction in left ventricular afterload and elevation of diastolic arterial pressure) to the same extent as the intra-aortic balloon.[9] Therefore balloon pumping performs a unique role in the treatment of patients with cardiovascular compromise.

Coronary perfusion pressure is increased with the use of peripheral vasoconstrictive agents (alpha adrenergics) but usually at the expense of increasing myocardial work and oxygen consumption and thereby reducing cardiac output. The intra-aortic balloon's inflation in diastole elevates aortic pressure and potentially increases coronary perfusion. Rapid deflation of the balloon during isovolumic contracton reduces the aortic end-diastolic pressure or the resistance to left ventricular ejection (the balloon puts rollers under the left ventricle [Fig. 8-9, C]). Therefore left ventricular work load and myocardial oxygen consumption are reduced (Fig. 9-1).

Systolic unloading with intra-aortic balloon counterpulsation

In spite of the overwhelming clinical evidence of the beneficial effects of the IABP, the underlying mechanisms have not been totally resolved.[5] Dr. Akyurekli and researchers[1] at the University of Ottawa undertook a study to determine the systolic unloading effects of the IABP, independent of diastolic augmentation. This was accomplished by counterpulsating dogs while their coronary arteries were perfused from an extracorporeal source. The perfusion pressure was lowered to produce acute cardiac failure. When intra-aortic balloon counterpulsation was instituted, systolic unloading (a reduction in left ventricular systolic pressure) was only evident at normotensive states (coronary perfusion pressure of 80 mm Hg). Employment of IABP during acute coronary insufficiency and subsequent left ventricular failure did not result in systolic unloading or a reduction in oxygen consumtion.

These results suggest that balloon unloading responses may be intimately related to the functional status of the circulatory system before balloon pumping. For example, an increase in aortic compliance at lower aortic pressures reduces the aortic volume.[3] A lower arterial pressure has been demonstrated to cause the aortic wall to move with the balloon so that changes in balloon volume do not accompany changes in aortic blood volume.[4]

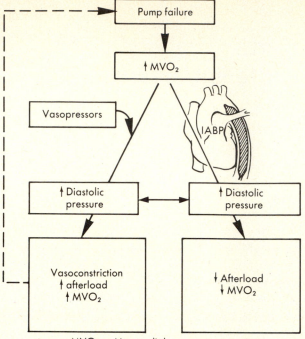

MVO$_2$ = Myocardial oxygen consumption

FIG. 9-1 Comparison of treatment of pump failure with vasopressors and intra-aortic balloon counterpulsation. Elevation of diastolic pressure occurs with both modalities. Vasopressors, however, cause vasoconstriction and increased afterload, ventricular work, and myocardial oxygen consumption. Balloon counterpulsation decreases afterload, myocardial work, and oxygen consumption.

Coronary perfusion with balloon diastolic augmentation

Coronary perfusion is potentially increased as the balloon inflates in diastole. Effective augmentation of coronary perfusion is, however, dependent on the degree of vasodilation within the coronary bed. Myocardial ischemia is a potent stimulus for increasing blood flow and oxygen delivery to the myocardium through vasodilation; coronary flow then becomes pressure dependent.[8] The process of autoregulation involves coronary vasodilation, occurring as a means to maintain a balance between myocardial oxygen supply and demand.[6,19,23]

Balloon inflation displaces blood proximally, potentially increasing coronary perfusion. If the coronary arteries are already maximally dilated by an autoregulatory response to myocardial ischemia, little if any increase in coronary flow will occur. Autoregulatory vasodilation of coronary vessels is impaired by atherosclerosis. Augmentation of coronary perfusion pressure by balloon blood volume displacement proximally in diastole may therefore significantly improve flow through atherosclerotic coronary vessels and establish collateral pathways of perfusion.

Increases in coronary blood flow ranging from 7% to 50% with balloon counterpul-

TABLE 9-1 Hemodynamic factors monitored following balloon pumping in patients with and without ischemia at onset of counterpulsation

	Continuing ischemia Group I N = 12	No ischemia Group II N = 14
Hours lapse from onset of symptoms to initiation of CP*		
Median	19	57
Range	5-72	8-456
Heart rate		
Before CP	119 ± 13 SD†	117 ± 18 SD
After 24 hours of CP	101 ± 14	107 ± 18
At termination of CP	81 ± 10	101 ± 9
Pulmonary artery pressure (mm Hg)		
Before CP	33 ± 7	31 ± 8
After 24 hours of CP	18 ± 5	20 ±
At termination of CP	12 ± 3	10 ± 4
Duration of CP (days)	8.9	6.3

Modified from O'Rourke, M.F., et al.: Am. J. Cardiol. **47**:8, 1981.
*CP, Counterpulsation.
†SD, Standard Deviations.

sation have been demonstrated in a number of experiments.[28] Experiments described by Powell and associates[19] illustrated the improvement in coronary flow with balloon counterpulsation in nonhypovolemic, hypotensive animals. Balloon augmentation in normal animals did not significantly improve coronary flow. This finding was subsequently confirmed by Weber and Janiche.[26]

O'Rourke and others[16] suggested that counterpulsation was often initiated so late after an acute infarction that myocardial ischemic damage had become irreversible. The University of Australia, under O'Rourke's direction, tested the effects of counterpulsation on 26 patients who had refractory heart failure without shock complicating acute myocardial infarction. Patients were divided into a group of 12 with continuing myocardial ischemia, evidenced by anginal pain and associated with abnormal S-T segment elevation, and a group of 14 without continuing ischemia.

Though all patients demonstrated improvement in hemodynamic areas with the initiation of balloon pumping, those with sustained ischemia (Group I) exhibited more pronounced hemodynamic improvement, reflected by pulmonary artery pressure and heart rate (Table 9-1). The effect on ischemia was impressive; pain was abolished within minutes for 11 patients and within 12 hours for one person in Group I.

Of the 12 patients in Group I there was only one hospital death attributed to low cardiac output failure 27 days after termination of counterpulsation. Eight of the 14 patients in Group II died in the hospital—three from late ventricular fibrillation and five from cardiac failure.

The fact that improvement in morbidity and mortality was associated with prompt relief of anginal pain suggests that such improvement resulted directly from relief of myocardial ischemia and preservation of reversibly damaged muscle. Patients with myocardial ischemia underwent counterpulsation much earlier than those without continued ischemia. This factor alone may have been more important than the presence of ischemia in determining a favorable outcome. Counterpulsation was most effective when applied early after onset of symptoms because there was usually more ischemia and reversible damage present at that time.

Lorente and associates[13] formulated a decision-making algorithm for use in treatment of patients with cardiogenic shock. Clinical and hemodynamic data were extrapolated from patients with cardiogenic shock secondary to myocardial infarction, compared to a 1-month survival rate. Survival and nonsurvival zones were defined within the algorithm. Patients who fell within the nonsurvival zone, following onset of cardiogenic shock, were placed in a study. Group I underwent balloon pumping, and Group II continued with pharmacological management of their pump failure. At 1 month there were seven survivors in Group I (N = 26) and no survivors in Group II (N = 17). Of the seven 1-month survivors, only three lived for more than a year.

Effects on infarct size

O'Rourke and associates[16] continued their work with balloon pumping and evaluation of its effect on the failing myocardium in a later study. Thirty patients received the treatment, following infarction, but ischemic pain had subsided by the time the patients were placed on the balloon pump (an average of 7.1 hours after the onset of symptoms). No benefit was apparent from counterpulsation in this sample population. It was anticipated that infarct size could be limited with interventions initiated up to 24 hours after the onset of symptoms. This view was based largely on the time course of enzyme release from the myocardium after infarction.

Other studies have shown that early institution of measures to reduce infarct size is vital. Administration of propranolol leads to a decrease in enzyme release (and presumably, limitation of infarct size) only when administered within 4 hours after the onset of symptoms.[15] Limitation of infarction and improvement in survival have been demonstrated in dogs when IABP was begun within minutes after coronary artery occlusion.[20]

The conclusion of these researchers was that it was unrealistic to expect that counterpulsation begun an average of 7.1 hours after the onset of symptoms would limit infarct size and improve ischemia. In this study counterpulsation was most likely begun too late; myocardial ischemia had become irreversible.[15]

The study of Laas and co-workers[12] has enhanced our understanding of the role and limitations of IABP. Without developed collateral circulation, balloon pumping did not reduce the area of myocardial infarction. However, with total or subtotal coronary occlusion, but developed collateral circulation, IABP suggested a decrease in the ischemic area. The authors concluded that much more research was needed on the use of the IABP for treatment of myocardial ischemia.

IABP for cardiogenic shock following acute myocardial infarction

The Department of Surgery at Kobe University School of Medicine studied the effect of IABP in cardiogenic shock following acute myocardial infarction in 94 dogs.[14] Significant increases of 40% in aortic diastolic pressure, 30% in cardiac output, and 30% in coronary blood flow were recorded. Left ventricular pressure decreased 20%, and left ventricular end-diastolic pressure fell 15%. These favorable effects of IABP were not observed in dogs that had infarcted areas, involving more than 50% of the free wall of the left ventricle.

DeWood and associates[5] compared 40 patients who were treated with balloon pumping for cardiogenic shock. Group I was treated with intra-aortic balloon counterpulsation, and Group II was treated with counterpulsation and coronary artery bypass grafting. The in-hospital mortality between groups was not significantly different. The difference in long-term mortality between Groups I and II was substantially impressive (71.4% versus 47.3%). The subset of Group II that underwent reperfusion and counterpulsation within 16 hours from the onset of symptoms had a lower mortality (25.0%) than the subset that underwent surgery more than 18 hours after the onset of symptoms (71.4%).

Sweden's Karolinska Institute reversed cardiogenic shock, following myocardial infarction, in 80% of their study group with the use of IABP. Thirty-three percent were successfully weaned off the balloon pump and discharged from the cardiac care unit. However, only 13% were long-term survivors.

Classification of patients with impending or definitive left ventricular power failure and indications for intra-aortic balloon assist

Fig. 9-2 depicts a schema for classification of patients with subsequent acute myocardial infarction. Stroke index and mean arterial pressure are multiplied to plot a point on the vertical axis. By plotting this point against mean wedge pressure, patients fall into one of

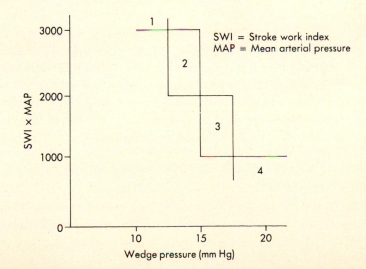

FIG. 9-2 Schema for classification of severity of pump failure and application of balloon pump (see text for discussion).

four arbitrary classes. The schema is used to aid in early diagnosis of hemodynamic deterioration following myocardial infarction and to establish a protocol for use of balloon assist.[3]

In Groups I and II, close observation of the patient's hemodynamic status is maintained for ongoing signs of medically refractory angina. Intra-aortic balloon assist is indicated in Group III patients if:

1. Blood pressure is falling, and the patient is not responding to increasing catecholamines.
2. Pulmonary capillary wedge pressure is increasing.
3. Urine output is decreasing.
4. Myocardial irritability occurs while hemodynamic status is pharmacologically controlled.

The significant factor in the care of this subset of patients is to determine the point at which aggressive medical therapy is failing and when balloon pumping should begin. Physiological effects of the balloon are weighed against the drug effects, and the intervention that allows the heart to function most efficiently is selected.

Group IV consists of patients who have cardiogenic shock. Intra-aortic balloon counterpulsation is indicated if within 1 to 2 hours vigorous medical therapy has failed to reverse the following:

1. Urine output less than 20 ml per hour
2. Pulmonary capillary wedge pressure greater than 18 mm Hg
3. Cold, clammy skin
4. Obtundation

Combination of dobutamine and intra-aortic counterpulsation

The Department of Cardiac Surgery, University of Munich,[20] researched the benefits of combined dobutamine and balloon pumping for pump failure and found that the combined effects of these two agents offered a very positive hemodynamic gain. The IABP has been demonstrated to be relatively ineffective in patients with low peripheral pressures (mean aortic pressures of 50 mm Hg and below).[11] Use of dobutamine for treatment of low cardiac output improves contractility but at the expense of producing a rise in heart rate and myocardial oxygen consumption. Therefore a combination of dobutamine and intra-aortic counterpulsation, as observed by the Munich researchers, provided a symbiosis; dobutamine increased peripheral blood pressure and improved cardiac output, whereas balloon augmentation improved coronary flow and reduced afterload.

Combination of dopamine and nitroprusside therapy in conjunction with IABP

Sturm and associates[24] have demonstrated that once preload has been optimized with volume loading, administration of nitroprusside improves ventricular performance beyond that already being provided by intra-aortic balloon augmentation in postoperative low cardiac output states. These researchers have found that adding dopamine further increases cardiac index as a result of an increase in stroke volume and a modest increase in heart rate. The advantage of combined therapy of nitroprusside and dopamine over nitroprusside therapy alone in postoperative patients receiving balloon assist is that once impedance to left ventricular ejection is reduced by nitroprusside, cardiac index is augmented to a greater degree by the addition of dopamine. Each pharmacological infusion can be titrated individually to achieve maximum physiological effects.

REFERENCES

1. Akyurekli, M.D., et al.: Effectiveness of intra-aortic balloon counterpulsation on systolic unloading, Can. J. Surg. **23**:122, 1980.
2. Angerpointer, T.A., et al.: The long term effect of intra-aortic balloon counterpulsation of left ventricular performance, J. Cardiovasc. Surg. **21**:399, 1980.
3. AVCO Medical Products: Guide to the physiology and operation of the AVCO intra-aortic balloon pump, Everett, Mass.
4. Brown, B.G., et al.: Diastolic augmentation by intra-aortic balloon. Circulatory hemodynamics and treatment of severe, acute left ventricular failure in dogs, J. Thorac. Cardiovasc. Surg. **53**:798, 1967.
5. Chaterjee, S., and Rosensweig, J.: Evaluation of intra-sortic balloon counterpulsation, J. Thorac. Cardiovasc. Surg. **61**:405, 1971.
6. Chilian, W.L., and Marcus, M.L.: Phasic coronary blood flow velocity in intramural and epicardial coronary arteries, Circ. Res. **50**:775, 1982.
7. DeWood, M.A., et al.: Intra-aortic balloon counterpulsation with and without reperfusion for myocardial infarction shock, Circulation **61**:1105, 1980.
8. Flopa, M., et al.: Intra-aortic balloon pumping (IABP) at different levels of experimental acute left ventricular failure, Chest **59**:68, 1971.
9. Forssel, G., et al.: Intraaortic balloon pumping in the treatment of cardiogenic shock complicating acute myocardial infarction, Acta. Med. Scand. **206**:189, 1979.
10. Haston, H.H., and McNamara, J.J.: The effects of intraaortic balloon counterpulsation on myocardial infarct size, Ann. Thorac. Surg. **28**:335, 1979.
11. Irnich, W., et al.: Die physiologischen und technischen Grundlagen der balloon Pulsationsmethode, 2 Schr. Kreislaufforschung **61**:339, 1972.
12. Laas, J.: Failure of intra-aortic balloon pumping to reduce experimental myocardial infarct size in swine, J. Thorac. Cardiovasc. Surg. **80**:85, 1980.
13. Lorente, P., et al.: Multivariate statistical evaluation of intra-aortic counterpulsation in pump failure complicating acute myocardial infarction, Am. J. Cardiol. **46**:124, 1980.
14. Miura, M., et al.: The effect of delay in propranolol administration on reduction of myocardial infarct size after experimental coronary artery occlusion in dogs, Circulation **60**:1148, 1979.
15. Okada, M. et al.: Experimental and clinical studies on the effect of intra-aortic balloon pumping for cardiogenic shock following acute myocardial infarction, Artif. Organs **3**:271, 1979.
16. O'Rourke, M.F., et al.: Randomized controlled trial of intra-aortic balloon counterpulsation in early myocardial infarction with acute heart failure, Am. J. Cardiol. **47**:8, 1981.
17. Oster, N., et al.: Regional blood flow after intra-aortic balloon pumping before and after cardiogenic shock, Trans. Am. Soc. Artif. Intern. Organs **20**:721, 1974.
18. Peter, T., et al.: Reduction of enzyme levels by propranolol after acute myocardial infarction, Circulation **57**:1091, 1978.
19. Powell, W.J., Jr., et al.: Effects of intra-aortic balloon counterpulsation on cardiac performance, oxygen consumption, and coronary blood flow in dogs, Circ. Res. **26**:753, 1970.
20. Reichart, B.: Treatment of acute left heart failure using dobutamine and intra-aortic counterpulsation, Intensive Care Medicine **7**:135, 1981.
21. Ruleto, R., et al.: Regulation of coronary blood flow, Prog. Cardiovasc. Dis. **18**:105, 1975.
22. Sammel, N.L., and O'Rourke, M.F.: Arterial counterpulsation in continuing myocardial ischemia after acute myocardial infarction, Br. Heart J. **42**:579, 1979.
23. Sonnenblick, E.H., and Shelton, C.L.: Myocardial energetics: basic principles and clinical implications, N. Engl. J. Med. **285**:668, 1971.
24. Sturm, J.Y., et al.: Combined use of dopamine and nitroprusside therapy in conjunction with intra-aortic balloon pumping for the treatment of post-cardiotomy low-output syndrome, J. Thorac. Cardiovasc. Surg. **82**:13, 1981.

25. Tyberg, J.V., et al.: Effectiveness of intra-aortic balloon counterpulsation in the experimental low output state, Am. Heart J. **80:**89, 1970.
26. Weber, K.T., and Janicki, J.S.: Intraaortic balloon counterpulsation. A review of physiological principles, clinical results, and device safety, Ann. Thorac. Surg. **17:**602, 1974.
27. Wolsinski, H., et al.: Structural basis for the static mechanical properties of the aortic media, Circ. Res. **14:**400, 1964.
28. Yahr, W.Z., et al.: Cardiogenic shock: dynamics of coronary blood flow with intra-aortic phase shift balloon pumping, Surg. Forum **19:**142, 1968.

CHAPTER 10 Extended medical indications for balloon pumping

As discussed in the previous chapter, balloon counterpulsation has received notoriety in the treatment of patients with refractory left ventricular pump failure.[16] Other medical uses include treatment of papillary muscle dysfunction with mitral regurgitation and/or ventricular septal defect (VSD) as a complication of myocardial infarction, angina preceding or following infarction, recurrent ventricular arrhythmias, in combination with thrombolytic therapy, and in miscellaneous conditions in which coronary artery disease coexists with other serious medical emergencies.

Acute mitral regurgitation and VSD

Acute mitral regurgitation from papillary muscle rupture following a myocardial infarction may lead to rapid clinical deterioration with pulmonary edema, hypotension, and death. Pressor agents that increase afterload and resistance to left ventricular ejection can aggravate mitral regurgitation[4] (Fig. 10-1). Vasoconstriction occurs with infusion of vasopressor agents, thereby directing more of the stroke volume out the lesser resistant regurgitant mitral valve pathway, rather than through the aortic valve to the systemic circulation.

A VSD may arise following an anterior septal myocardial infarction if wound healing has failed to transform the infarct into a stable scar. Necrotic septal tissue may actually rupture, creating a hole between the right and left ventricles.[5,19] The diagnosis of a VSD can be made at the bedside with the passage of a Swan-Ganz catheter (Chapter 30). Oxygen samples from the right atrium, a pulmonary artery, and a systemic artery identify the presence of a VSD. Pulmonary artery oxygen saturation is unusually high compared to the systemic arterial sample, as oxygenated blood from the left ventricle is shunted to the right ventricle through the VSD.[10] Infusion of an agent that strengthens contraction, an inotropic agent, may increase systemic output in the presence of a VSD. However, a concomitant increase in left-to-right shunting also occurs with a resultant increase in left ventricular work (Fig. 10-2).

Gold and associates[11] used IABP in patients who deteriorated into cardiogenic shock following sudden onset of a VSD after infarction or mitral regurgitation. Although counterpulsation produced clinical and hemodynamic improvement in all patients, a completely

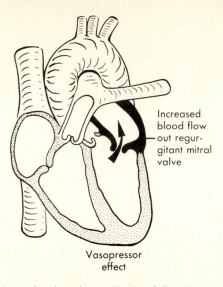

FIG. 10-1 Mitral regurgitation—developed complication following myocardial infarction, second-ary to papillary muscle rupture. Hypotension may ensue as a consequence. Using a vasopressor agent to raise blood pressure may increase afterload to left ventricular ejection (vasoconstriction) thereby actually forcing more of left ventricular stroke volume to flow out regurgitant mitral valve pathway (pathway of lesser resistance).

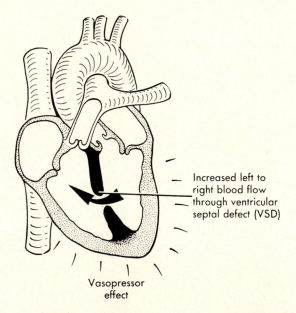

FIG. 10-2 Ventricular septal defect—developed complication, following myocardial infarction. Oxygenated blood is shunted through septal defect from left ventricle to right ventricle, which decreases stroke volume pumped to systemic circulation. Infusion of agent to strengthen force of contraction increases left-to-right shunt and causes increase in left ventricular work.

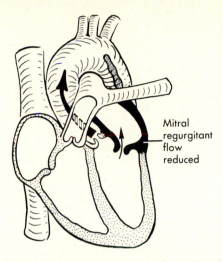

FIG. 10-3 Balloon's effect on improving hemodynamics in mitral regurgitation. Balloon's inflation in diastole elevates intra-aortic pressure; deflation just before systole reduces aortic end-diastolic pressure, thereby reducing afterload or resistance to left ventricular ejection. Greater stroke volume is ejected out aortic valve rather than through regurgitant mitral valve.

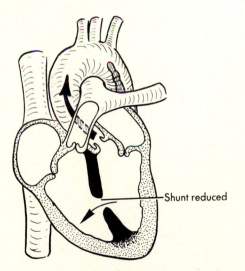

FIG. 10-4 Balloon's effect on improving hemodynamics with presence of a VSD. By reduction of afterload with balloon's counterpulsation effect, left-to-right shunting of blood is reduced, and greater stroke volume is ejected out aortic valve.

satisfactory correction of the impaired circulatory dynamics could not be obtained. The peak improvement occurred within the first 24 hours of pumping. In no patient did prolonged pumping produce further benefit. Intra-aortic balloon counterpulsation did afford a sufficient level of hemodynamic stability to permit left ventricular cineangiography in these critically ill patients. Reduction of afterload, as achieved with intra-aortic balloon assistance, lowers the impedance to left ventricular ejection. Stroke volume is thereafter more easily ejected out the aorta, rather than through the regurgitant mitral valve (Fig. 10-3) or VSD (Fig. 10-4).

At Kobe University in Japan[20] the effect on IABP in dogs with induced mitral regurgitation and VSD was studied. The hemodynamic changes after creation of a VSD secondary to myocardial infarction included decreases of 29% in mean aortic pressure, 20% in left ventricular systolic pressures, and 46% in cardiac output. The researchers observed an increase of 13% in right ventricular pressure and 11% in pulmonary artery pressure related to the size of the VSD. Initiation of the intra-aortic balloon assist produced a 7% increase in mean aortic pressure and a 13% increase in cardiac output. Right ventricular pressure decreased by 10%, and pulmonary artery pressure decreased by 7%.

Hemodynamic deterioration after iatrogenic creation of mitral regurgitation included a reduction in mean aortic pressure by 35% and a 36% reduction in left ventricular pressure and cardiac output. Mean left atrial pressure rose 300%, and pulmonary artery wedge pressure rose 50%. Initiation of balloon pumping produced increases of 9% in mean aortic pressure and 18% in cardiac output and decreases of 7% in left ventricular pressure, 13% in mean left atrial pressure, and 9% in pulmonary wedge pressure. This study concluded that IABP was effective in improving hemodynamics for both VSD and mitral regurgitation following acute myocardial infarction, except when the mean left atrial pressure was greater than 30 mm Hg.

Angina preceding infarction

For many years it has been appreciated that myocardial infarction is frequently preceded by angina that develops abruptly, progresses rapidly, or occurs at rest. Many different terms are used to describe this clinical condition, including *impending infarction, preinfarction angina,* and *premonitory phase of coronary occlusion.*[15,18] Contained in all of these terms is the indication that without treatment myocardial infarction is inevitable. It follows that the recognition and treatment of the condition may prevent infarction and favorably influence survival.

Criteria established for angina preceding infarction include ST-T wave changes on the electrocardiogram during pain, no electrocardiographic evidence of infarction, no elevation in the serum level of cardiac muscle enzymes, chest pain continuing and relieved only by opiates, and clear evidence of coronary disease on angiography.[15] IABP is ideally suited for the treatment of angina preceding infarction. By improving coronary blood flow and reducing the work of the left ventricle, chest pain and electrocardiographic changes may be ameliorated.[11,24] In the short term further ischemic damage is unlikely to occur.

In a report by Mundth, and others[19] 24 patients who had accelerating chest pains and ST-T wave abnormalities were treated with balloon counterpulsation. Pain was abolished, and ST-T wave changes were reversed in 20 of the patients.

In the long term IABP alone is unlikely to provide a complete answer to the problem, since the risk of infarction reoccurs once treatment is discontinued. Coronary arteriography, followed by coronary artery bypass grafting, can be carried out with comparative safety, sustaining the patient hemodynamically with balloon pumping. Twenty-five patients in Harris's study were treated with combined balloon pumping and bypass grafting. All patients met the established criteria for angina preceding infarction. Twenty-two of the 25 patients who were treated with the combined technique made a complete recovery. Three patients sustained definitive myocardial infarctions, and one patient died. Of five patients treated by bypass grafting alone, they all suffered infarction, and three died.

Ischemia

Effects of balloon pumping on myocardial blood flow distal to a severe coronary artery stenosis

Gerwitz and associates[9] examined the effect of counterpulsation in controlling myocardial ischemia in patients with unstable angina. The study was performed by creating an artificial proximal coronary stenosis in the left anterior descending coronary arteries of nine pigs and assessing whether or not balloon pumping could increase flow distal to this severe stenosis. Pressure distal to the stenosis was recorded along with measurements of arterial and great cardiac vein oxygen content, regional myocardial blood flow distal to the stenosis, and hemodynamic areas of control (no balloon pumping) after 20 minutes of full volume balloon inflation followed by another period without balloon pumping.

Heart rate was held constant with atrial pacing. In response to balloon counterpulsation, regional myocardial blood flow (RMBF) in the endocardium distal to the stenosis remained unchanged when compared with the control; epicardial RMBF declined. Myocardial oxygen consumption distal to the stenosis also declined when compared with the control. Diastolic pressure augmentation was documented proximal to the lesion, but no increase was noted distally. The authors concluded the following: (1) counterpulsation reduces myocardial oxygen demand but does not augment RMBF distal to a severe stenosis; (2) RMBF may not increase because balloon pumping may fail to increase distal coronary pressure, and the distal coronary bed tends to autoregulate in response to a decrease in oxygen demand during balloon pumping.

Restoration of oxygen supply and demand balance

During balloon pumping a favorable balance between myocardial oxygen supply and demand can be restored by simultaneous increases in coronary perfusion pressure and the reduction of cardiac work. If conventional modes of therapy have failed to reverse ischemia, including bed rest, nitrates, and propranolol, balloon pumping can be successfully employed to salvage viable ischemic myocardium when ischemia is diagnosed by clinical, hemodynamic, and electrocardiographic criteria.[7]

Angina following infarction

Some patients continue to experience severe angina following infarction, despite aggressive medical therapy. Bardet's group[1] in France studied counterpulsation combined with revascularization surgery in 21 patients whose chest pain reappeared after a pain-free interval of more than 24 hours but less than 15 days following the initial episode, accentuation, or reappearance of ST-T wave electrocardiographic abnormalities. These patients underwent a period of stabilization with balloon pumping, followed by coronary angiography. Fifteen of the patients achieved a totally pain-free status following revascularization when balloon pumping was used to stabilize them at the time of recurrence of angina following myocardial infarction. Such success depends on whether the coronary lesions are amenable to surgery.

The Cardiovascular Division[4] of the Department of Surgery at the University of California in San Francisco takes a different perspective. The IABP is not used to treat angina following infarction but rather is used to maintain hemodynamic stability. After evaluating operative mortality in patients who underwent revascularization secondary to accelerating angina without balloon pumping (9.1%) compared to operative mortality with IABP used preoperatively (8.8% in Levine's group[17] and 5.9% in Bardet's group[2]), the authors concluded that most of these potentially high-risk patients can undergo coronary angiography and surgery, if appropriate, without intra-aortic balloon support.

Ventricular irritability following infarction

Researchers at Massachusetts General Hospital[14] undertook a study of 22 patients with medically refractory ventricular irritability after myocardial infarction. These patients underwent IABP in an attempt to control ventricular irritability. Ventricular irritability was improved in 19 of the 22 patients and totally resolved in 12.

Combination of IABP and intracoronary thrombolysis therapy for acute myocardial infarction

Rentrop and associates[22] demonstrated that the acutely occluded coronary artery could be recanalized by the direct intracoronary administration of streptokinase. The restoration of antegrade flow was accompanied by relief of the signs and symptoms of ischemia and improvement in overall left ventricular performance as judged by contrast ventriculography. Intra-aortic balloon counterpulsation and its dual mechanism of potentially increasing coronary diastolic perfusion while simultaneously reducing left ventricular oxygen demand has substantial promise in conjunction with thrombolytic therapy for treatment of acute myocardial infarction.

Approximately 90% of patients with acute myocardial infarction have total thrombotic occlusion of the infarcted vessel as demonstrated on early angiography.[6,13] Myocardial cells damaged by interruption of this coronary blood flow undergo necrosis at a rate that depends on the time elapsed after the interruption of flow and the degree of hypoperfusion. Less reduction of blood flow occurs at the periphery of the hypoperfused zone than at the center. Cells in this peripheral area evolve to necrosis more slowly. Myocardial cells completely deprived of flow develop irreversible ischemia in 30 minutes; myocardium that is residually perfused through collateral channels following infarction resists necrosis for several hours. The ultimate extent of necrosis can be reduced by increasing myocardial oxygen supply and decreasing myocardial oxygen demand. Restoration of antegrade flow through this infarcted vessel can often be achieved by thrombolytic therapy with reduction of oxygen demand through balloon pumping.

Goldberg and associates[13] of Thomas Jefferson University in Philadelphia are currently assessing the efficacy of coronary recanalization plus IABP in patients with an evolving myocardial infarction. To assess the efficacy of combination therapy in acute myocardial infarction, patients with definitive evidence of acute myocardial infarction within 5 hours of the onset of symptoms are selected. After the insertion of the percutaneous balloon (percutaneous insertion is selected because of the expediency of initiating pumping over the surgical insertion method), the occluded vessel is identified with coronary angiograms. Intracoronary thrombolysis is performed using streptokinase, and coronary angiograms are repeated every 10 minutes. The infusion of streptokinase is continued for a total of 90 minutes. Repeat assessment of left ventricular function by contrast ventriculogram, echocardiogram, and electrocardiogram of ischemic injury is obtained before and after the infusion of streptokinase. Balloon pumping is continued for a variable length of time. If a high grade fixed stenosis remains at the completion of the thrombolysis and the patient is judged to be a candidate for early percutaneous angioplasty or coronary bypass surgery, the intra-aortic balloon is left in place for the subsequent procedure. If no subsequent procedure is likely and the clinical course is stable, the balloon is removed after 48 to 72 hours. The most recently published data reveal this technique, used in 15 patients in the acute phase of myocardial infarction. There has been improvement in left ventricular performance and concomitant reduction in signs of ischemic injury. No serious complications have been directly related to this aggressive combined form of therapy.

Miscellaneous applications

Balloon pumping has been successfully used to treat patients with septic shock and pulmonary embolus. Stroke work index improved, and less tissue damage was observed in the liver and small bowel of animals with septic shock that were treated with IABP when compared to a control group with septic shock that was not treated with balloon pumping.[3,23] Intra-aortic balloon counterpulsation has demonstrated its positive outcome by increasing left ventricular performance following myocardial contusion, particularly when applied early after injury.[24] The presence of a ventricular aneurysm can produce significant mechanical dysfunction; malignant ventricular arrhythmias can also develop. Use of balloon counterpulsation in these patients has been documented to stabilize ventricular arrhythmias and improve cardiac output.[2]

REFERENCES

1. Bardet, J., et al.: Treatment of post-myocardial infarction angina by intra-aortic balloon pumping and emergency revascularization, J. Thorac. Cardiovasc. Surg. 74:299, 1977

2. Bardet, J., et al.: Treatment of early postinfarction ventricular aneurysm by intra-aortic balloon pumping and surgery, J. Thorac. Cardiovasc. Surg. 78:445, 1979.

3. Berger, R.L., et al.: The use of diastolic augmentation with the intra-aortic balloon in human septic shock with associated coronary artery disease, Surgery 74:601, 1973.

4. Brundage, B.H., et al.: The role of aortic balloon pumping in post-infarction angina—a different perspective, Circulation **62**(suppl. 1):119, 1980.
5. Daggett, W.M., et al.: Surgery for post-myocardial infarction ventricular defect, Ann. Surg. **186**:260, 1977.
6. DeWood, M.A., et al.: Prevalence of total coronary occlusion during the early hours of transmural myocardial infarction, N. Engl. J. Med. **303**:897, 1980.
7. Ford, P.J., and Buckley, M.J.: Circulatory assistance. In Kinney, M.R., et al.: AACN's clinical reference for critical care nursing, New York, 1981, McGraw-Hill Book Co.
8. Gaudiani, V., et al.: Surgical management of acute myocardial infarction. In Eliot, R., et al., editors: Cardiac emergencies, ed. 2, Mount Kisco, N.Y., 1982, Futura Publishing Co., Inc.
9. Gerwitz, H., et al.: Effect of intra-aortic balloon pumping on myocardial blood flow distal to a severe coronary artery stenosis, Am. J. Cardiol. **49**:969, 1982.
10. Gold, H.K., et al.: Editorial: wedge pressure monitoring in myocardial infarction, N. Engl. J. Med. **285**:230, 1971.
11. Gold, H.K., et al.: Intra-aortic balloon pumping for control of recurrent myocardial ischemia, Circulation **47**:1197, 1973.
12. Gold, H.K., et al.: Intra-aortic balloon pumping for ventricular septal defect or mitral regurgitation complicating acute myocardial infarction, Circulation **47**:1191, 1973.
13. Goldberg, S.: Combination therapy for acute myocardial infarction intracoronary thrombolysis and percutaneous intra-aortic balloon counterpulsation, Cardiac Assist, **1**:1, 1982.
14. Hanson, E.C., et al.: Control of post-infarction ventricular irritability with the intra-aortic balloon pump, Circulation **62**(suppl. 1):130, 1980.
15. Harris, P.L., et al.: The management of impending myocardial infarction using coronary artery by-pass grafting and an intra-aortic balloon pump, J. Cardiovasc. Surg. **21**:405, 1980.
16. Kantrowitz, A., et al.: Initial clinical experience with intra-aortic balloon pumping, JAMA **203**:113, 1968.
17. Levine, F.H., et al.: Safe early revascularization for continuing ischemia after myocardial infarction, Circulation **60**(suppl. 1):5, 1979.
18. Master, A.M.: The treatment of "impending infarction" (premonitory phase of coronary occlusion), Dis. Chest **43**:302, 1963.
19. Mundth, E.D., et al.: Surgical treatment of cardiogenic shock and of mechanical complications following myocardial infarction, Cardiovasc. Clin. **8**:273, 1977.
20. Okada, M., et al.: Experimental and clinical studies on the effect of intra-aortic balloon pumping for cardiogenic shock following acute myocardial infarction, Artif. Organs **3**:271, 1979.
21. O'Rourke, M.F., and Sammel, N.L.: Arterial counterpulsation in severe refractory heart failure complicating acute myocardial infarction, Br. Heart. J. **41**:308, 1979.
22. Rentrop, P., et al.: Selective intra-coronary thrombolysis in acute myocardial infarction and unstable angina pectoris, Circulation **63**:307, 1981.
23. Talpins, N.L., et al.: Counterpulsation and intra-aortic balloon pumping in cardiogenic shock: circulatory dynamics, Arch. Surg. **97**:991, 1968.
24. Weintraub, R.M., et al.: Treatment of pre-infarction angina with intra-aortic balloon counterpulsation and surgery, Am. J. Cardiol. **34**:809, 1974.
25. Wood, P.: Therapeutic application of anticoagulants, Trans. Med. Soc. Lond. **66**:80, 1948.

CHAPTER 11 Surgical indications for balloon pumping

Since its inception in the care of the postoperative cardiac patient, the indications for supportive use of the IABP with surgical patients have greatly expanded. Use of the IABP in conjunction with surgical patient management either preoperatively, intraoperatively, or postoperatively dates back to the early 1970s. Mundth[24] introduced the balloon as a means of stabilizing patients with cardiogenic shock in preparation for emergency coronary artery bypass surgery following myocardial infarction. Several publications in the middle of the 1970s confirmed the beneficial effects of interim balloon support in patients who could not be successfully weaned from cardiopulmonary bypass.[2,4,18]

Balloon pump support has been endorsed for cardiac surgery before anesthesia induction, specifically for patients with left main coronary artery disease[9] and/or patients with poor left ventricular function.[12] Counterpulsation has been suggested and implemented successfully in the clinical setting as a means of lowering the formidable surgical mortality observed in patients with acute myocardial injury who require emergency noncardiac surgery.[6] The most recent application concerns patients requiring abdominal aortic aneurysm resection. IABP used after resection of the aneurysm has favorably influenced mortality in these patients.[17]

Balloon support before cardiac surgery

Intra-aortic balloon counterpulsation provides an adjuvant for the high-risk cardiac surgical patient with angina preceding infarction or poor left ventricular performance.[5,10,19] Bolooki and associates[2] at the University of Miami demonstrated that elective intraoperative balloon augmentation employed during cardiac surgery diminished mortality, based on specific criteria that defined impaired left ventricular function. Hemodynamic subsets were retrospectively evaluated in a large group of patients with moderate-to-severe cardiac dysfunction who developed complications after cardiac surgery. Bolooki's group concluded that patients with high-risk pathological conditions, such as severe aortic and coronary obstruction, left main coronary lesion with concomitant right coronary disease, or presence of acute infarction and its complications, could greatly benefit from elective balloon pumping before surgery. The presence of this type of pathological condition as an indication for IABP has also been outlined by Goldman[11] and Bregman.[3] The previously described populations were observed to have a high incidence

---

Criteria for elective use of IABP before cardiac surgery

1. Severe left ventricular dysfunction (CI* < 1.8, EF† < 30%, EDP‡ 22)
2. Presence of moderate left ventricular dysfunction (CI < 2.2, EF 40%, EDP > 18) in patients with the following:
   a. Severe aortic stenosis (gradient > 80 mm Hg)
   b. Acute myocardial infarction or its complications
   c. Intermediate coronary syndrome (especially caused by LMC§)
   d. Valvular heart disease and coronary obstruction

Data summarized from Sturm, J.T., et al.: Am. J. Cardiol. 45:1333, 1980.
*CI, Cardiac index in liters per minute per square meter.
†EF, Ejection fraction.
‡EDP, End-diastolic pressure of left ventricle in millimeters of mercury.
§LMC, Left main coronary stenosis.

of postoperative cardiac failure; elective preoperative employment of the balloon improved survival. Bolooki's criteria for selection of patients who would benefit from elective counterpulsation before and during cardiac surgery are outlined in the above box.

Another study performed at Charing Cross Hospital in London[13] compared two groups of patients who underwent coronary artery bypass grafting for impending myocardial infarction, which was defined by (1) anginal pain continuing despite bed rest, sedation, coronary vasodilators, and beta blockade; (2) ST-T wave changes on an electrocardiogram (ECG) during pain; (3) no ECG evidence of infarction; (4) no elevation in the serum level of cardiac muscle enzyme; (5) clear evidence of coronary disease on an angiogram. One group of patients was treated with a combination of coronary artery bypass grafting and IABP. The positive value of cardiac support by IABP before revascularization for impending myocardial infarction was suggested by this study. Those patients in the group (88%) who were treated with combined balloon support and revascularization successfully recovered from surgery and were discharged without evidence of infarction. In the second group of patients managed by coronary artery grafting alone because IABP was not possible, 62% suffered a myocardial infarction.

Therefore the combined regimen of IABP and coronary grafting seems to offer certain advantages.

1. It protects against ischemic damage as soon as counterpulsation is instigated and reduces the need for extreme urgency in further management.
2. Counterpulsation affords protection during the critical period of anesthetic induction before the patient is placed on cardiopulmonary bypass.

Left main coronary disease and balloon pumping

Left main coronary disease carries a significant risk factor for operative mortality and perioperative myocardial infarction in coronary bypass surgery. Operative mortality has been reported to be two to five times higher and perioperative myocardial infarction over 50% more common in patients with left main lesion.[22,28] Tahan and associates[27] from Yale University have documented a reduction in perioperative infarction in patients with left main coronary disease who underwent bypass surgery. These researchers did a retrospective analysis of 91 patients who underwent revascularization for an angiographically defined left main coronary lesion of 50% or greater luminal narrowing. The preoperative establishment of balloon pumping yielded a significantly lower incidence of perioperative myocardial infarction (3%) as compared to patients who underwent correction of a left main coronary lesion without pumping (23% incidence of perioperative myocardial infarction).

In contrast, Kaplan and associates[20] from Emory University proclaimed that elective preoperative insertion before cardiopulmonary bypass is most controversial. Kaplan did not concur that the routine use of the balloon in the period before bypass for all patients with left main coronary disease, angina (before infarction or unstable), or moderately depressed left ventricular function was necessary. Conservative use of the balloon was proposed by Kaplan, who argued that most patients with the above surgically treatable disorders can be safely anesthetized with the careful use of modern monitoring and anesthetic techniques without the complications associated with balloon pumping.

Windle and Farha[30] supported Kaplan's position of selective use of counterpulsation in the period before bypass, taking the stance that it was unnecessary to initiate elective prophylactic balloon assist routinely in all patients with left main disease, unstable angina, or decreased left ventricular function. They supported conservative use of the balloon with careful anesthetic management, adequate monitoring, and appropriate pharmacological intervention.

Postoperative balloon support

Buckley and colleagues[4] reported on the success of IABP as an interim organ support for patients who were unable to be weaned from cardiopulmonary bypass in 1973. Since Buckley's early employment of counterpulsation after bypass, postoperative low-output syndrome has been successfully corrected with balloon assist. The Texas Heart Institute[27] has reported 419 cases of low-output syndrome following cardiac surgery treated with IABP between 1972 and 1979. Overall, 226 patients (54%) were weaned from the balloon, and 188 (45%) were subsequently discharged from the hospital. Patients who underwent aortocoronary bypass surgery had significantly better survival rates than patients who underwent combined aortocoronary bypass and valve procedures. Hemodynamic classifying of the patients is represented in Table 11-1.

Class A hemodynamic status patients (cardiac index [CI] greater than 2.1 liters/min and systemic vascular resistance [SVR] less than 21,000 dynes/sec/cm^{-5}) were all successfully weaned from the pump. The mortality of Class B hemodynamic status patients (CI greater than 1.2 but less than 2.1 liters/min and SVR less than 2100 dynes/sec/cm^{-5}) was 46.3%. Class C hemodynamic status patients failed to progress beyond a CI less than 1.2 liters/min or SVR greater than 2100 dynes/sec/cm^{-5}. The mortality of this class of patients was 96.6% during balloon pumping. The differences in survival rates among patient classifications of A, B, and C during balloon pumping were statistically significant ($p < 0.001$).

The duration of support averaged 60.2 ± 44.7 hours in survivors compared to 10.9 ± 21.1 hours in nonsurvivors, suggesting an early high attrition rate for unsuccessful post-

TABLE 11-1 Successful treatment of postoperative low cardiac-output syndrome with balloon pumping in 263 patients at the Texas Heart Institute

Class	N	Highest hemodynamic level achieved with balloon pumping	Outcome
A	134	CI* > 2.1 SVR† < 2,100	All successfully weaned from balloon pump
B	41	CI 1.2-2.1 SVR < 2,100	Mortality 46.3%
C	88	CI < 1.2 SVR > 2,100	Mortality 46.3%

Sturm, J.T., et al.: Am. J. Cardiol. **45**:1033, 1980.
*CI, Cardiac index, liters per minute per meter^2.
†SVR, Systemic vascular resistance dynes per second per centimeter^{-5}.

operative support. Patients receiving assist with balloons of 30 and 40 cc demonstrated significantly better survival rates (52% and 67%, respectively) than patients with 20 cc balloons (47%). Thus survival in postoperative low-output syndrome treated with IABP correlates with postoperative hemodynamic classification and trajectories of improvement or deterioration.

A review of Stanford University's[7] postoperative use of the balloon pump over 7 years revealed the following stringent indications: (1) unsuccessful discontinuation of cardiopulmonary bypass, (2) postoperative low cardiac output, or (3) intractable ventricular tachyrhythmias. These patients were compared to a control group similar in postoperative symptoms except for a mean older age and ejection fraction in the control group. Operative mortality was 45% and 62% for the group who received IABP and the control group respectively. Two years postoperatively the actuarial survival was 45 ± 3% for the group who had balloon assist and 23 ± 20% for the control group.

In the group with balloon assistance, the time of insertion appeared to influence the outcome significantly. Patients in whom balloon support was instituted before discontinuation of cardiopulmonary bypass was attempted sustained a lower operative mortality than those in whom balloon support was begun after an unsuccessful attempt at weaning (34% versus 54%, $p < 0.01$). A cause-and-effect relationship could not be imputed. These researchers concluded that balloon counterpulsation was a therapeutic adjunct in the surgical management of some patients, but the long-term survival was poor and warranted continued development of more effective methods of mechanical circulatory assist and heart replacement.

The need for escalating the degree of mechanical support after cardiopulmonary bypass in certain patients was documented by the Texas Heart Institute in a 44-month study of patients undergoing balloon pumping for failing circulation after cardiopulmonary bypass. Three percent of their population (N = 14,168) required more profound mechanical support (i.e., use of the left ventricular assist device) after being weaned from cardiopulmonary bypass.[8]

Combined use of dopamine and nitroprusside therapy in conjunction with IABP for the treatment of postcardiotomy low-output syndrome

According to the Texas Heart Institute's criteria for a successful outcome with balloon pump management of postcardiotomy low-output syndrome, the best results were achieved if the SVR was maintained less than 2000 dynes/sec/cm^{-5} and the CI maintained greater than 2.0 liters/min/m^2.[27]

The Texas Heart Institute's research documented the efficacy of combined nitroprusside and dopamine therapy as adjuncts to balloon pump therapy of postcardiotomy low-output syndrome.[26] The rationale for this approach is that nitroprusside provides a vasodilator and afterload reduction effect but should not be initiated until intravascular volume is sufficient. If this precaution is not taken, the cardiac index can decrease and profound hypotension may ensue. If volume loading and nitroprusside therapy do not increase cardiac index to more than 2.0 liters/min/m^2, it is recommended that dopamine be added to augment the cardiac index with its inotropic effects.[23]

This classification for hemodynamic performance has been used to predict the likelihood of success of balloon pumping for postcardiotomy low-output syndrome and to assess the efficacy of individual therapeutic interventions. When combined balloon pumping and nitroprusside/dopamine pharmacological support failed to improve the hemodynamic status above Class C (CI 1.2 liters/min/m^2 or SVR 2000 dynes/sec/cm^{-5}) within 12 to 24 hours postoperatively, mortality was greater than 95%. If hemodynamic performance could be improved to Class B (CI 1.2 but 2.1 liters/min/m^2 and SVR 2000 dynes/sec/cm^{-5}), mortality would be approximately 45%. Patients who achieved Class A status (CI 2.1 liters/min/m^2 and SVR 2000 dynes/sec/cm^{-5}) were usually able to be weaned from both mechanical and pharmacological support.

Effect of intra-aortic counterpulsation on renal function

Experimental studies have suggested several possible effects of intra-aortic balloon support on renal function. Increased renal blood flow has been demonstrated in sheep, but in other studies no change in renal blood flow was observed in dogs.[21,30] Following 1 week of canine balloon counterpulsation in animals with mild to moderate failure, renal blood flow increased 9% to 25%. No change in serum creatinine level was observed, but after 1 week of pumping, pathological kidney examination revealed renal infarcts involving 6% to 16% of the kidney surface area.[1]

Stanford University, under the direction of Hilberman, has meticulously investigated the effect of postoperative balloon pumping in humans.[16] Protracted depression of cardiac performance was the most common antecedent of acute renal failure postoperatively.[15] Balloon support often dramatically improves cardiac performance; therefore renal failure could presumably be averted by temporary balloon counterpulsation. Pressure measurements recorded above and below the balloon (i.e., radial and femoral arterial tracings) suggested that blood flow below the balloon was not interfered with by the presence of the balloon.

Renal failure was documented as occurring in 17% of the population undergoing cardiac surgery. Acute increases in the level of balloon support (i.e., increasing from a ratio of 1:4 assistance to 1:1 assistance) did not demonstrably improve poor renal function.

When impaired renal function develops after initiation of balloon pumping, the following two specific anatomical disasters should always be considered in evaluating the pathogenesis of diminished urine output: (1) aortic dissection by the balloon and (2) juxtarenal balloon placement. Renal emboli have been documented but found to contribute in a minor way to renal functional deterioration. After balloon insertion, onset of renal failure not attributed to iatrogenic causes is best explained by the observation that a persistent low cardiac output, despite balloon assist, is the antecedent of postoperative acute renal failure. Therefore in patients who fail to improve hemodynamically after cardiac surgery, despite the assistance rendered with balloon counterpulsation, the development of renal failure can be anticipated. Treatment of postoperative persistent low cardiac output in these situations may need to be extended to include the use of dopamine to improve myocardial contraction and renal perfusion.

Balloon pumping as an adjunct to abdominal aortic aneurysmectomy in high-risk patients

Surgical indications for the use of balloon pumping have expanded to include trials as an adjunct to abdominal aortic aneurysmectomy. Patients with coronary artery disease that is not amenable to bypass grafting face an operative mortality approaching 80% for elective resection of an abdominal aortic aneurysm.[25] Attempts to reduce this mortality have centered primarily on coronary artery bypass performed before the aneurysmectomy.[14] There remains a population of patients who require emergency aneurysmectomy, which does not allow for coronary grafting before the surgery; other patients simply have severe inoperable coronary disease. The IABP may afford a margin of safety for these patients who otherwise would be subjected to unacceptable surgical risk associated with the aneurysm resection procedure.

Hollier and associates[17] at Mayo Clinic recently began using balloon assist after abdominal aortic aneurysm resection. Balloon pumping is activated as a supportive measure after resection of the abdominal aortic aneurysm, replacement of that segment of the aorta, and declamping of the aorta with a graft prosthesis. The balloon is inserted via a Dacron side-arm graft through the femoral artery, passed through the segment of aorta prosthesis, and positioned in the thoracic aorta just distal to the left subclavian artery (Fig. 11-1). Improvement has been documented with a 1:1 balloon assist ratio until the patient can eventually be completely weaned.

Balloon support in noncardiac surgery

The spectrum of balloon pumping in the surgical field has broadened beyond interim organ support after discontinuation of extracorporeal circulation. Counterpulsation has also been suggested as playing a useful role in lowering the formidable surgical mortality observed in patients with acute myocardial injury who require emergency noncardiac

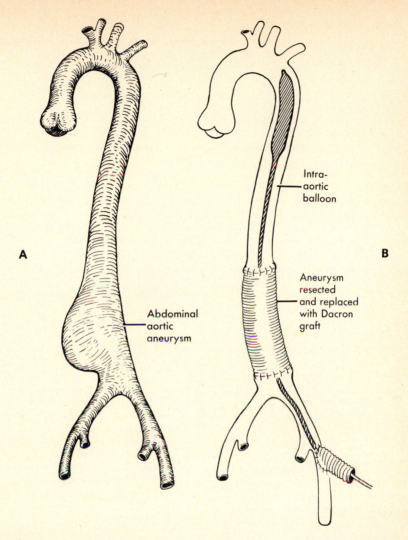

A

B

Intra-
aortic
balloon

Abdominal
aortic
aneurysm

Aneurysm
resected
and replaced
with Dacron
graft

FIG. 11-1 A, Presence of abdominal aortic aneurysm. **B,** Aneurysm resected and replaced with Dacron graft. After resection of aneurysm, intra-aortic balloon is inserted through femoral artery Dacron side-arm graft and passed up through segment of aortic graft into descending thoracic aorta to reset just distal to left subclavian artery.

operations. Such a case has been reported by the Beth Israel Hospital.[6] A major abdominal procedure was required for a patient who had suffered a myocardial infarction 5 days earlier. Anticipating that cardiac work would be substantially increased by the stress of anesthesia and surgery, the surgeon elected to use balloon pumping before laparotomy. With the initiation of IABP, a marked improvement occurred in all factors that represented a shock state preoperatively. The application of balloon counterpulsation for patients with myocardial ischemia who require any major surgery seems logical and an impressive approach to lower the mortality in these high-risk surgical candidates.

REFERENCES

1. Blatt, S.J., et al.: Hematologic, biochemical and pathologic effects of intra-aortic balloon counterpulsation in the calf, Surg. Gynecol. Obstet. **137:**238, 1973.
2. Bolooki, H., et al.: Clinical and hemodynamic criteria for use of the intra-aortic balloon pump in patients requiring cardiac surgery, J. Thorac. Cardiovasc. Surg. **72:**756, 1976.
3. Bregman, D., et al.: Intraoperative unidirectional intra-aortic balloon pumping in the management of left ventricular power failure, J. Thorac. Cardiovasc. Surg. **70:**1010, 1975.
4. Buckley, M.J., et al.: Intra-aortic balloon pump assist for cardiogenic shock after cardiopulmonary bypass, Circulation **48**(suppl. 3):90, 1973.
5. Cleveland, J.C., et al.: The role of intra-aortic balloon counterpulsation in patients undergoing cardiac operation, Ann. Thorac. Surg. **20:**652, 1975.
6. Cohen, S.F., and Weintraub, R.: A new application of counterpulsation: Safar Laparotomy after recent myocardial infarction, Arch. Surg. **110:**116, 1975.
7. Downing, T.P., et al.: Therapeutic efficacy of intra-aortic balloon pump counterpulsation: analysis with concurrent "control" subjects, Circulation **64**(suppl. 2):108, 1981.
8. DuBaky, M., et al.: Retrospective analysis of the need for mechanical circulatory support (intra-aortic balloon pump/abdominal left ventricular assist device or partial artificial heart) after cardiopulmonary bypass, Am. J. Cardiol. **46:**135, 1980.
9. Garcia, J.M., et al.: Surgery management of life-threatening coronary artery disease, J. Thorac. Cardiovasc. Surg. **72:**593, 1976.
10. Golding, L.R., et al.: Use of intra-aortic balloon pump in cardiac surgical patients; the Cleveland Clinic experience, 1975-1976, Cleve. Clin. Q. **43:**117, 1976.
11. Goldman, B.S., et al.: Increasing operability and survival with intra-aortic balloon pump assist, Can. J. Surg. **19:**69, 1976.
12. Goldman, B.S., et al.: Intra-aortic balloon pump as an adjunct to surgery for left ventricular dysfunction, J. Surg. **19:**128, 1976.
13. Harris, P.L., et al.: The management of impending myocardial infarction using coronary artery bypass grafting and an intra-aortic balloon pump, J. Cardiovasc. Surg. **21:**405, 1980.
14. Hertzer, N.R., et al.: Routine coronary angiography prior to elective aortic reconstruction: results of selective myocardial revascularization in patients with peripheral vascular disease, Arch. Surg. **114:**1336, 1979.
15. Hilberman, M., et al.: Sequential pathophysiological changes characterizing the progression from renal dysfunction to acute renal failure following cardiac surgery, J. Thorac. Cardiovasc. Surg. **79:**838, 1980.
16. Hilberman, M., et al.: Effect of the intra-aortic balloon pump upon postoperative renal function in man, Crit. Care Med. **9:**85, 1981.
17. Hollier, L.H.: Intra-aortic balloon counterpulsation as adjunct to aneurysmectomy in high-risk patients, Mayo Clin. Proc. **56:**565, 1981.
18. Houseman, L.B., et al.: Counterpulsation for intraoperative cardiogenic shock: successful use of the intra-aortic balloon, JAMA **224:**1131, 1973.
19. Kaiser, G.C., et al.: Intra-aortic balloon assistance, Ann. Thorac. Surg. **21:**487, 1976.
20. Kaplan, J.A., et al.: The role of the intra-aortic balloon in cardiac anesthesia and surgery, Am. Heart J. **98:**580, 1979.
21. Kondratovitch, M.A., and Ursulinko, V.I.: The effect of intra-aortic balloon counterpulsation on regional circulation, Kardiologiia, **19:**122, 1978.
22. Langou, R.A., et al.: Incidence and mortality of perioperative myocardial infarction in patients undergoing coronary artery bypass grafting, Circulation **55**(suppl. 2):54, 1977.
23. Miller, C.D., et al.: Postoperative enhancement of left ventricular performance by combined inotropic-vasodilator therapy with preload control, Surgery **88:**108, 1980.
24. Mundth, E.D., et al.: Circulatory assistance in emergency direct coronary artery surgery for shock complicating acute myocardial infarction, N. Engl. J. Med. **283:**1382, 1970.
25. Myhre, I.A., et al.: Clinical problems in the use of the intra-aortic balloon, Int. Surg. **64:**57, 1979.
26. Sturm, J.T.: Combined use of dopamine and nitroprusside therapy in conjunction with intra-aortic balloon pumping for treatment of postcardiotomy low-output syndrome, J. Thorac. Cardiovasc. Surg. **82:**13, 1981.

27. Sturm, J.T., et al.: Treatment of postoperative low output syndrome with intra-aortic balloon pumping: experience with 419 patients, Am. J. Cardiol. **45:**1033, 1980.
28. Tahan, S.R., et al.: Bypass surgery for left main coronary artery disease—reduced perioperative myocardial infarction with preoperative intra-aortic balloon counterpulsation, Br. Heart J. **43:**191, 1980.
29. Takaro, T., et al.: The VA cooperative randomized study of surgery for coronary arterial occlusive disease II. Subgroup with significant left main lesions, Circulation **53**(suppl. 3):107, 1976.
30. Talpin, N.L., et al.: Hemodynamics and coronary blood flow during intra-aortic balloon pumping, Surg. Forum **19:**122, 1967.
31. Windle, R., and Farha, S.J.: Intra-aortic balloon pump. Limited use for maximum effectiveness in cardiac surgery, J. Kans. Med. Soc. **82:**229, 1981.

CHAPTER 12 **Contraindications**

Contraindications to balloon placement involve anatomical disorders such as aortic aneurysms, aortic valve insufficiency, and peripheral vascular atherosclerosis or vessel tortuosity. The presence of an aortic aneurysm (Fig. 12-1) precludes balloon insertion because of the risk of aortic wall rupture from elevated aortic pressure in diastole. Aortic insufficiency is a contraindication as well because elevation of diastolic pressure by balloon inflation worsens the retrograde blood regurgitation through the aortic valve. The degree of aortic insufficiency is considered before totally eliminating the possibility of balloon pumping in an individual patient. With relatively minor degrees of aortic insufficiency, the decision may be made to use counterpulsation on a patient by employing intra-aortic balloon placement. The rationale is that the benefits of balloon augmentation outweigh the possible risks of worsening the aortic insufficiency.

Atherosclerosis in the peripheral arterial vessels may prevent passage of the balloon catheter through the femoral artery and may increase the possibility of peripheral embolization. The double-lumen balloons have allowed insertion under fluoroscopy via a guide wire in many cases in which atherosclerosis previously would have prevented insertion

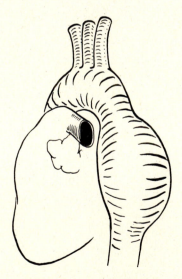

FIG. 12-1 Aortic aneurysm. Contraindications to balloon pumping.

through a conventional femoral artery cutdown. The inability to insert an intra-aortic balloon because of peripheral vascular diseases decreases the usefulness of the device, which may potentially relieve cardiogenic shock or allow a patient to be weaned from cardiopulmonary bypass. Concomitantly, the peripheral vessel may be too small or tortuous to accommodate both the balloon in situ and blood flow. Lefemine and colleagues[2] noted a failure of femoral or iliac passage of the intra-aortic balloon in 12.8% of the patients in whom placement was attempted.

Bahn and associates[1] at Tacoma Washington General Hospital have identified a subgroup of patients undergoing cardiac catheterization with increased likelihood of needing balloon counterpulsation. Criteria established include the following:

1. Multiple coronary artery lesions (three or more possible bypass sites)
2. Ejection fraction less than 40%
3. Valvular and coronary artery disease
4. Previous coronary artery operation
5. Previous myocardial infarction
6. Hypertension
7. Claudication
8. Weak or unequal femoral pulses

Patients who meet the criteria at the time of cardiac catheterization receive one aortoiliac injection of contrast material at the time of cardiac catheterization. Impressive degrees of vessel irregularity and atherosclerotic disease have been noted in the groups studied by Bahn. Such information gathered at little additional risk is most useful in the subsequent selection of a site for transfemoral balloon insertion or may rule out the transfemoral approach.

Aside from avoiding femoral arteries with poor pulsation or diagnosed claudication, no satisfactory femoral artery screening procedure has been available before balloon passage. Bahn and associates have impressively demonstrated how a single injection through the catheter in place for cardiac study can reveal significant iliofemoral artery abnormalities that discourage balloon passage by one or both femoral routes. Aortoiliac arteriograms are not indicated routinely on all patients before balloon insertion; the seriousness of cardiac illness often precludes this study. When prophylactically performed, however, the information obtained greatly assists in the choice of balloon insertion site, if the need for balloon pumping should arise.

REFERENCES

1. Bahn, C., et al.: Vascular evaluation for balloon pumping, Ann. Thorac. Surg. **27**:474, 1979.
2. Lefemine, A., et al.: Results and complications of intra-aortic balloon pumping in surgical and medical patients, Am. J. Cardiol. **40**:416, 1977.

CHAPTER 13 Retrograde and antegrade insertion of balloon

Most balloon insertions are performed electively in the operating room, recovery room, intensive care unit, cardiac catheter laboratory, and occasionally in the emergency room. The standard intra-aortic balloon insertion requires a femoral arteriotomy and attachment of an end-to-side prosthetic graft. Rarely antegrade insertion through the aorta is performed in the operating room when femoral artery disease prevents a femoral arteriotomy approach. Percutaneous balloon insertion using the Seldinger catheterization technique provides a simple nonsurgical procedure that can be employed at the bedside by a physician who is not a surgeon.

Femoral arteriotomy and retrograde insertion

After moderate sedation, preferably with an analgesic such as morphine, a length of 2-inch tape is placed across the patient's legs proximal to his knees to provide immobilization. His hands are restrained to prevent contamination of the sterile field. Following the preparation of the selected side, a plastic sterile drape is placed over the groin area, which is then infiltrated with a local anesthetic. An incision is made over the course of the femoral artery, and dissection is undertaken to expose it. One suggested method of femoral insertion requires a second stab wound incision 1 cm long over the femoral artery, 6 to 8 cm below the main incision.[6] A tunnel is constructed between the stab incision and the subcutaneous layer in line with the vessel and enlarged to admit one finger. A 10 mm Dacron graft long enough to reach from the artery to the skin stab wound is prepared. An arteriotomy is performed in the femoral artery, and the graft is sutured to the arteriotomy. On completion of the anastomosis, the graft is brought out through the subcutaneous tunnel to the skin at the stab incision (Fig. 13-1).

A clamp is applied at the femoral bifurcation below the graft anastomosis, and the common femoral artery above the anastomosis is occluded by umbilical tape. Following aspiration of the graft segment to remove any clots, the open-end segment of the graft is grasped with a hemostat for countertraction. The balloon is introduced through the graft and passed into the artery system. The occluding tape and clamp above the graft are released to facilitate retrograde advancement of the balloon.

Once the balloon has been advanced into the descending thoracic aorta, the graft at the skin level is tied firmly around the catheters by umbilical tape. Pumping is begun, followed by immediate fluoroscopy or chest x-ray films to verify balloon position. The

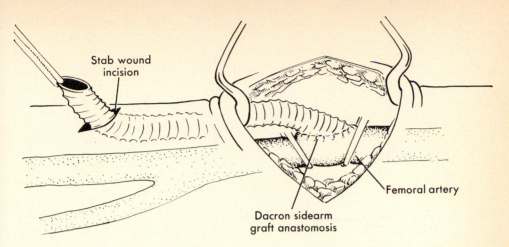

Stab wound
incision

Femoral artery

Dacron sidearm
graft anastomosis

FIG. 13-1 Retrograde insertion of balloon through femoral arteriotomy and Dacron side-arm graft, which is brought out through subcutaneous tunnel to skin through stab wound incision.

incision is closed, and the balloon catheter is secured at the skin level of the stab incision with a heavy gauge tie to prevent movement. Some physicians routinely insert the balloon under fluoroscopy to avoid left common carotid artery obstruction.

Alternative technique

An alternative technique of retrograde femoral artery insertion is suggested in emergency situations when the patient's condition is deteriorating and insertion must be completed as expediently as possible.[4] Local anesthetic is infiltrated; a longitudinal incision is made over the femoral artery, and dissection to the vessel is employed. Thereafter the femoral artery is clamped distally and secured with a tape proximally. The balloon is selected, and a 10 mm Dacron graft is threaded over the balloon onto its catheter. A longitudinal femoral arteriotomy is performed, and the balloon is introduced into the femoral artery on release of the clamp and umbilical tie (Fig. 13-2). Once the balloon is in position, balloon pumping commences while the Dacron graft is anastomosed to the femoral artery, and the wound is closed.

Pericardial graft rather than Dacron graft. Zapolanski and others [10] in the Division of Cardiovascular Surgery at Toronto General Hospital use a pericardial patch with its visceral side in, rather than a Dacron graft. They believe this facilitates the management of a potential groin infection if prolonged postoperative balloon pumping is necessary. A pericardial patch is obtained while the sternum is open and is sutured to a common femoral arteriotomy. A 6-0 Prolene mattress stitch is inserted at the heel of the graft, anastomosing the patch of pericardium to the femoral artery. The suturing is continued along the sides to construct a tube of pericardium over the balloon catheter (Fig. 13-3). Thrombus has not been present in the pericardial patch, as it commonly occurs inside the Dacron tube. Since pericardium is autologous tissue, the problem of infection from foreign material (Dacron) in the groin can be avoided.

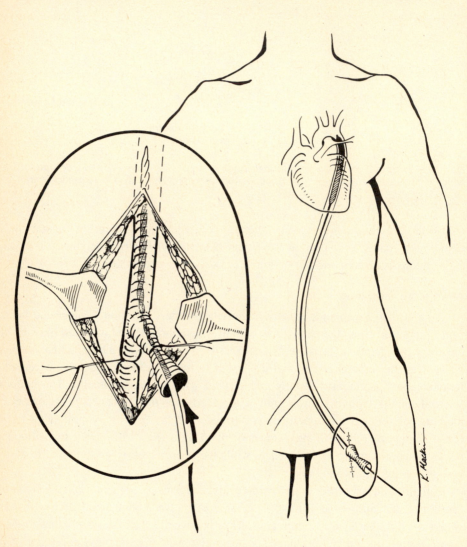

FIG. 13-2 Introduction of balloon catheter directly into femoral artery; thereafter Dacron graft is sutured to femoral artery insertion site.

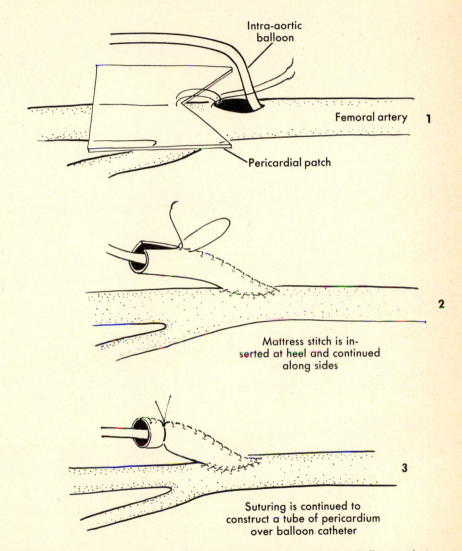

FIG. 13-3 Use of pericardial patch rather than Dacron graft in inserting balloon catheter retrogradely through femoral artery. (Modified from Zapolanski, A., et al.: Ann. Thorac. Surg. 33:516, May 1982.)

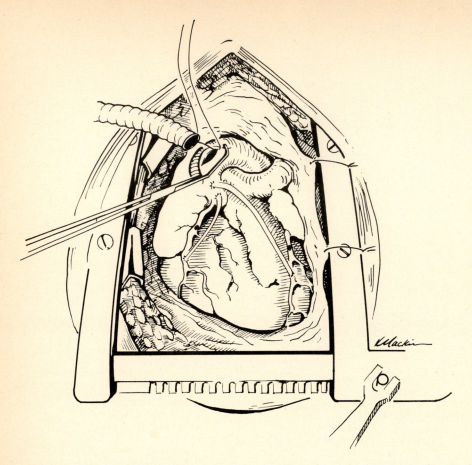

FIG. 13-4 Antegrade insertion of balloon through ascending aorta. Chest is retracted with rib spreaders.

Transaortic balloon insertion through the ascending aorta

Transaortic insertion can only be undertaken in the operating room when the aortic arch is exposed. This method of insertion of the balloon through the ascending aorta has been used when balloon counterpulsation was required at the conclusion of cardiopulmonary bypass and transfemoral insertion of the balloon was not possible as a result of atherosclerotic obstruction of the peripheral vessels.[3,5] A partial occlusion clamp is applied to the anterior wall of the aorta. The aortic wall is incised, and a Dacron graft is anastomosed end-to-side to the entire aortic wall.[2] The balloon is introduced through the graft into the aorta and advanced to the desired position in the descending thoracic aorta distal to the left subclavian artery (Fig. 13-4).

Patients with a short aorta, aortic valve replacement, and multiple aorta-saphenous vein anastomoses have little room to apply a partial occlusion clamp to the ascending aorta. Techniques are described in which the graft is anastomosed just to the right of the aortic annula and through the left lateral wall of the aortic arch in such situations.[8]

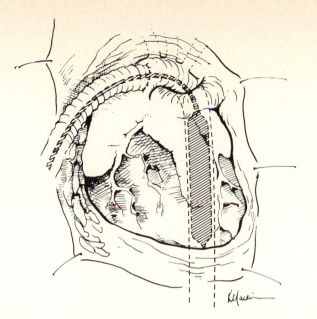

FIG. 13-5 After balloon catheter has been inserted antegradely through ascending aorta, balloon catheter is brought out through Dacron woven graft at about level of second intercostal space.

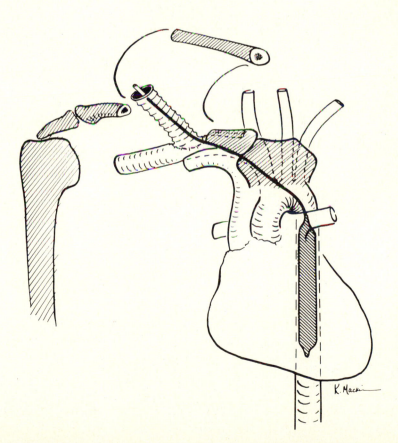

FIG. 13-6 Insertion accomplished through subclavian artery.

Umbilical tapes are tied over the graft and the catheter in a manner similar to the technique for femoral artery. The balloon catheter is brought out via the Dacron graft through a stab wound incision at about the level of the second intercostal space (Fig. 13-5).[1]

Counterpulsation with antegrade insertion

Antegrade counterpulsation, as opposed to retrograde counterpulsation, is produced when a balloon is inserted antegradely through the aorta.[1] This method has demonstrated a satisfactory increase in cardiac output.[9]

Subclavian artery approach for insertion

In an effort to avoid major surgical intervention for balloon placement when aortoiliac stenosis prevents femoral retrograde advancement, Mayer (1978) reported use of the sub-clavian artery approach. A longitudinal incision is made over the middle third of the right clavicle with use of local anesthetic. A 2- to 3-inch segment of the clavicle is resected. The third portion of the subclavian artery, lying between the anteriorly located subclavian vein and posteriorly located brachial plexus, is mobilized. The balloon is then passed in an antegrade fashion with the usual end-to-side graft placement (Fig. 13-6).

REFERENCES

1. Bleifeld, W., et al.: Improved cardiac assistance with an aortic arch balloon, Cardiovasc. Res. **7:**115, 1973.
2. Cooley, D.S., and Norman, J.C.: Techniques in cardiac surgery, Houston, 1975, Texas Medical Press.
3. Gueldner, T.L., and Lawrence, G.H.: Intra-aortic balloon assist through cannulation of the ascending aorta, Ann. Thorac. Surg. **19:**88, 1975.
4. Kantrowitz, A., et al.: Technique of femoral artery cannulation for phase-shift balloon pumping, J. Cardiovasc. Surg. **56:**219, 1968.
5. Krause, A.H., Jr.: Transthoracic intra-aortic balloon cannulation to avoid repeat sternotomy for removal, Ann. Thorac. Surg. **21:**562, 1976.
6. Maggs, P.R.: Technical aspects of intra-aortic balloon insertion, Surg. Clin. North Am. **60:**545, 1980.
7. Mayer, J.H.: Subclavian artery approach for insertion of intra-aortic balloon, J. Thorac. Cardiovasc. Surg. **76:**61, 1978.
8. Nunez, A., et al.: Transaortic cannulation for balloon pumping in a "crowded aorta," Ann. Thorac. Surg. **40:**400, 1980.
9. Pooley, R.W., et al.: Increased cardiac output by downstream pumping with a reversed unidirectional intra-aortic balloon, J. Cardiovasc. Surg. **73:**647, 1977.
10. Zapolanski, A., et al.: Pericardial graft for intraoperative balloon insertion, Ann. Thorac. Surg. **33:**516, May 1982.

CHAPTER 14 Percutaneous balloon insertion

Need for percutaneous technique

Inability to insert the balloon catheter through a femoral arteriotomy incision and into the descending thoracic aorta because of severe vessel tortuosity or obstructive atherosclerosis has prevented implementation of balloon counterpulsation in a surprising number of patients. Specifically, Bregman and associates[5] encountered this difficulty in 29% of their attempts. Ten years later, Lundell and associates[11] reported inability to successfully complete femoral artery cutdown insertion in 28% of their patient group.

Since 1979,[17] the percutaneous insertion method has become a popular means of employing intra-aortic counterpulsation, offering less inherent delays in application and greater ease of removal compared to the surgical insertion method. The new central lumen guide wire frequently affords insertion of the percutaneous balloon into atherosclerotic and tortuous vessels. Pressure monitoring and injection of a contrast medium can be accomplished through the capabilities of this central lumen catheter. An intrinsic wrapping knob allows the percutaneous balloon to be evenly wrapped around its catheter before insertion. Because of the ease of insertion, physicians who are not surgeons can insert the percutaneous balloon, thereby extending the possible application of balloon pumping into the community hospitals. This technique has been greeted with great enthusiasm. Limitations and complications must however be recognized.

Preparation of percutaneous balloon for insertion

Preparation should be undertaken in compliance with specific manufacturer's instructions. General preparation consists of lubricating the balloon in saline solution. The deflated balloon is furled by wrapping it around the balloon catheter, starting at the distal end and proceeding proximally (Fig. 14-1). Any residual air remaining in the balloon is completely evacuated with a syringe and stopcock.

Insertion

Under local anesthetic, percutaneous insertion is carried out according to the Seldinger technique.[15] The femoral artery is punctured percutaneously with an 18-gauge angiographic needle, and a 0.0135-inch diameter spring guide wire with a J tip is advanced through the needle into the abdominal aorta. The needle is then removed from the guide

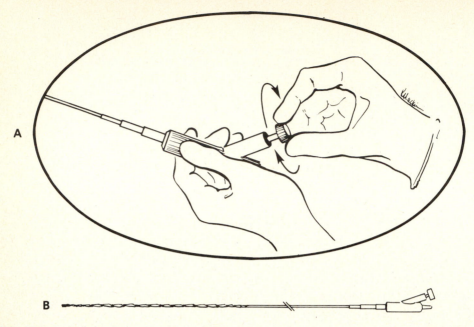

FIG. 14-1 A, Balloon is wrapped around support wire. **B,** Percutaneous balloon completely wrapped before insertion.

wire and the common femoral artery is dilated with an 8 F dilator. A 12 F dilator-sheath assembly, 11 inches long, is inserted over the guide wire, leaving only the 12 F sheath in situ in the femoral artery. The wrapped percutaneous balloon is then inserted through the sheath into the descending thoracic aorta (Fig. 14-2). When pumping commences, the balloon immediately unwraps and functions as a standard intra-aortic balloon. Once the proper position is obtained, the sheath and the balloon catheter are snared with a ligature, and the assembly is sutured to the skin. The puncture site and the sheath-balloon assembly are dressed, and the position is confirmed by a chest x-ray film or fluoroscopy.

Central lumen percutaneous balloon

Percutaneous insertion may be hampered by atherosclerotic disease of the femoral artery (Fig. 14-3) and/or tortuosity of the vessel. A percutaneous balloon design is available that provides a central lumen for passage of a guide wire to facilitate difficult insertion around atherosclerotic plaques (Fig. 14-4). The double-lumen design allows direct monitoring of arterial pressure and injection of contrast medium to define obstructions and/or to ensure proper balloon positioning.[11]

Technical detail

Neither the guide wire nor the catheter should be forced into the artery if resistance is encountered. The cannula and balloon catheter must be securely taped to the groin because

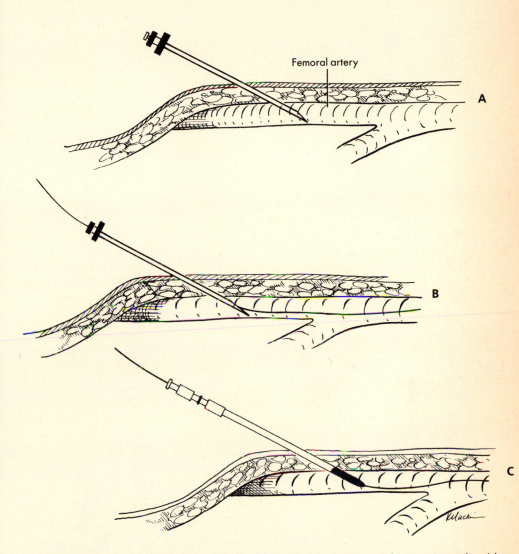

FIG. 14-2 Percutaneous balloon insertion. **A,** Femoral artery is punctured percutaneously with 18-gauge angiographic needle. **B,** Guide wire is advanced, 18-gauge needle is removed, and femoral artery is dilated. **C,** Dilator (12F) is inserted over guide wire, leaving only sheath in situ. Percutaneous balloon is inserted through sheath.

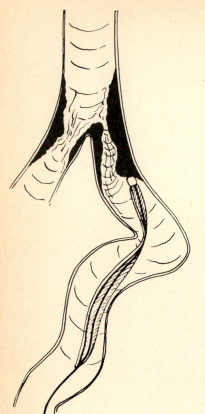

FIG. 14-3 Percutaneous insertion impossible because of atherosclerotic disease of femoral artery.

FIG. 14-4 Insertion of percutaneous balloon through J wire to guide balloon past atherosclerotic plaques.

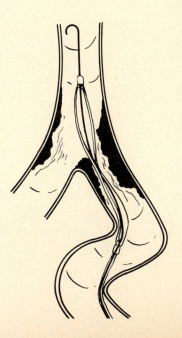

accidental removal of the balloon catheter could cause serious hemorrhage.

Vignola and associates[19] recommended using a longer 15-inch introducer sheath after successful passage of the guide wire in all balloon placements performed without fluoroscopic guidance, assuring successful balloon passages into the thoracic aorta without risking potentially lethal aortoiliac dissection. The use of a 16-inch introducer sheath has more recently received favorable review.[2]

Clots that can form on the catheter may be sheered off as the balloon is pulled through the femoral puncture site. Although the complication may be unavoidable, Vignola and associates[19] further suggested that the wound be allowed to bleed vigorously for 1 to 2 seconds while pressure is applied proximal and then distal to the actual puncture site. Pressure is applied directly to the puncture site to control bleeding. A mechanical clamp is used to achieve hemostasis when the balloon catheter is removed. Once the balloon catheter is wrapped, it is flexible; therefore accidental insertion of the balloon into any of the major visceral arteries or the ascending aorta can occur. Proper attention must be paid to the positioning of the balloon and to the correct measuring of the distance that it is to be inserted.

Although percutaneous insertion can be accomplished without the use of fluoroscopy, Bregman and associates[4] recommended fluoroscopy to permit more precise positioning of the balloon in the aorta, which obviates the risk of balloon occlusion of arterial branches.

Direct ascending aorta insertion of percutaneous catheter

Direct insertion of the balloon catheter into the ascending aorta (Chapter 12) is an alternative insertion approach employed when iliofemoral arteriosclerosis prevents retrograde insertion of the balloon. The catheter is usually inserted into the ascending aorta through a segment of Dacron graft, which requires application of a partial occlusion clamp to the aorta.

Bonchek and Olinger[3] listed the following limitations to aortic insertion of the balloon through a Dacron graft:
1. The technique can impose undesirable delay in a deteriorating patient.
2. The aorta may already be crowded with coronary artery bypass grafts, an arterial perfusion cannula, and possibly an aortotomy incision.
3. The time required to perform the technique may impose an undesirable delay in the care of the patient whose condition is deteriorating.

The aforementioned researchers used the percutaneous balloon for direct insertion into the aorta, which can be done quickly in a crowded aorta because a partially occluding clamp is not required. Safe positioning of the balloon catheter is facilitated by the flexibility of the distal portion of the balloon catheter.

Heparinization

Thrombus accumulated on the percutaneous catheter could be "stripped" off as it is withdrawn through the aortic wall; embolization could potentially ensue. Shirkey and

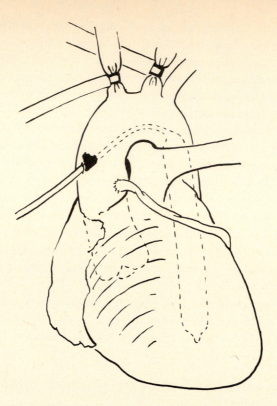

FIG. 14-5 Removal of percutaneous balloon from aortic arch. Innominate and left carotid arteries are occluded with tourniquets to prevent embolization of thrombus to vessels as catheter is removed. (Modified from Bonchek, M.D., and Olinger, G.: Ann. Thorac. Surg. **32:**512, 1981.)

associates[16] recommended that patients be totally heparinized as long as a balloon remains in the aortic arch to prevent thrombus formation.

Bonchek and Olinger[3] found total heparinization undesirable postoperatively. They suggested that during removal of the percutaneous balloon from the aortic arch, the innominate and left carotid arteries be occluded with tourniquets (Fig. 14-5). Following removal of the balloon, the catheter insertion site is allowed to bleed momentarily before reclosing the arch vessel, releasing the tourniquets, and securing the wound.

In view of the present effectiveness and efficacy demonstrated by use of the percutaneous method of balloon insertion, expansion of this technique is anticipated to be included in the armamentarium of the community hospital's available services.

Percutaneous technique in clinical situations
Advantages

Use of the percutaneous intra-aortic balloon catheter has broadened the application of balloon pumping in both medical and surgical fields. The percutaneous technique offers greater facility of insertion and removal compared to the surgical method. Bregman and associates[5] related the following clinical situations, which were more successfully treated because of the prompt institution of balloon pumping with the percutaneous technique:

1. Patients with refractory angina after acute myocardial infarction, undergoing coronary arteriography. Percutaneous balloon insertion was employed in this group of patients in the catheterization laboratory just before coronary arteriography. This approach potentially augments coronary circulation during the angiographic study,[9] and the balloon is left in place to provide circulatory support for the patient during induction of the anesthetic and in the immediate postoperative period.

2. Patients experiencing myocardial ischemia or a myocardial infarction during coronary arteriography. The coronary catheter can be rapidly exchanged for the balloon pump through the same puncture site in the femoral artery. Five patients in Bregman's series, who experienced acute myocardial infarction during coronary arteriography, received percutaneous intra-aortic balloon placement and pumping that rapidly reversed cardiogenic shock and supported them during emergency revascularization.

3. Mechanical circulatory support of patients during cardiac arrest. Conventional arteriotomy balloon insertion is not optimal during resuscitation because of the time required for surgical insertion. Rapid insertion by the percutaneous technique does not interfere with chest massage.

Using conventional surgical techniques, an experienced surgeon requires a minimum of 30 to 45 minutes to insert the intra-aortic balloon and must perform a second operative procedure to remove the balloon. The insertion of the percutaneous intra-aortic balloon precludes dependence on cardiovascular surgeons; it can be performed by any physician skilled in catheterization techniques.

Complications

Early optimism for a lower complication rate, using the percutaneous technique, was expressed by Bregman and associates[5] who encountered no major complications in 27 percutaneous balloon insertions. However, when Harvey and others[7] reviewed 89 consecutive patients who underwent percutaneous balloon insertion at Cornell Medical Center, they found that 23 of the patients exhibited major complications, including limb ischemia in 12, bleeding at the puncture site in three, permanent foot drop in three, aortic dissection in three, renal embolism in one, and false aneurysm at the puncture site in one. Fourteen patients had the following minor complications: asymptomatic loss of pedal pulses in eight, transient bacteremia in two, and wound hematoma in two. No patient experienced free perforation, balloon rupture, or wound infection. Harvey concluded that the rate and severity of complications of percutaneous balloon pumping were similar to those of conventional IABP.

Bregman and associates[5] reported the complication of a patient complaining of abdominal pain after percutaneous placement of the intra-aortic balloon. Mesenteric angiography disclosed that the distal aspect of the balloon was intermittently interrupting the arterial inflow of a stenotic superior mesenteric artery. Following repositioning of the balloon, the patient's abdominal pain was relieved. An isolated case of failure of the balloon to unwrap has also been reported.[6]

Bregman's experience suggests that the vascular complications associated with conventional surgical intra-aortic balloon insertion may be diminished by the use of the percutaneous technique. None of the patients in his series experienced hematoma of the groin, aortic dissection, compromised distal pulses, or late wound complications after percutaneous insertion of the intra-aortic balloon.

The Miami Heart Institute[19] documented femoral arterial thrombosis in 10.2% of the patients, and an asymptomatic pulse loss in the ipsilateral leg developed in one patient. There were no cases of pseudoaneurysm, groin hematoma, aortic dissection, or infection related to percutaneous balloon employment. The percutaneous balloons were kept in place an average of 3.1 days. The lowest platelet counts reported ranged from 55,000 to 308,000.

Mason and associates[12] reported complications no greater but no lesser with conventional balloon pumping. The most recent study of percutaneous intra-aortic balloon counterpulsation was undertaken by Hauser and associates.[8] Their 18.6% complication rate with the percutaneous technique was similar to their 21% complication rate with the surgical technique and comparable to other reported complication percentages with the surgical technique.[9,13,14] Thus the original anticipation of reduced complications with this method has not been realized. Continued scrutiny of new balloon catheters and judicious selection of patients continue to be mandatory criteria for current percutaneous insertion and for any further developments in balloon catheter design and insertion techniques.

New advances that reduce hazards

Recently Dr. David Bregman, Chairman of the Department of Surgery at St. Joseph's Hospital and Medical Center in Patterson, New Jersey, summarized his observations and advances made in the percutaneous technique. Bregman recommended attention be paid to the following details to reduce the potential morbidity associated with the percutaneous technique[4]:

1. The percutaneous intra-aortic balloon *must* be inserted by a physician skilled in the Seldinger technique of cardiac catheterization.
2. Ideally the insertion procedure should be carried out under fluoroscopic control.
3. The advent of the long dilator sheath has significantly increased the success of insertion.
4. In critically ill patients undergoing cardiac catheterization who have poor ventricular function, study of the aortoiliac system is highly desirable as a guide for subsequent balloon insertion.
5. In high-risk cardiac surgical patients undergoing open heart surgery, in whom an intra-aortic balloon was not inserted before anesthetic induction, femoral artery access should be obtained with an arterial needle and then a guide wire, which are maintained in the sterile operative field. If IABP is subsequently required for separation from cardiopulmonary bypass, arterial access is then already established for IABP insertion.
6. A major advance in percutaneous balloon technology has been the advent of the dual-lumen percutaneous balloon. This balloon can follow a guide wire into the

aorta, virtually eliminating aortic dissection. In addition, arterial pressure monitoring can be performed through the balloon.

7. Finally, balloon removal should be carried out in the following manner. The balloon is deflated and pulled down to (but not into) the sheath. The femoral artery immediately distal to the balloon is tightly compressed, and the balloon and sheath are then removed as a unit. Blood is allowed to spurt from the artery for a few seconds, and then the compression is shifted over the puncture site for 30 minutes. Distal pulses are monitored with a Doppler apparatus, and manual compression is adjusted so that an audible pulse is registered. With this technique we have occasionally retrieved specimens of thrombus that have come out of the femoral artery and therefore have not embolized distally.

By following the above guidelines, the morbidity in Bregman's recent study has been reduced to no more than 5%. Bregman suggested that if these guidelines are followed, percutaneous IABP will remain as the temporary mechanical assist treatment of choice for the management of medically refractory left ventricular power failure and other ischemic cardiovascular states.

REFERENCES

1. Beckman, C.B., et al.: Results and complications of intra-aortic balloon counterpulsation, Ann. Thorac. Surg. **24:**550, 1977.
2. Bemis, C.E., et al.: Comparison of techniques for intra-aortic balloon insertion (abstract), Am. J. Cardiol. **47:**417, 1981.
3. Bonchek, M.D., and Olinger, G.: Direct ascending aortic insertion of the "percutaneous" intra-aortic balloon catheter in the open chest: advantages and precautions, Ann. Thorac. Surg. **32:**512, 1981.
4. Bregman, D.: Percutaneous intra-aortic balloon pumping: a time for reflection, Chest **82:**397, 1982.
5. Bregman, D., and Goetz, R.H.: Clinical experience with a new cardiac assist device—the dual chambered intra-aortic balloon assist, J. Thorac. Cardiovasc. Surg. **62:**577, 1971.
6. Grotte, G.J., and Butchart, E.G.: Impaction of the intra-aortic balloon due to dislocation of central stylet, J. Thorac. Cardiovasc. Surg. **80:**232, 1980.
7. Harvey, J.C., et al.: Complications of percutaneous intra-aortic balloon pumping, Circulation **64**(suppl. 2):114, 1981.
8. Hauser, A.M., et al.: Percutaneous intra-aortic balloon counterpulsation, Chest **82:**422, 1982.
9. Lefemine, A.A., et al.: Results and complications of intra-aortic balloon pumping in surgical and medical patients, Am. J. Cardiol. **40:**416, 1977.
10. Leinbach, R.C., et al.: Selective coronary and left ventricular cineangiography during intra-aortic balloon pumping for cardiogenic shock, Circulation **45:**845, 1972.
11. Lundell, D.C., et al.: Randomized comparison of the modified wireguided and standard intra-aortic balloon catheters, J. Thorac. Cardiovasc. Surg. **81:**297, 1981.
12. Mason, D.T., et al.: Diagnosis and management of myocardial infarction shock. In Eliot, R.S., et al.: Cardiac emergencies, ed. 2, Mount Kisco, N.Y., 1982, Futura Publishing Co.
13. McCabe, J.C., et al.: Complications of intra-aortic balloon insertion and counterpulsation, Circulation **57:**769, 1978.
14. McEnany, M.T., et al.: Clinical experience with intra-aortic balloon support in 728 patients, Circulation **58**(suppl.[1]):124, 1978.
15. Seldinger, S.I.: Catheter replacement of the needle in percutaneous arteriography: a new technique, Acta Radiol. **39:**368, 1953.
16. Shirkey, A.L., et al.: Insertion of the intra-aortic balloon through the aortic arch, Ann. Thorac. Surg. **21:**560, 1976.
17. Subramanian, V.A.: Percutaneous intra-aortic balloon pumping, Ann. Thorac. Surg. **29:**102, 1980.
18. Subramanian, V.A., et al.: Preliminary clinical experience with percutaneous intra-aortic balloon pumping, Circulation **62**(suppl. 1):123, 1980.
19. Vignola, P.A., et al.: Guidelines for effective and safe percutaneous intra-aortic balloon pump insertion and removal, Am. J. Cardiol. **48:**660, 1981.

CHAPTER 15 Counterpulsation timing: arterial pressure waveform

Timing defined

Timing of the IABP deals with the beat-to-beat interaction of the balloon's inflation-deflation sequence and the arterial circulatory system of the patient. Proper timing is conceived as the appropriate interaction between the electrical activity of the heart, the hemodynamic activity of the left ventricle and the great vessels, and the mechanical activity of the inflating balloon.

Delay between electrical and mechanical events

A delay exists between the electrical and mechanical events of the heart. Braunwald and associates[2] constructed a schematic representation of the timing of electrical and mechanical events based on data collected from 13 patients during exposure of the heart while undergoing chest surgery. Permutation of simultaneous pressure recordings was obtained from the four chambers of the heart. Left ventricular systole began .052 (standard deviation $\pm$ .0067) second after electrical depolarization (Fig. 15-1). This electrical-mechanical delay is essential in understanding the importance of examining the arterial pressure waveform rather than the electrocardiogram (ECG) to achieve proper timing.

Arterial pressure waveform

The R wave of the ECG is the reference point for inflation and deflation of the intra-aortic balloon. A fail-safe mechanism commands the pump to automatically deflate on sensing of an R wave or a waveform that meets voltage criteria for sensing of the particular console in use. The automatic deflation safety feature assures that the balloon does not inflate in full systole. The timing of inflation and deflation with respect to an R-wave reference point is controversial.[6] In general, inflation occurs at the dicrotic notch and deflation at the R wave. Bemis and associates,[1] however, have suggested that inflation should occur during a significant portion of systole to increase coronary flow at the expense of a slight decrease in stroke volume.

Manual inflation-deflation controls allow the operator to fine tune the timing sequence of inflation and deflation to afford the patient the best possible hemodynamic gain from counterpulsation. Because of the delay between electrical depolarization of the heart and

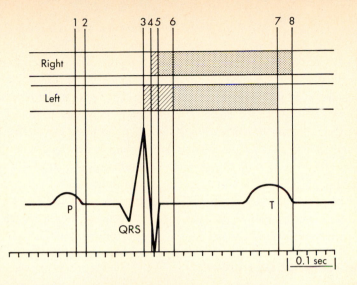

FIG. 15-1 Diagrammatic representation of average timing of electrical and mechanical events on both sides of heart during atrial and ventricular systole in normal subjects. *(1)* Onset of right atrial contraction, *(2)* onset of left atrial contraction, *(3)* onset of left ventricular contraction, *(4)* onset of right ventricular contraction, *(5)* onset of right ventricular ejection, *(6)* onset of left ventricular ejection, *(7)* end of left ventricular ejection, *(8)* end of right ventricular ejection. Striped areas represent ventricular isometric contraction. Stippled areas represent ventricular ejection. (From Braunwald, E., et al.: Circ. Res. **4:**100, 1956. Reproduced by permission.)

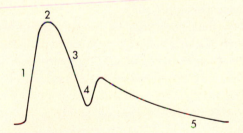

FIG. 15-2 Normal arterial pressure waveform. *(1)* Anacrotic limb, *(2)* peak systolic pressure, *(3)* dicrotic limb, *(4)* dicrotic notch, *(5)* aortic end-diastolic pressure.

mechanical contraction, the arterial waveform is used to reflect the hemodynamic impact of counterpulsation. It is necessary to become familiar with the elements of the arterial pressure curve and to associate the physiological action of the balloon with the systolic and diastolic components of the arterial pressure.

The normal arterial pressure waveform exhibits several points of reference that are easily understood if related to the cardiac cycle (Fig. 15-2). Aortic pressure rises at the moment the aortic valve opens and ejection begins. This steeply rising component of the arterial pulse curve is termed the *anacrotic limb* (Greek, ''upbeat''). Peak systolic pressure is the highest point on the arterial curve, representing left ventricular ejection. During this rapid ejection phase about 75% of the stroke volume for that beat is ejected. The descending limb is termed the *dicrotic limb* (Greek, ''double beat''). The pressure in the aorta decreases as the left ventricle relaxes, and blood perfuses out the arterial system. This decrease in pressure is interrupted by the *dicrotic notch* (or incisura, Latin, ''cutting into''), the incursion on the trailing edge of the systolic waveform that represents closure of the aortic valve.[4] The dicrotic notch is an extremèly important landmark for timing.

Left ventricular diastole begins following closure of the aortic valve. This filling phase is characterized by a continuous fall in the aortic pressure as the blood is perfused peripherally without further supply from the left ventricle until the next systole. The lowest aortic diastolic pressure point (end-diastolic pressure) signifies the afterload component of cardiac work or the resistance against which the left ventricle must work during isovolumic contraction. Accurate location of the peak systolic pressure, dicrotic notch, and aortic end-diastolic pressure (AoEDP) is essential to achieve proper timing.

Functional range of safe timing

There is probably no such thing as absolutely perfect timing. There is evidence that, depending on the state of the cardiovascular system and the hemodynamic variables measured, no single timing setting produces optimal results for all variables.[3] Timing can best be thought of in terms of the following three descriptive ranges for each complete ejection cycle of the left ventricle: (1) safe, (2) unsafe, and (3) optimum effectiveness (Fig. 15-3). The safe range is that segment of the ejection cycle in which the balloon can be inflated and deflated without competing with normal cardiac physiological events. This period is between the time of closure and opening of the aortic valve. Inflation and deflation during any part of this period does not cause harm to the patient. However, the most effective hemodynamic support may not be afforded. Late inflation provides less optimal augmentation and coronary perfusion. Deflation could occur early and be considered safe but ineffective. Early deflation reduces the AoEDP (afterload reduction) too early in the cardiac cycle, and the AoEDP equalizes with the patient's end-diastolic pressure before ejection. Therefore the work of systole is not reduced.

The unsafe range is that segment of the ejection cycle in which the inflated balloon could possibly cause harm to the heart. This unsafe range is the period of time between the opening of the aortic valve at the beginning of systole and closure of the aortic valve at the

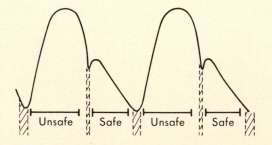

FIG. 15-3 Functional range of safe timing.

beginning of diastole. The balloon must complete its total augmented cycle during diastole because inflation during systole would constitute unsafe balloon timing. Balloon pumps are engineered with a safety feature that prevents inflation during full systole.

The concept of the most effective timing range must be discussed in terms of inflation and deflation of the counterpulsation mechanism. Again emphasis is placed on the need for balloon timing from the arterial waveform. The electrical event of the heart does not reflect the hemodynamic activity of the left ventricle. Thus the discussion of effective timing centers around the arterial pressure waveform.

Physiologically effective timing

A delay in waveform propagation exists between the aortic root and peripheral vessels. This delay is caused by the following:
1. Aortic valve closure actually occurs centrally before it manifests as a dicrotic notch on the peripheral arterial trace.
2. Similarly there exists a delay in retrograde transmission of the balloon assisted pressure pulse back to the aortic root.[5]

In absolute timing the reference point for balloon placement is always the ascending aorta. The central site is ideal, since there is no need to compensate for timing delays. However, aortic root pressure monitoring is not convenient except during cardiac catheterization or open heart surgery. Therefore the arterial pressure is usually monitored from a long radial artery indwelling catheter or a double-lumen or central lumen balloon that lies at the junction of the left subclavian artery and the aortic arch (Fig. 15-4). Because the balloon is not positioned precisely at the aortic valve and the monitoring site is not directly from the aortic root, the slightly induced time delays between actual physiological events and transmission to the catheter must be recognized. The essence of proper timing centers around allowing for the waveform propagation delay from the aortic root to the periphery and transmission of the balloon assisted pressure pulse back to the aortic root.

Waveform propagation delays

Approximately 20 to 25 msec are required for the pressure pulse to travel from the aortic valve, across the aortic arch, and to the subclavian artery (the extra time required for this pulse to reach the radial artery is insignificant).[4] Approximately 20 to 25 msec lapse before the augmented diastolic balloon pressure waveform reaches the aortic root. The two delays in this configuration are additive so that the total delay considered is 40 to 50 msec (Fig. 15-5).[5] Instructions are given on how to achieve proper timing, allowing for this 40 to 50 msec delay in waveform propagation, in the discussion of conventional timing— inflation.

Augmented arterial pressure waveform

Balloon inflation in diastole produces a diastolic pressure that is higher than systole. Rapid inflation of the balloon with helium or carbon dioxide just after the aortic valve has closed markedly elevates or augments the diastolic pressure. Fig. 15-6 illustrates the

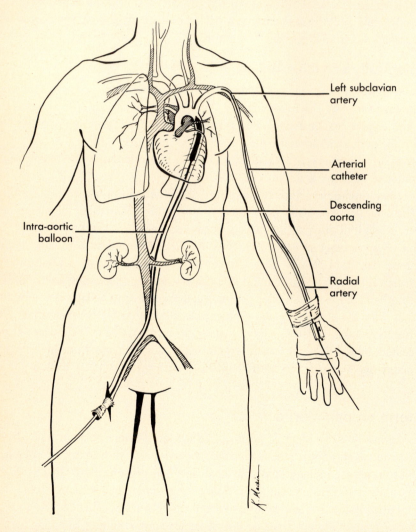

FIG. 15-4 Position of radial artery monitoring catheter and balloon in situ in descending aorta just distal to left subclavian artery.

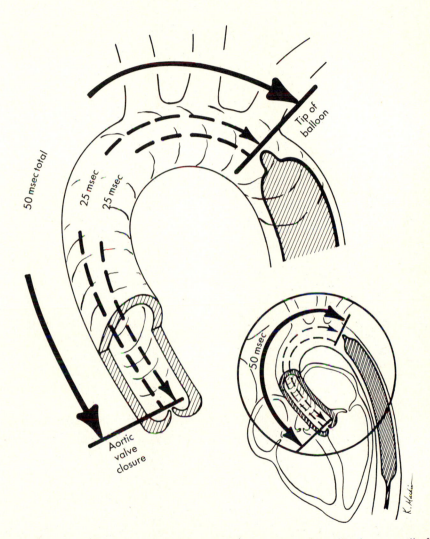

FIG. 15-5 Delay of approximately 25 msec occurs from time of aortic valve closure until effect is realized at subclavian artery. An equal delay also exists from balloon inflation at bifurcation of subclavian artery (elevation of aortic pressure at that point) until that pressure is appreciated at aortic root.

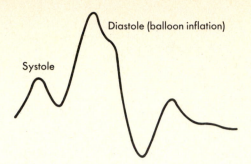

FIG. 15-6 Arterial pressure curve illustrating increased diastolic pressure with balloon inflation.

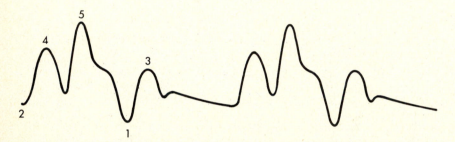

FIG. 15-7 Arterial pressure curve contour changes with balloon inflating on every other beat. *(1)* Balloon assisted aortic end-diastolic pressure, *(2)* patient aortic end-diastolic pressure, *(3)* balloon assisted systole, *(4)* patient systole, *(5)* peak diastolic augmented pressure.

arterial pressure curve with balloon inflation. Proper timing of the balloon is achieved with the balloon inflating on every other beat; a comparison is then made of the augmented and unaugmented arterial waveforms. The following five points of reference should be noted:

1. Patient (or unassisted) systole
2. Peak diastolic augmented pressure
3. Balloon AoEDP
4. Assisted systole
5. Patient AoEDP (Fig. 15-7)

Timing with Datascope, Hoogstraat, Kontron, and SMEC pumps

Imperative to proper pump placement is a thorough understanding of pump operation. Resource representatives from each manufacturer should be contacted for indepth instruction on timing for that particular pump. Principles of conventional timing are applicable to

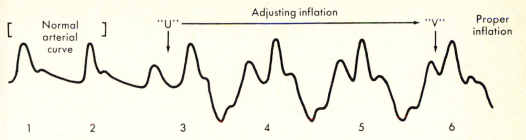

FIG. 15-8 Beats 1 and 2 represent normal arterial pressure curve. Beats 3, 4, 5, and 6 represent adjustment of inflation (adjusted to gradually occur earlier with each beat) so that U shape of dicrotic notch forms V, signifying proper inflation by beat 6.

Datascope, Hoogstraat, and Kontron pumps. The SMEC pump, however, employs an alternative approach to timing. The operator must therefore become thoroughly acquainted with timing differences before beginning operation.

Conventional timing

Inflation. The balloon must be able to generate the maximum amount of pressure for the longest safe period in diastole. The further into diastole that inflation begins, the lower the diastolic augmentation pressure, and thus the hemodynamic advantages of augmentation are compromised. Effective augmentation is achieved if inflation begins just after the aortic valve closes. The dicrotic notch on the arterial waveform usually exhibits a U-shaped appearance. Once balloon pumping begins, inflation should be adjusted with the appropriate knob or slide, according to the manufacturer's instructions. Inflation should begin at the dicrotic notch creating a V appearance rather than a U shape (Fig. 15-8). This change in waveform from a U to a V configuration accounts for the 40 to 50 msec delay in waveform propagations from the aortic root to the monitoring site.

Effects (Fig. 15-9). The aortic pressure is increased, and blood volume is displaced. Desired effects of inflation in diastole include the following:

1. Coronary blood flow is potentially increased.
2. Perfusion is augmented to the aortic arch and distal systemic circulation.
3. Coronary collateral circulation is potentially increased.

Deflation. Balloon deflation is set to occur just before the aortic valve opens or during isovolumic contraction. AoEDP is markedly reduced, thereby lowering the resistance against which the left ventricle must eject in systole (Fig. 15-10). Deflation has two rules.

1. Balloon AoEDP should be lower than patient AoEDP.
2. Balloon assisted systole should be lower than patient systole. If afterload is reduced, less pressure is required for ejection.

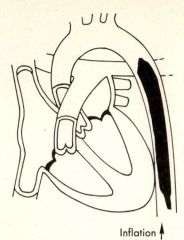

Inflation: Aortic pressure
    is increased, and blood
    volume is displaced

Desired effects of inflation

1. Coronary blood flow potentially ↑.
2. Perfusion is augmented to the
   aortic arch and distal
   systemic circulation
3. Coronary collateral circulation is potentially ↑.

Inflation ↑

FIG. 15-9 Effects of proper inflation.

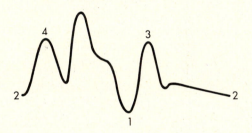

FIG. 15-10 Proper deflation. Balloon assisted aortic end-diastolic pressure *(1)* should be lower than patient aortic end-diastolic pressure *(2)*; balloon assisted systole *(3)* should be lower than patient systole *(4)*.

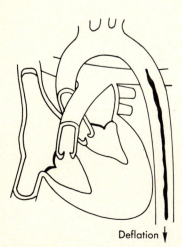

Desired effects of deflation

1. Reduction of aortic end-diastolic
   pressure reduces afterload
2. Systole following balloon inflation
   should be lower than unassisted
   systole
3. Myocardial oxygen consumption (MVO_2)
   is decreased
4. Cardiac output is increased
5. Reduction in peak systolic pressure
   reduces left to right shunting
   in ventricular septal defects
   and regurgitant blood flow
   in mitral insufficiency

Deflation ↓

FIG. 15-11 Effects of proper deflation.

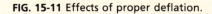

Effects (Fig. 15-11)

1. Reduction of AoEDP achieved by the balloon's deflation just before the next systole enables the left ventricle to eject against a lower resistance (afterload reduction).

2. The systole following balloon inflation should be lower than unassisted systole. Maximum tension required in systole is reduced because the afterload is decreased.

3. Myocardial oxygen consumption (MVO_2) is decreased because cardiac work during isovolumic contraction is reduced.

4. Cardiac output is increased.

5. Reduction in peak left ventricular pressure generated during systole reduces left-to-right shunting secondary to ventricular septal defects and reduces the amount of regurgitation in mitral insufficiency.

Comparison of unaugmented and augmented arterial waveforms. Examination of the unaugmented (balloon off) and augmented (balloon inflation in diastole) cycles reveals significant differences (Fig. 15-12). The arterial pressure waveform and cuff pressure take on a different meaning with balloon pumping. A blood pressure taken off the balloon pump and recorded as 100/70 mm Hg represents the onset of Korotkoff's sounds at 100 mm Hg. Hence the actual physiological pressures of the cardiac cycle are recorded. With balloon inflation the peak diastolic augmented pressure is an artificially produced pressure. The initial Korotkoff's sounds heard at 100 mm Hg represent this balloon inflation pressure, which is higher than systole (Fig. 15-13). The correct description of this event is to state that the patient has an augmented peak diastolic pressure of 100 mm Hg.

Timing from the femoral artery. The differences observed between radial and femoral artery tracings in the timing of the balloon pulse seem best explained by the spatial relationship between these catheters, the aortic valve, and the balloon itself. Specifically the balloon is closer to the femoral catheter, and the balloon and the aortic valve are aproximately the same distance from the radial catheter (Fig. 15-14). The femoral artery poses a more difficult problem for proper timing as a result of waveform distortion and significant time delays. The total time delay involved is approximately 120 msec, which compensates for the fact that the monitoring site is distal to both the aortic valve and the balloon. If the balloon is properly timed from a femoral site, inflation appears to occur at peak systole (Fig. 15-15). Operators who do not understand that necessary time delays, when pumping from the femoral artery, may compensate for what appears to be a dangerous situation may inflate the balloon too late. This could significantly decrease the effectiveness of the augmentation; therefore timing from a radial artery site is preferable.

Summary of conventional timing. In summary the following events ensue during counterpulsation. Following aortic valve closure and the onset of diastole, a gas is rapidly propelled into the intra-aortic balloon, creating a peak diastolic augmented pressure. The volume of blood in the aorta at this moment (see Chapter 8, Windkessel effect) is displaced proximally to potentially increase coronary and aortic arch perfusion and distally to the sytemic circulation. The balloon is rapidly deflated at the end of diastole, just before the next systole, or during isovolumic contraction. Deflation markedly lowers the AoEDP (afterload reduction) and decreases the work of the next systole.

The ability to compare timing on the balloon to a normal configuration is critical.

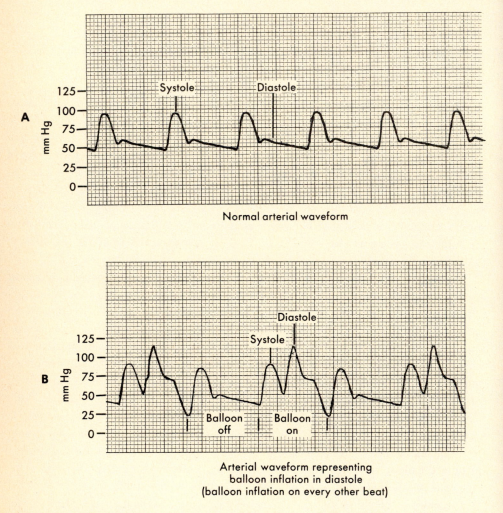

Normal arterial waveform

Arterial waveform representing
balloon inflation in diastole
(balloon inflation on every other beat)

FIG. 15-12 Comparison of arterial pressure waveform without balloon assistance. **B,** Arterial pressure waveform with balloon inflation in diastole, which elevates or augments diastolic pressure higher than systolic pressure.

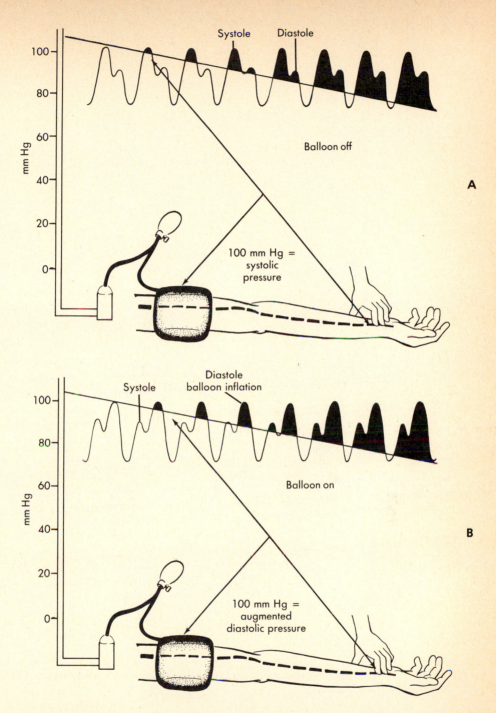

FIG. 15-13 Numerical millimeter of mercury blood pressure recorded has different meaning when recorded while patient receives balloon pump assist **A,** Traditional blood pressure recording *without* balloon assistance; initial Korotkoff's sounds heard (100 mm Hg) are recorded as patient's systolic pressure. Normal arterial pressure curve is also noted. **B,** Blood pressure recorded *with* balloon assistance. In this example, 100 mm Hg point of onset of Korotkoff's sounds is not systolic pressure but rather diastolic augmented pressure caused by balloon inflation, which nets higher pressure than patient's systole.

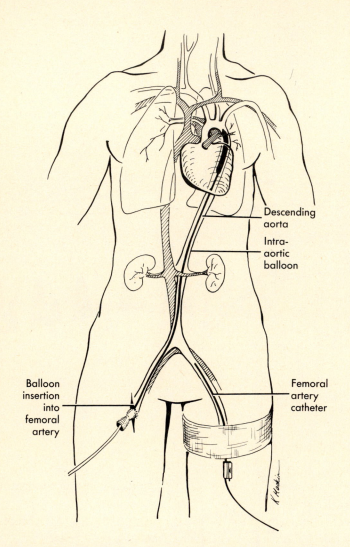

FIG. 15-14 Placement of femoral artery monitoring catheter with intra-aortic balloon positioned in situ in descending thoracic aorta.

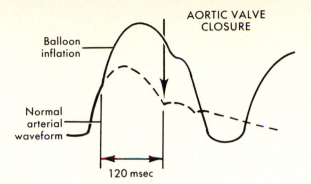

FIG. 15-15 Balloon inflation-deflation timed from femoral artery tracing. Inflation "appears" early, allowing for approximately 120 msec delay total for aortic valve closure to be realized at monitoring catheter and retrograde transmission of balloon inflation pressure to aortic root.

Therefore the balloon should be timed on 1:2 (inflation on every other beat). This method is even more critical when timing from a femoral arterial waveform. Sometimes the timing may look correct but if examined according to the previously described protocols, it may in fact be incorrect, and the effect of the balloon is diminished. The nurse or technician must be certain that the arterial pressure waveform meets the criteria for safe and effective augmentation. The clinician should never assume that because the arterial waveform looks correct, timing is correct or that because the arterial waveform appears incorrect in morphology, timing is incorrect! The patient's balloon arterial pressure curves should be compared to the theoretical model of timing as outlined in this discussion, and the hemodynamic status should be observed in conjunction with the timing established. Balloon timing should be rechecked whenever the following occur: rate change ± 10 beats per minute, arrhythmias, a change in volume or pressure status, a change between wall current and portable power, hemodynamic deterioration of the patient, and at least twice during a shift as routine nursing care.

Timing of the SMEC pump[8,9,10]

SMEC's rationale for timing is based on the following principles:
1. The delay from the R wave to the left ventricular contraction does not change significantly with rate changes.
2. The duration of systole does not change significantly with rate changes.
3. The period of diastole does not change with changes in rate.

The SMEC console is triggered by the immediately preceding R wave for a predetermined period of inflation (Fig. 15-16). The machine triggers the balloon to deflation at point *a*. The duration of deflation is manually selected, and the console inflates the balloon at point *b*. Thereby the balloon is inflated at all times and is simply triggered to deflation by an R wave. The entire sequence of events would be repeated at point *c*. Myocardial contraction is not anticipated with the SMEC system to create end-diastolic unloading. Instead the balloon deflates rapidly and is timed to coincide with myocardial contraction.

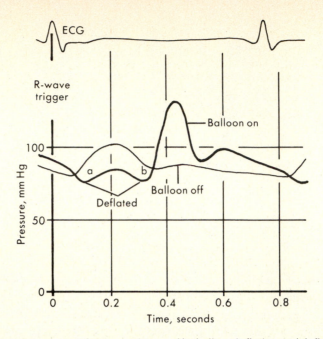

FIG. 15-16 Arterial pressure waveform superimposed by balloon inflation and deflation timed with SMEC pump. (Courtesy SMEC, Cookeville, Tenn.)

Removal of gas volume from the aortic balloon exceeds dv/dt* of the left ventricle. By comparison, conventional timing sets the duration of inflation to correspond with cardiac diastole. The pump is triggered by an R wave to inflate the balloon for a predetermined interval of inflation. The balloon thereby deflates in anticipation of the next systole, timed from the previous R wave.

The very fast balloon response necessitates timing the balloon with the onset of systole and diastole for deflation and inflation, rather than anticipating these by earlier deflation and inflation as in conventional timing.

The "balloon on" arterial pressure waveform is superimposed over the "balloon off" arterial pressure on the scope of the SMEC console. This allows an immediate assessment of the timing and effectiveness of the balloon. This feature is especially valuable in recognizing the assist for low arterial pressure and irregular rates.[10]

---

*dv/dt, Acceleration of blood sustained during early ejection.[4]

REFERENCES

1. Bemis, C.E., et al.: A comparison of techniques of intra-aortic balloon insertion (abstract), Am. J. Cardiol. **47**:417, 1982.
2. Braunwald, E., et al.: Time relationship of dynamic events in the cardiac chambers, pulmonary artery and aorta in man, Circ. Res. **4**:100, 1956.
3. Bregman, D., et al.: Percutaneous intra-aortic balloon insertion, Am. J. Cardiol. **46**:261, 1980.

4. Burton, A.C.: Physiology and biophysics of the circulation, ed. 2, Chicago, 1972, Year Book Medical Publishers, Inc.
5. Cohn, J.J.: Blood pressure and cardiac performances, Am. J. Med. **55:**351, 1973.
6. Ohley, W.: Measuring the performance characteristics of an IABP system, Cardiac Assists **2:**6, 1982.
7. Rushmer, R.F.: Cardiovascular dynamics, Philadelphia, 1976, W.B. Saunders Co.
8. Schiff, P., President, SMEC, Inc.: Personal Communication, Sept. 1982.
9. SMEC Newsletter, vol. 10, Jan. 1979, Cookeville, Tenn.
10. SMEC Newsletter, vol. 14, Jan. 1982, Cookeville, Tenn.

CHAPTER 16 Improper timing

The nurse must learn to recognize improper timing from a hemodynamic perspective rather than from rote. One of the most important components of nursing care of the patient requiring the balloon pump is to set the balloon's counterpulsation mechanism with the patient's cardiac cycle through the proper timing of the inflation-deflation sequence.

Although all balloon pumps have safety mechanisms to prevent inflation during peak systole, which would compete with natural ejection, safe timing may not necessarily be the most effective and beneficial timing for hemodynamic improvement of the patient's status.

The previous chapter carefully outlined the identifying components of proper timing but as a review they are the following (Fig. 16-1):

Proper inflation: Dicrotic notch assumes a V shape.

Proper deflation: Balloon assisted aortic end-diastolic pressure (AoEDP) (B) is lower than patient AoEDP (A). Assisted systole (D) is lower than patient systole (C).

Recognizing improper inflation and deflation: conventional timing
Early inflation

Early inflation is easily recognizable; inflation appears to be encroaching on the previous systole. The dicrotic notch landmark is no longer visible because of the early rise of the augmented pressure as the balloon inflates (Fig. 16-2).

Effects

1. Diastolic augmentation seems to be encroaching on the systolic wave.
2. Can cause regurgitation of blood into the left ventricle.
3. Can raise the pressure in the aorta, which closes the aortic valve prematurely and does not allow the ventricle to completely empty.
4. Decreases cardiac output and increases intraventricular volume and pressure (preload).

Late inflation

Inflation occurs well after the aortic valve closes. Less effective augmentation occurs because the balloon inflates later in diastole, rather than just after the aortic valve closes (represented by the dicrotic notch, (Fig. 16-3).

Effects

1. May lower diastolic augmentation pressure.
2. May reduce coronary artery perfusion pressure.

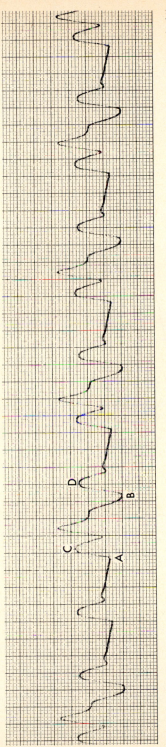
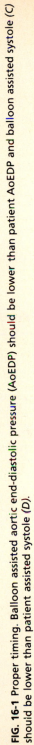

FIG. 16-1 Proper timing. Balloon assisted aortic end-diastolic pressure (AoEDP) should be lower than patient AoEDP and balloon assisted systole (C) should be lower than patient assisted systole (D).

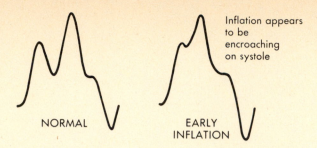

FIG. 16-2 Early inflation. Inflation of balloon causes augmented diastolic pressure to appear to be encroaching on systole. Dicrotic notch landmark is no longer visible because of early rise of diastolic augmented pressure.

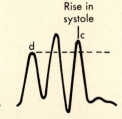

FIG. 16-3 Late inflation. Inflation occurs well after aortic valve closes. Dicrotic notch widens, giving appearance of plateau.

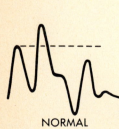

FIG. 16-4 Early deflation. Drop in balloon assisted AoEDP occurs too soon to reduce work of next systole. Assisted systole may rise (c) in comparison to patient systole (d). Pressure drop in aorta that occurs early attempts to equilibrate. Retrograde flow can be identified by plateau arising on upstroke of assisted systole. Retrograde flow that equilibrates AoEDP can perfuse from coronary arteries or any branch of arterial tree.

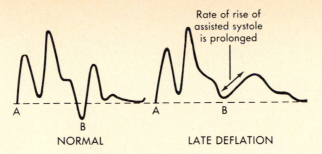

FIG. 16-5 Late deflation. Assisted AoEDP is increased. Because of the increased afterload to left ventricular ejection, rate of rise of assisted systolic pressure (dp/dt) may be increased. Assisted AoEDP is equal to or higher than patient AoEDP.

Early deflation

The drop in balloon assisted AoEDP occurs too early in the cycle to effectively reduce afterload. The AoEDP equilibrates, which may result in retrograde flow from the coronary arteries (Fig. 16-4).

Effects

1. Level of the patient systole affected by the balloon may rise in comparison with the level of systole unaffected by the balloon. The work effort of systole following balloon augmentation is not reduced.
2. Afterload reduction is reduced or nonexistent.
3. There are increased oxygen demands on an already ischemic myocardium.
4. Hemodynamic deterioration results unless improper timing is corrected to the following:
   Rising pulmonary artery wedge pressure and left atrial pressure.
   Falling arterial pressure.
5. AoEDP equilibrates following early deflation. Retrograde flow may occur from the coronary arteries, causing the patient to experience angina, or from other branches of the arterial tree.

Late deflation

The afterload is increased, since the left ventricle must eject against a greater resistance (Fig. 16-5).

Effects

1. There is no reduction in balloon assisted AoEDP compared to patient AoEDP.
2. Left ventricle must eject against a greater resistance; thus the work effort of systole is increased.
3. Isovolumic contraction phase is prolonged, and myocardial oxygen consumption is increased.
4. Rate of rise of systolic pressure may be prolonged (dp/dt) because of increased resistance to ventricular ejection.

Recognizing improper timing with the SMEC System[1]

1. Balloon is not deflated for systole (*not* rate dependent).
2. Deflation occurs before systole (causes retrograde flow in aorta from the coronary arteries).
3. Inflation occurs before the dicrotic notch (interrupts ejection caused by fast balloon response).

REFERENCE

1. Schiff, P., President, SMEC, Inc.: Personal communication, Sept. 1982.

CHAPTER 17 Exercises in mastering proper timing

The following exercises are intended to provide practical experience in recognizing improperly timed (early or late inflation-deflation) arterial waveform tracings. All tracings are examples of the balloon inflating on every other beat. Each strip is accompanied by a blank space for comments on inflation and deflation (early or late). A line is also provided for additional comments (i.e., hemodynamic consequences of the representative timing error and/or corrective action). The strips are reproduced beginning on page 162 with answers and discussions. Key:

A, Patient aortic end-diastolic pressure (AoEDP)
B, Balloon assisted AoEDP
C, Unassisted systole
D, Balloon assisted systole

No. 1

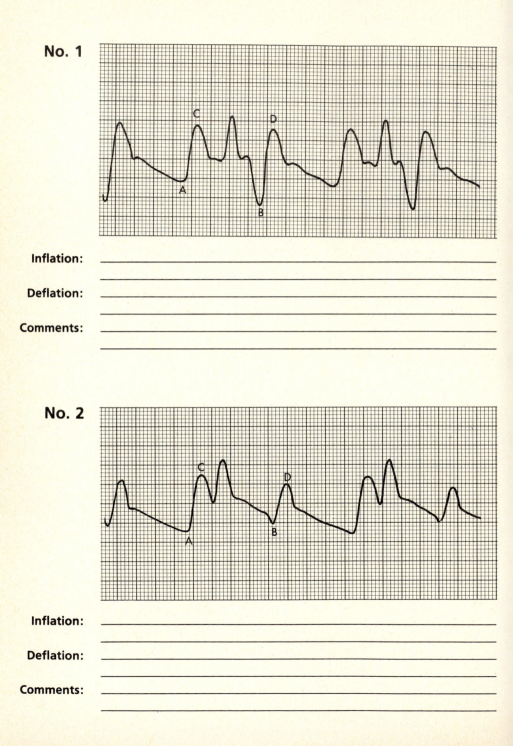

Inflation: _____
_____

Deflation: _____
_____

Comments: _____
_____

No. 2

Inflation: _____
_____

Deflation: _____
_____

Comments: _____
_____

No. 3

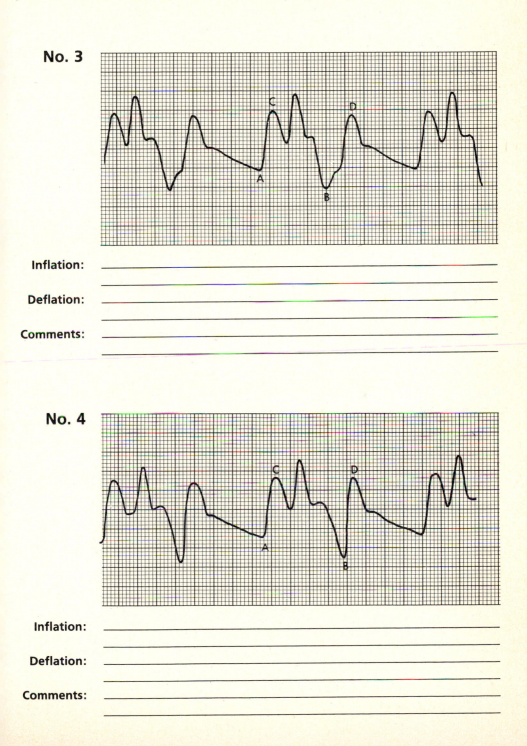

Inflation: _____

Deflation: _____

Comments: _____

No. 4

Inflation: _____

Deflation: _____

Comments: _____

No. 5

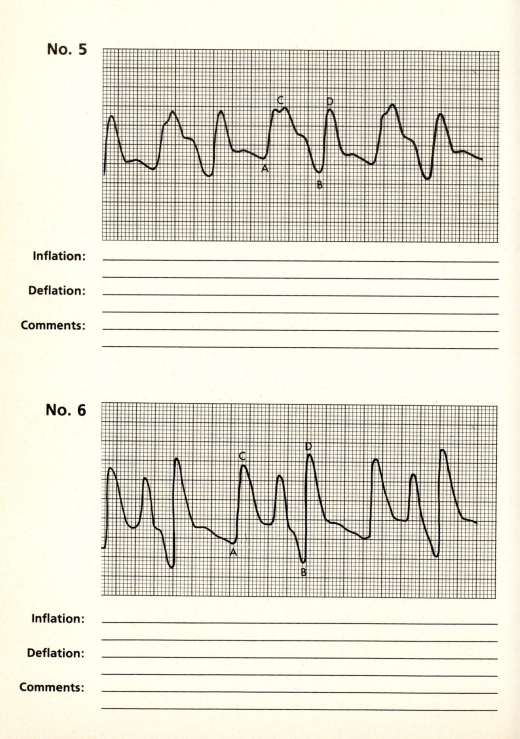

Inflation: _____

_____

Deflation: _____

_____

Comments: _____

_____

No. 6

Inflation: _____

_____

Deflation: _____

_____

Comments: _____

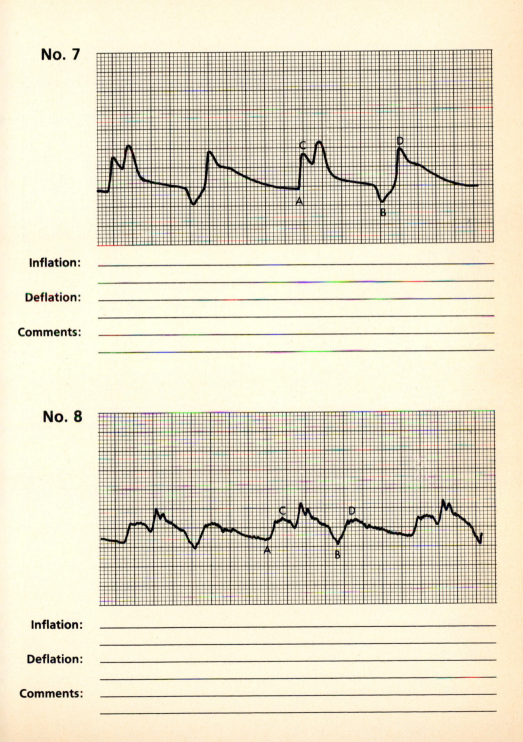

No. 7

Inflation: _____

Deflation: _____

Comments: _____

No. 8

Inflation: _____

Deflation: _____

Comments: _____

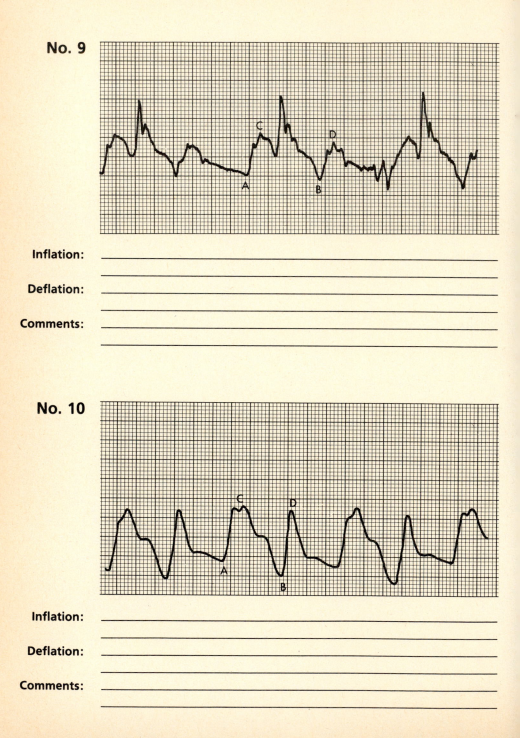

No. 9

Inflation: _____

_____

Deflation: _____

_____

Comments: _____

_____

No. 10

Inflation: _____

_____

Deflation: _____

_____

Comments: _____

_____

No. 11

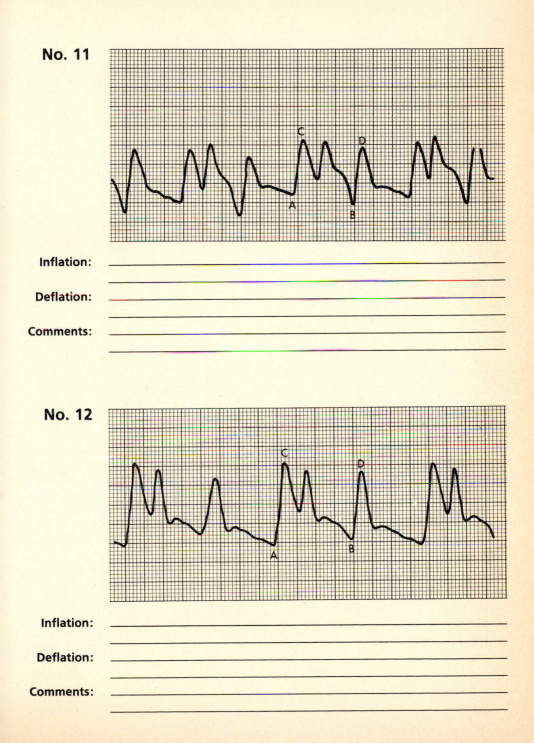

Inflation: _____

_____

Deflation: _____

_____

Comments: _____

_____

No. 12

Inflation: _____

_____

Deflation: _____

_____

Comments: _____

_____

No. 13

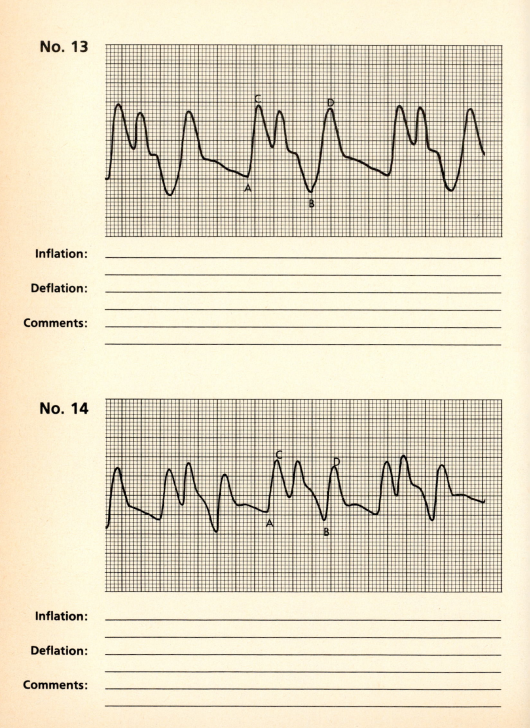

Inflation: _____

_____

Deflation: _____

_____

Comments: _____

_____

No. 14

Inflation: _____

_____

Deflation: _____

_____

Comments: _____

_____

No. 15

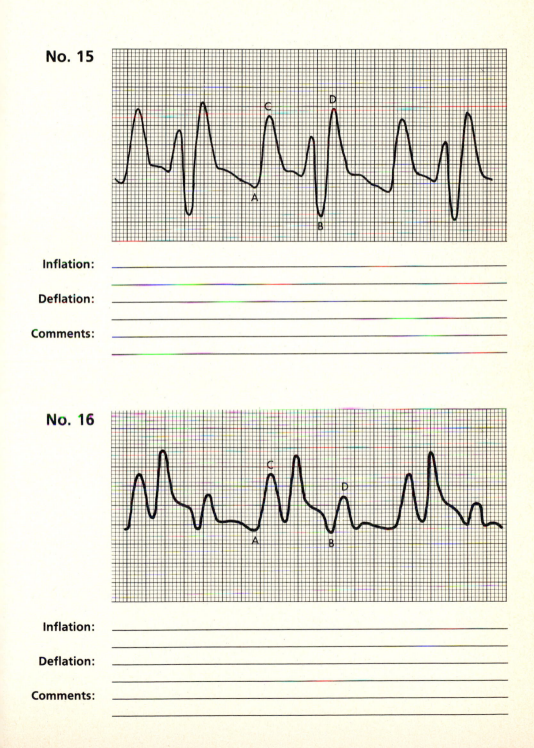

Inflation: _____

Deflation: _____

Comments: _____

No. 16

No. 17

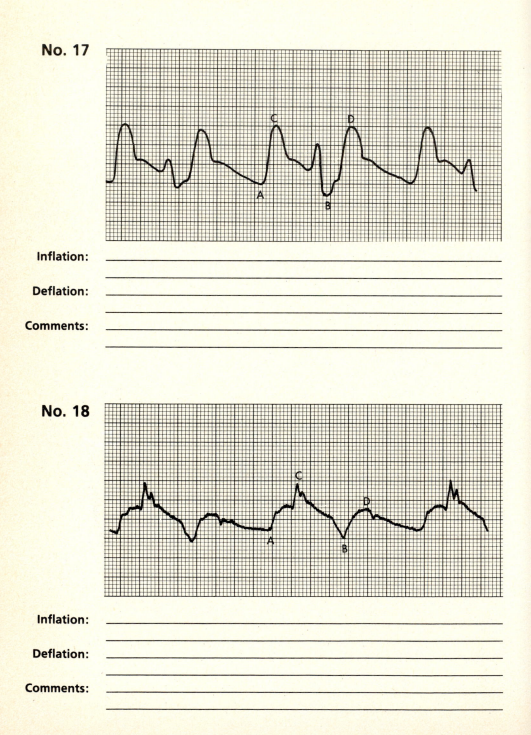

Inflation: _____

_____

Deflation: _____

_____

Comments: _____

_____

No. 18

Inflation: _____

_____

Deflation: _____

_____

Comments: _____

_____

No. 19

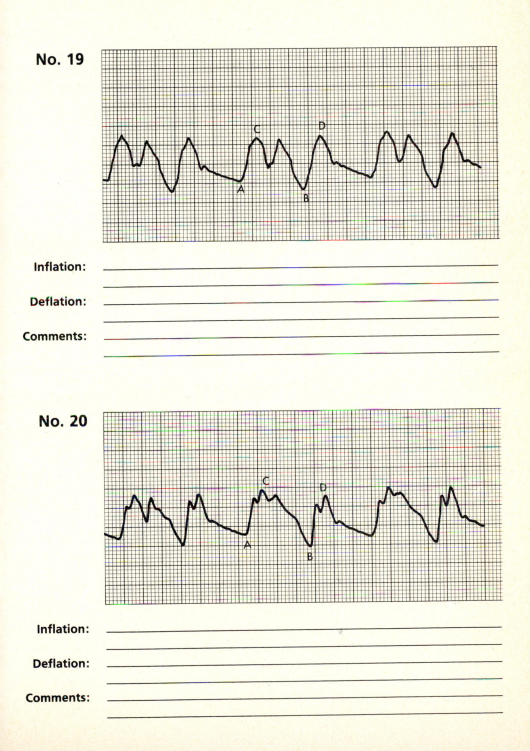

Inflation: _____
_____
Deflation: _____
_____
Comments: _____
_____

No. 20

Inflation: _____
_____
Deflation: _____
_____
Comments: _____
_____

ANSWERS AND DISCUSSION ON TIMING ARTERIAL TRACINGS

No. 1

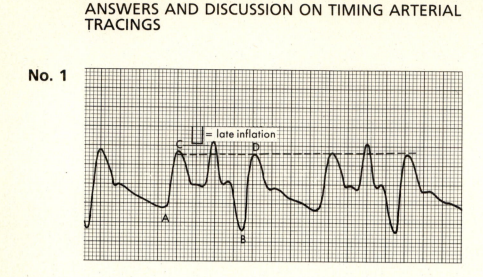

Inflation:	Very late. Note square wave of dicrotic notch rather than V appearance.
Deflation:	Possibly slightly early. Assisted systole (D) is not appreciably lower than unassisted systole (C).
Comments:	Try adjusting deflation to occur slightly later in an attempt to reduce assisted systole further.

No. 2

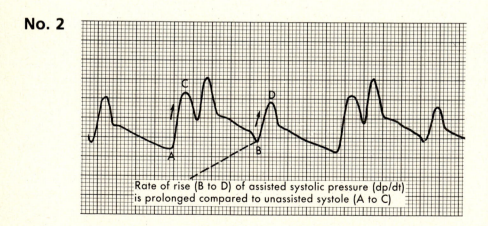

Inflation:	Okay. Nice V appearance to dicrotic notch.
Deflation:	Very late. Balloon assisted AoEDP (B) is greater than patient AoEDP (A).
Comments:	The left ventricle must eject against a greater AoEDP. Afterload is increased, isometric contraction is prolonged, and the rate of rise of systolic pressure (dp/dt) is prolonged.

No. 3

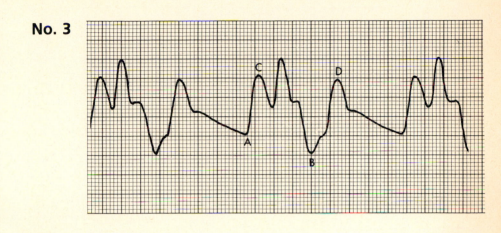

Inflation:	Okay. Nice V appearance to dicrotic notch.
Deflation:	Okay.
Comments:	Balloon AoEDP (B) is lower than patient AoEDP (A); Balloon assisted systole (D) is lower than patient systole (C); afterload reduction is achieved.

No. 4

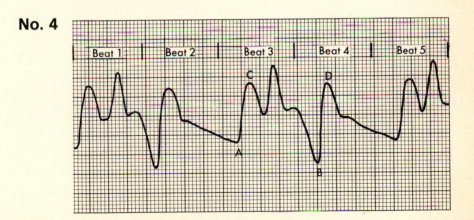

Inflation:	First beat is late and then adjusted for proper inflation (dicrotic notch assumes a V shape by beat 5).
Deflation:	Okay. D < C; B < A.
Comments:	Examine several beats when assessing timing. An isolated beat can appear improperly timed, when the other beats are actually properly timed. A premature beat can throw off the timing for that one beat.

No. 5

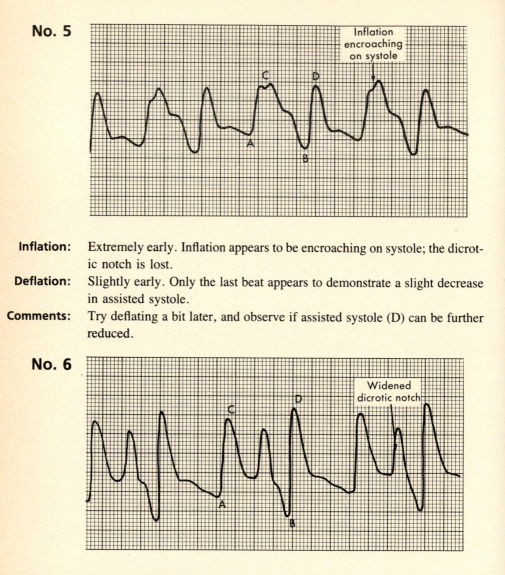

Inflation:	Extremely early. Inflation appears to be encroaching on systole; the dicrotic notch is lost.
Deflation:	Slightly early. Only the last beat appears to demonstrate a slight decrease in assisted systole.
Comments:	Try deflating a bit later, and observe if assisted systole (D) can be further reduced.

No. 6

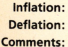

Inflation:	Very late. Note plateau at area of dicrotic notch.
Deflation:	Very early. Assisted systole (D) is greater than patient systole (C).
Comments:	Early reduction of aortic pressure has no effect on reducing the work of the next systole (afterload reduction comes too early). More work is required for the next systole D > C. With early deflation the balloon assisted AoEDP equilibrates. Retrograde filling could occur from the coronary arteries, and the patient could develop angina. Balloon counterpulsation is not helping this patient. Note the very poor augmentation in diastole caused by late inflation and early deflation.

No. 7

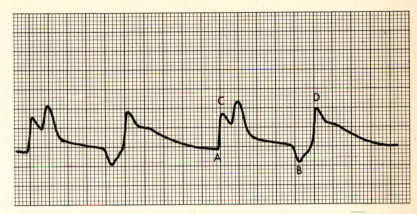

Inflation:	Okay.
Deflation:	Early. Assisted systole (D) is greater than patient systole (C).
Comments:	Go back to strip 6, and review the consequences of early deflation. This strip is probably not as detrimental as strip 6, where (D) is actually greater than (C). Attempt to deflate a bit later.

No. 8

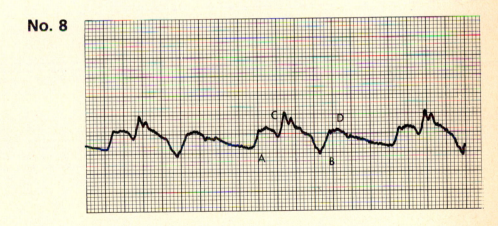

Inflation:	Okay.
Deflation:	Slightly late. Balloon assisted AoEDP (B) is equal to or only slightly lower than patient AoEDP (A).
Comments:	Try deflating a bit earlier, and observe if balloon assisted AoEDP (B) is further reduced.

No. 9

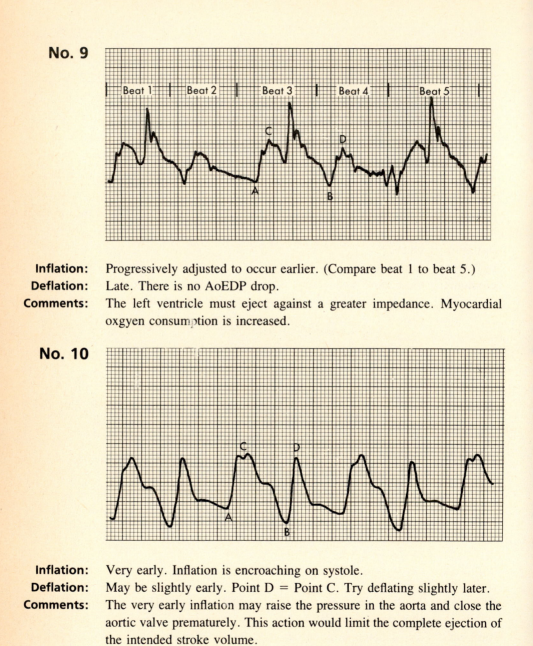

Inflation:	Progressively adjusted to occur earlier. (Compare beat 1 to beat 5.)
Deflation:	Late. There is no AoEDP drop.
Comments:	The left ventricle must eject against a greater impedance. Myocardial oxgyen consumption is increased.

No. 10

Inflation:	Very early. Inflation is encroaching on systole.
Deflation:	May be slightly early. Point D = Point C. Try deflating slightly later.
Comments:	The very early inflation may raise the pressure in the aorta and close the aortic valve prematurely. This action would limit the complete ejection of the intended stroke volume.

No. 11

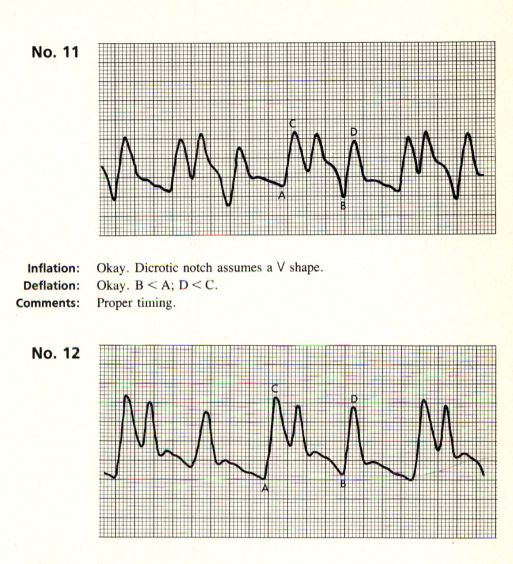

Inflation: Okay. Dicrotic notch assumes a V shape.
Deflation: Okay. B < A; D < C.
Comments: Proper timing.

No. 12

Inflation: Okay.
Deflation: Late. B ≥ A, rather than B < A.
Comments: No afterload reduction is occurring. The work load of the myocardium is actually increased with late deflation. Correct by deflating earlier. Note lack of comparatively higher diastolic augmentation. Unassisted patient systolic pressure appears excellent; therefore less impressive diastolic augmentation is to be anticipated. From assessment of this arterial waveform alone (no clinical data available) it appears that this patient could begin more progressive weaning from the pump.

No. 13

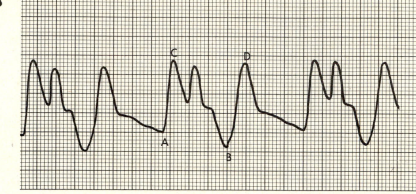

Inflation: Okay.
Deflation: B < A; D is slightly lower than C.
Comments: Deflation appears good, but try deflating a bit later in an attempt to further reduce assisted systole (D).

No. 14

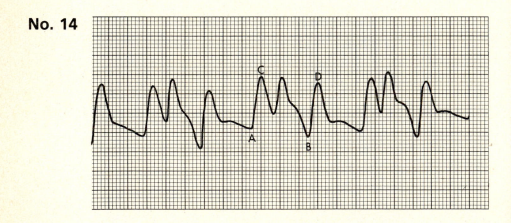

Inflation: Okay.
Deflation: B < A, and D < C.
Comments: Try deflating a bit earlier to determine if the assisted AoEDP can be lowered further.

No. 15

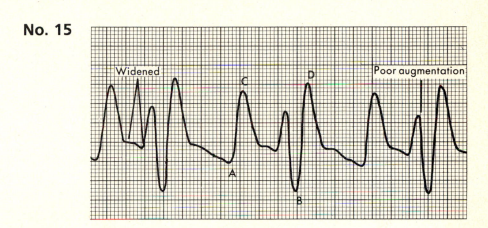

Inflation:	Very late.
Deflation:	Very early. D > C. The drop in AoEDP comes too early to effectively reduce the ensuing systole.
Comments:	Note very poor diastolic augmentation. When the balloon is timed to inflate very late and deflate very early, there is little time available in the cycle for augmentation. Note that assisted systole (D) is actually higher than unassisted systole (C). The patient would probably be better off without the balloon than with this poorly timed counterpulsation.

No. 16

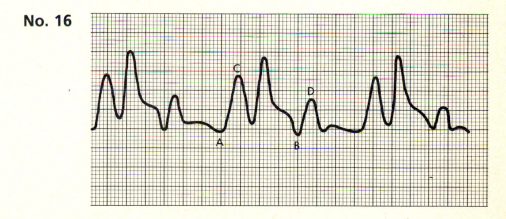

Inflation:	Okay.
Deflation:	Assisted AoEDP (B) = Patient AoEDP (A). Balloon is deflated too late.
Comments:	There is increased impedance to ejection because the balloon is deflating at the point that systole occurs, rather than before systole begins. Myocardial oxygen consumption is increased.

No. 17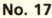

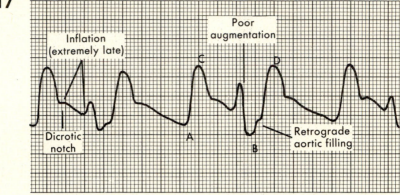

Inflation:	Extremely late. A long trough is present after the dicrotic notch.
Deflation:	Early. Assisted systole (D) = Patient systole (C).
Comments:	1. This tracing illustrates a very important point about early deflation. Note the plateau at point B. This small plateau actually represents retrograde filling as the aortic pressure attempts to equilibrate after its temporary drop caused by rapid deflation.
	2. The retrograde filling that occurs may be from the coronary or renal arteries.
	3. Because this deflation occurs early, it does not reduce the work of the next systole (D).
	4. Late inflation and early deflation produces a very poor diastolic augmentation.

No. 18

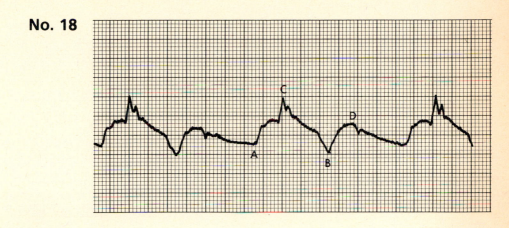

Inflation:	Early.
Deflation:	Late. Assisted AoEDP (B) is not effectively decreased.
Comments:	The patient has poor perfusion pressure to begin with in addition to some artifact. Try to deflate earlier to achieve better afterload reduction. This timing may be as good as you will get.

No. 19

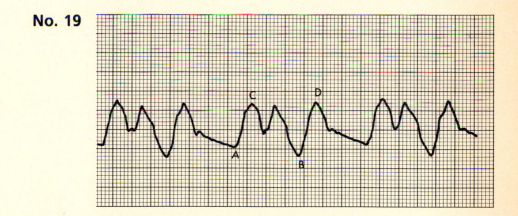

Inflation:	First beat, late inflation. Remainder are okay.
Deflation:	Early. Assisted systole (D) = Patient systole (C).
Comments:	Drop in AoEDP occurs too early to be effective.

No. 20

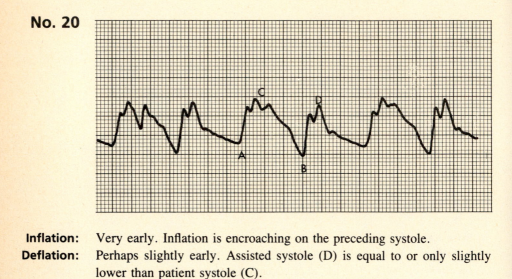

Inflation: Very early. Inflation is encroaching on the preceding systole.

Deflation: Perhaps slightly early. Assisted systole (D) is equal to or only slightly lower than patient systole (C).

Comments: The early inflation of the balloon may raise aortic pressure to a point that closes the aortic valve prematurely. The notching of the systolic peaks may be caused by catheter fling.

CHAPTER 18 **Balloon gas pressure waveforms**

Select balloon consoles display a tracing representative of gas propulsion into the balloon during inflation and withdrawal of the gas during deflation. The normal balloon pressure curve configuration is presented in Fig. 18-1.

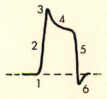

FIG. 18-1 Normal balloon pressure curve configuration.

Points of recognition are the following:
1. Zero baseline
2. Inflation
3. Peak inflation
4. Plateau (period of full inflation)
5. Deflation
6. Peak deflation

Variations in this balloon pressure curve have been identified by clinicians at Beth Israel Hospital in Boston.* Awareness of alterations in balloon gas pressure curves and the underlying cause should be part of the nurse's data base in the management of patients requiring the balloon pump assistance.

---

*Tracings courtesy Beth Israel Hospital, Boston.

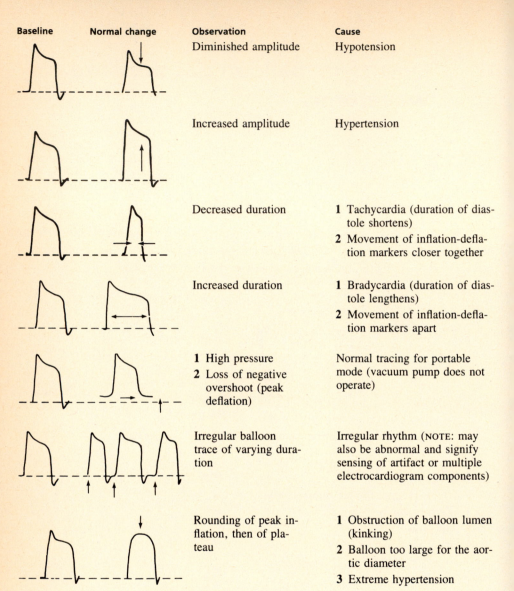

Baseline	Normal change	Observation	Cause
		Diminished amplitude	Hypotension
		Increased amplitude	Hypertension
		Decreased duration	1 Tachycardia (duration of diastole shortens) 2 Movement of inflation-deflation markers closer together
		Increased duration	1 Bradycardia (duration of diastole lengthens) 2 Movement of inflation-deflation markers apart
		1 High pressure 2 Loss of negative overshoot (peak deflation)	Normal tracing for portable mode (vacuum pump does not operate)
		Irregular balloon trace of varying duration	Irregular rhythm (NOTE: may also be abnormal and signify sensing of artifact or multiple electrocardiogram components)
		Rounding of peak inflation, then of plateau	1 Obstruction of balloon lumen (kinking) 2 Balloon too large for the aortic diameter 3 Extreme hypertension

The cause of the rounding can be differentiated by reducing the volume of the balloon 5 to 7 cc.

1. Pattern reverts to normal if balloon is too large.
   a. Aortic rupture may result if balloon is run at full volume.
   b. Therefore a smaller balloon must be inserted or balloon must be run at reduced volume (55 minutes of pumping at reduced volume should be alternated with 5 minutes of pumping at full volume to reduce the hazard of clot formation in balloon folds).
2. Pattern remains rounded if balloon catheter is kinked internally or externally.

Baseline	Normal change	Observation	Cause
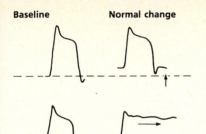		High pressure	Balloon may be overfilled; follow specific vendor's instructions for overfilled balloon
		Sustained inflation	Consoles have safety factors that should prevent sustained inflation, but if it occurs, balloon should be manually deflated with a syringe
		Loss of zero baseline	Duration of diastolic augmentation is too long
		Low pressure	Balloon may need to be refilled
			System may have leak; follow individual's protocol for leak detection

CHAPTER 19 Electrocardiogram and balloon pump

Although timing of the balloon pump can only be accurately achieved from the arterial waveform, the efficacy of balloon pumping is dependent on the quality and reliability of the electrocardiographic signal. Therefore the goal of electrocardiographic monitoring for timing of the balloon pump is to maximize the amplitude of the R wave, to minimize the amplitude of all other waves, and to avoid signal interference by other electrical equipment.

All balloon pumps recognize the R wave of the electrocardiogram (ECG) as the reference point for inflation-deflation. Manual adjustments are thereafter made following inspection of the arterial waveform to achieve proper timing. The electrocardiographic signal is most critically important in balloon pumping, and attention should be directed toward achieving a satisfactory tracing and gaining an understanding of the effect of the pacemaker artifact on the signal processing with the particular type of pump used.

Obtaining an optimum tracing

Trouble-free ECG monitoring depends to a large extent on site preparation before application of the electrodes. Each electrode site should be clean and dry and provide a smooth, even surface. Avoid bony protuberances, joints, and creases or folds in the skin. Excessive body hair should be shaved before applying the electrode. Electrode sites should be free of any oil film or residue that could affect electrode adhesion. Alcohol cleansing should be avoided, unless needed to remove previously applied oils, liniments, or lotions because alcohol that is trapped underneath the electrode is the frequent cause of patient skin irritation and adhesion loss. The film left by soap can impair electrode adhesion; in that case alcohol is used to remove the film, but care must be taken to allow the site to dry. Electrodes should be at room temperature to deliver their best performance. Pregelled electrodes should not be taken from the package until ready to use, since exposing the electrodes to air can cause evaporation of the electrolyte gel.[3]

Generally the R wave must be a minimum of 1.5 volts in amplitude to be sensed. Placement of electrodes parallel to the direction of ventricular activation (i.e., lead II) produces the tallest R-wave amplitude. R-wave voltage may be altered during the course of pumping if ventricular axis changes with position change of the patient. Therefore a safety factor should be maintained in monitoring; and the lead that affords just enough amplitude in R wave to be sensed should never be selected. The amplitude of the R wave should be maximized whenever possible.

Two options are usually available for input of the electrocardiographic signal into the balloon console. A direct patient cable attaches from the balloon console to electrodes positioned on the patient, or a telemetry unit that sends its signal into the console is attached to the patient; second, a phone jack cable is connected from the patient's bedside ECG module to the balloon console "monitor in" socket. A common practice consists of processing the ECG signal through the console via the bedside monitor. The direct patient cable is attached with electrodes to the patient, but the cable is kept disconnected from the console and coiled at the foot of the bed. It is available for hookup to the monitor in the event that the transmitted monitor signal is lost. This practice reduces the number of electrical devices connected directly to the patient, and the bedside monitor controls can be used to adjust the bedside and balloon signal quality simultaneously. However, some operators prefer the direct patient cable connection to the pump. Both methods are electrically safe.

Pacemaker signal and balloon pumping

The information included in this section is courtesy of the manufacturers—Datascope, Kontron, and SMEC. This section is not intended to be all inclusive, and the reader is encouraged to seek additional advice on the use of pacemakers and balloon pumping from the specific manufacturer.

Datascope[1]

Whenever the System 82 is triggered from the ECG, an internal fail-safe circuit causes an immediate command to apply vacuum to the cardiac assist device in the event that an R wave arrives before the selected deflation time occurs. This occurs in the presence of arrhythmias. In normal operation the vacuum is applied to the cardiac assist device at the end of the selected deflation time or at the arrival of the next R wave, whichever occurs first.

With atrial pacing, triggering of the System 82 may result from the pacer spike itself, rather than from the R wave. The pacer spike could cause an immediate command to apply vacuum to the cardiac assist device, resulting in a premature vacuum. This condition would not be unsafe, but the maximum presystole unloading could not be achieved. For this reason the fail-safe mechanism may be intentionally disabled with the rear panel *Pacer Timing Logic* control. When this control is set to the *Pacer Timing (IN)* position, the front panel *Pacer Timing* warning indicator flashes, alerting the operator to the fact that the fail-safe mechanism has been disabled. The System 82 should never be left unattended while operating in this mode.

Kontron[2]

The Kontron Model-10 uses the mechanism of pattern logic in which the QRS is recognized on a width basis. Analysis is made of the QRS partial width; that is, the

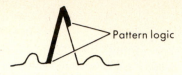

FIG. 19-1 Kontron Model-10 pattern logic mode recognizes QRS complex on width basis. Width of ascending limb over to ⅓ down descending limb should fall between 25 and 135 msec to be recognized as QRS complex. Pattern logic recognizes both positive and negative complexes based on above width criteria.

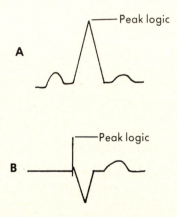

FIG. 19-2 Kontron Model-10 peak logic mode recognizes any positive waveform in electrocardiogram to trigger pump. In these two examples both amplitude of R wave (A) and pacer spike artifact (B) would trigger pump. There is no width criterion in peak logic.

upstroke and a third of the downstroke is recognized (Fig. 19-1). Any waveforms in the ECG must be greater than 25 msec and less than 135 msec to be recognized as a QRS complex. If the waveform does not meet this criterion, it is ignored, and the pump does not trigger. In this manner the pump can ignore all normal pacer spikes and much of the artifact that occurs. Pattern logic should be used with atrial, ventricular, or atrioventricular sequential pacemakers of normal milliamps. Extremely high milliamps on pacemakers can cause the pacer spike in the ECG to be greater than 25 msec; in that situation the pacer spike would be recognized as a QRS complex and trigger the pump.

Occasions may arise when the operator would want to omit the millisecond recognition specifications of pattern logic. Peak logic is therefore available as another option. Peak logic is the method whereby the Model-10 recognizes any positive waveform in the ECG to trigger the pump. A pacer spike and/or patient movement artifact are recognized as well as the QRS complexes (Fig. 19-2). If a negligible or extremely wide QRS complex occurs following a ventricular pacer spike, the machine may not recognize either as a trigger source in pattern logic. Therefore the peak logic mode that recognizes the amplitude of the pacemaker spike and triggers from that signal can be used.

Atrial pacemakers with an extremely high milliamp setting can provoke a unique

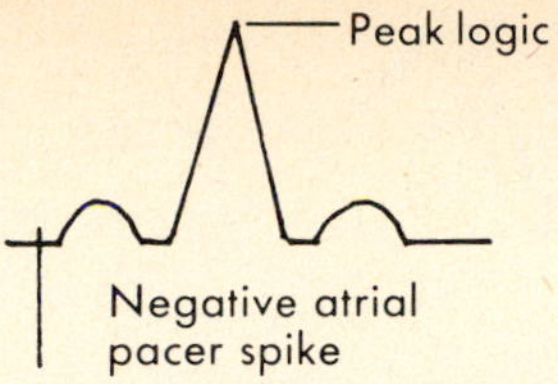

FIG. 19-3 Atrial pacemakers with extremely high milliamps setting could produce spike wider than 25 msec. Both atrial spike and QRS complex could trigger pump in pattern and peak logic modes. If polarity of pacemaker spike can be reversed, then peak logic mode only recognizes R wave of QRS complex (positive waveforms only are recognized in peak logic).

situation. The spike of the atrial pacemaker could be wider than 25 msec and be recognized as a QRS complex in both the pattern and peak logic modes. It is feasible for the pump to then double trigger. Rearranging patient electrodes to produce a negative pacemaker spike and a positive QRS complex is suggested (Fig. 19-3). Also, if the milliamps of the pacemaker are kept as low as possible, more effective signal processing is possible.

SMEC[5]

The recommendation is made to set up ECG monitoring to maximize the amplitude of the R wave for triggering and to minimize the pacer spike amplitude. For fixed rate pacing only, the red telewire terminal can be connected directly to the pacer output to synchronize with the pacemaker.

Ventricular demand pacemaker. With demand ventricular pacing, the console triggering may alternate between sensing the R wave and the ventricular pacemaker spike. The deflate period must be slightly extended so that the balloon is deflated for paced and nonpaced beats alike. The ECG triggered mode should be used, and there needs to be an attempt to maximize the R-wave amplitude for triggering.

Atrial pacing. ECG triggered mode should be used, and repositioning electrodes for R-wave triggering only (minimizes pacer spike amplitude) should be attempted, otherwise assist is asynchronous and detrimental if the patient is not in atrial capture from the atrial pacemaker spike. For demand atrial pacing the balloon timing is severely affected as the console alternates between the pacer spike and the R wave. Only as a last resort should the deflation be lengthened so that the balloon is deflated for either an R wave or pacer trigger.

Atrioventricular sequential pacing. The ECG electrode position must be changed to obtain a more distinct R wave. If double triggering persists, the balloon should be turned off, the rate limit pushed, the second unwanted trigger using fixed rate control tuned out, starting at 150 bpm (ECG triggered assist), and finally light pens should be used to retime.

Bipolar atrial pacing as an adjunct to simultaneous atrial pacing and balloon pumping. If a postoperative cardiac patient has a pacing wire that is connected to the negative terminal of the pacemaker sutured into the right atrium, a unipolar circuit exists with the ground or indifferent electrode placed into the pericardium or under the chest wall. The

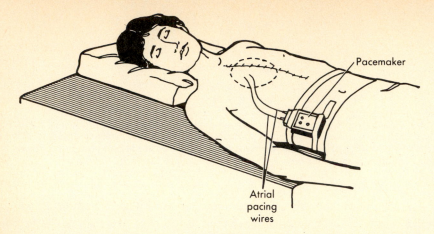

FIG. 19-4 Two pacing wires are sutured into right atrium to provide bipolar pacing circuit. Wires are brought out through chest incision and connected to external generator.

unipolar circuit produces a tall pacemaker artifact that presents a problem in balloon pumping, since this artifact may be sensed by the balloon pump, which causes the pump to trigger. Double trigger may occur if the pump is triggered again by the QRS complex.

One solution is to monitor the patient in an alternate lead, which maximizes the QRS complex and minimizes the amplitude of the atrial pacemaker spike. However, this cannot always be accomplished. Payne and Cleveland[4] from Tufts University have proposed another alternative. They suggested that at the conclusion of the open heart surgery procedure, two atrial wires can be sutured close together on the right atrial wall and brought out through the median sternotomy incision, and connected to the positive and negative poles of the pacemaker generator (Fig. 19-4). This bipolar system yields a much lower amplitude pacer spike in relation to the QRS complex and is usually ignored by the balloon pump console. Therefore the problem of double triggering is eliminated. Fig. 19-5 illustrates the double triggering problem observed with unipolar atrial pacing, which was corrected by bipolar atrial pacing.

Hoogstraat

No specific recommendations are available; the manufacturer should be contacted for advice.

Problem of atrial fibrillation

Atrial fibrillation with its inherent irregular cycles poses a problem for timing. With conventional timing (Datascope, Hoogstraat, and Kontron), regularity in the R wave is expected to ensure proper timing. Irregular rhythms can be followed. If, however, the R wave appears early (earlier than the cycle length for which the periods of inflation-

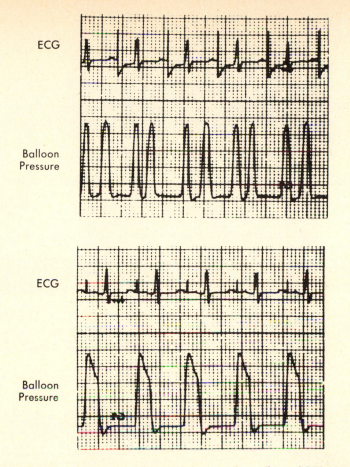

FIG. 19-5 A, Double triggering of pump from atrial pacemaker spike and QRS complex. **B,** Bipolar atrial pacing where pump triggers only from QRS complex. (From Payne, D., and Cleveland, R.: Ann. Thorac. Surg. **30**:191, 1980.)

deflation were preset), the pump commands the balloon to immediately deflate as a safety modality. Therefore this early R wave that results in immediate balloon deflation does not guarantee afterload reduction. Deflation does not always occur in isovolumetric contraction. It is recommended that the deflate control be pushed all the way to the left, which would coordinate deflation at the point of a sensed R-wave signal. The goal is to restore the irregular rhythm to a regular rhythm in which timing can be appropriately defined to facilitate afterload reduction.

The SMEC system is timed differently than the other balloon consoles. The machine is triggered by the immediately preceding R wave for a predetermined period of inflation. SMEC explains that since an R wave exists for every systolic contraction and because the interval from the R wave to left ventricular contraction and the duration of systole do not change significantly from beat to beat or with cardiac rate changes, the system does not have to be timed from the previous R wave. Therefore the SMEC system is promoted as being more effective in following the R-wave irregularity of atrial fibrillation.[6]

Timing and atrial fibrillation: afterload reduction

Adjustments in timing that are made for the irregular cycles of atrial fibrillation must be followed by a careful assessment of the arterial waveform. A trade-off is sometimes made in attempting to track this fast, irregular rhythm. Afterload reduction may be lowered or totally forfeited.

REFERENCES

1. Datascope, Inc.: Datascope System 82 intra-aortic balloon pump, operating instructions, Pub. No. 0070-00-0071, Paramus, N.J.
2. Kontron Cardiovascular, Inc.: Clinical application of peak pattern ECG recognition switch, user monograph, Everett, Mass.
3. NDM Corp.: Troublesome traces: prevention and cure of the most common ECG monitoring problems, Pub. No. 100, Dayton, Ohio.
4. Payne, D., and Cleveland, R.: Atrial pacing during intra-aortic balloon pumping, Ann. Thorac. Surg. **30:**191, 1980.
5. SMEC, Inc.: SMEC Model 1300i integrated balloon console, operating instructions outline, Cookeville, Tenn., Jan. 25, 1982.
6. SMEC Newsletter **19:**2, 1982.

CHAPTER 20 Clinical hemodynamic monitoring associated with balloon pumping

Hemodynamic monitoring is an essential adjunct to the care of the patient requiring the IABP. Prompt recognition and accurate assessment of the patient's circulatory status is imperative. Direct pressure measurement techniques, in which the cardiovascular system is invaded, have been in use in operating rooms and cardiac catheterization laboratories for quite some time. Early attempts to perform right and left heart catheterizations required moving the patient to a catheterization laboratory where fluoroscopy was available. Left heart pressures could be obtained only by positioning a catheter directly into the left-sided chambers in the operating room when the chest was opened for a thoracotomy procedure or by retrograde catheter placement through an arterial cutdown under fluoroscopy.

Central venous pressure (CVP): Inadequacies

In the late 1960s a more in-depth understanding of the complex series of phenomena surrounding myocardial infarction surfaced. Management of a variety of subsets grew to an appreciation of the need to assess the different elements of hemodynamic compromise associated with this taxonomic disease. Limited hemodynamic data can be obtained from a conventional CVP catheter that is inserted into the vena cava, reflecting right atrial pressure. Dependency on measurement of CVP as an index of left heart failure in acute myocardial infarction is imprecise and often misleading.[3] The value of the CVP is limited by the fact that it basically reflects the functional state of the right ventricle (RV), which frequently does not parallel that of the left ventricle (LV). CVP readings fluctuate with changes in the venous tone and compliance of the RV. Pressure readings recorded from a CVP catheter are reliable as an indicator of right heart function, systemic venous compliance, and intravascular volume only if the patient has no significant cardiopulmonary disease. This need to monitor left heart pressures finally prompted the initial trial of conventional cardiac catheterization techniques in the hemodynamic evaluation of patients critically ill after infarction.[33]

Advantages of a balloon-tipped, flow-directed catheter were noted by Lategola and Rahn[28] in an experimental investigation of the pulmonary circulation. The development of the flow-directed catheter by Swan and co-workers[38] facilitated right heart catheterization at the bedside and enabled catheters to be safely left in position for prolonged periods.

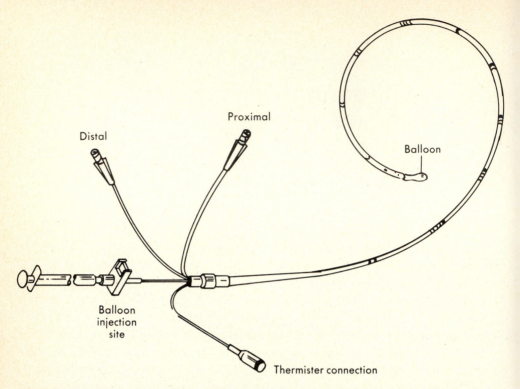

FIG. 20-1 Swan-Ganz double-lumen catheter. Distal port: monitors pulmonary artery pressures and used to draw a mixed venous blood gas sample. Proximal port: monitors right atrial pressure and is injection site for thermal dilution cardiac outputs. Smaller lumen terminates in latex balloon that is inflated to record pulmonary artery wedge pressure (PAWP). Thermister that measures changes in blood temperature after thermal dilution injectable instillation is housed 4 cm from distal tip.

Therefore left heart catheterization can be avoided in the acute setting, since the pulmonary artery end-diastolic pressure (PAEDP) and the pulmonary artery wedge pressure (PAWP) approximate the left ventricular end-diastolic pressure (LVEDP).

The pliable quadruple-lumen Swan-Ganz catheter (Fig. 20-1), fabricated from polyvinylchloride, is 110 cm long and is scored in 10 cm lengths. Catheter diameters are available as 5 and 7 french; the larger, major, lumen terminates at the distal catheter tip and is used to record PA pressure and to obtain mixed venous blood for oxygen content analysis. The smaller lumen terminates in a latex balloon that may be inflated with a recommended volume of air or carbon dioxide. The inflated balloon has a diameter of approximately 13 mm, which is sufficient to guide the soft catheter through the right atrium (RA) and tricuspid valve into the RV and from there into the main PA and into a branch of the PA, where its further progression is stopped by its impaction in a pulmonary vessel slightly smaller in diameter than the inflated balloon.[37] A proximal lumen is located 30 cm from the tip of the catheter and usually vents in the patient's RA. In addition to recording right atrial pressure, this port is used to deliver the injection to measure cardiac output (CO) by thermodilution technique. A thermister capable of measuring changes in

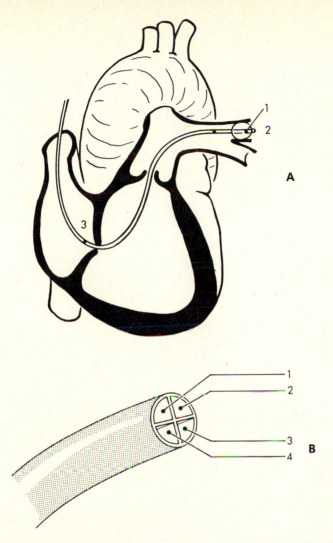

FIG. 20-2 A, Openings of lumens of Swan-Ganz catheter as it rests in situ in heart. **1,** Thermister lumen opening; **2,** inflated balloon in pulmonary artery branch; **3,** proximal lumen opening in right atrium. **B,** Cross section of Swan-Ganz catheter. **1,** Distal lumen; **2,** inflation lumen; **3,** thermister lumen; **4,** proximal lumen.

blood temperature is located 4 cm from the tip (Fig. 20-2). Thus with a single catheter in the right side of the heart, the effects of acute myocardial infarction on the patient's hemodynamic status can be easily monitored.

Catheter insertion

Before insertion the balloon should be inflated to check for integrity; the proximal and distal ports should be flushed with fluid to prevent the introduction of air into the central circulation. During balloon flotation catheterization, all patients must have electrocardio-

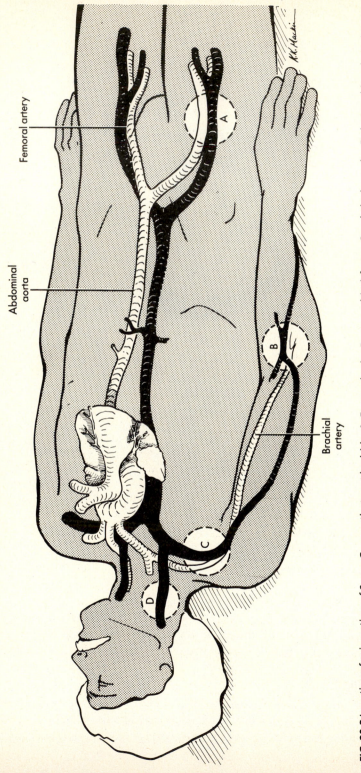

Femoral artery

Abdominal aorta

Brachial artery

FIG. 20-3 Locations for insertion of Swan-Ganz catheter at bedside. **A,** Femoral vein; **B,** antecubital fossa; **C,** subclavian vein; **D,** internal jugular vein.

graphic monitoring to detect any arrhythmia that may develop secondary to catheter insertion. Continuous pressure monitoring is essential as the catheter is passed through the various chambers. Percutaneous insertion is possible from the antecubital fossa, femoral vein, subclavian vein, or internal jugular vein (Fig. 20-3).

For the average patient an advancement of 35 to 40 cm from the right antecubital fossa places the catheter in the vena cava.[37.] The balloon is inflated, and as the catheter is advanced, pressures are continuously monitored; location of the catheter tip is identified by the proper waveform.[4]

Pressure waveform recognition

Each chamber of the heart and great vessels generate characteristic pressure waveforms. Verification of catheter tip location within the anatomical chambers of the heart is obtained by recognition of the waveform morphology characteristic of each chamber. An appreciation for the characteristics of the normal pressures recorded and continuously monitored in each chamber of the heart, as the catheter passes from the RA to the PA wedge position during insertion, must be mastered. An inflatable balloon located at the tip of the catheter provides the catheter with a flow-directed capability. During catheter insertion, the inflated balloon directs the catheter tip to sail with the flow of venous blood through the right heart chambers and out to the PA (Fig. 20-4). A principal requirement is to avoid the development of substantive forces at the catheter tip or in shaft loops in the atrium or ventricle. Subendocardial irritation has been demonstrated to be avoided by attention to the location of the balloon at the catheter tip. When inflated for passage through the RV, the balloon actually protrudes over the catheter tip, which comes to lie below its surface in ''the hole in the doughnut''[37] (Fig. 20-5). Forces that would ordinarily be concentrated at the catheter tip are dispersed over the wider surface of the flotation balloon. This flow-directed capability permits catheter insertion without the use of fluoroscopy.

Characteristics

Normal pressures recorded from each chamber of the heart have certain specific characteristics (Fig. 20-4). The low pressure atria may visibly produce three positive waveforms during each cardiac cycle. The A wave is produced by atrial contraction and therefore occurs just after the P wave (atrial depolarization). The V wave is produced by blood filling the atrium during ventricular contraction. A C wave may not be noted; if present between the A and V wave, it represents bulging to the atrioventricular (AV) valves into the atrium as the tricuspid valve closes.[9]

The X descent reflects pulling down of the AV valves' apparatus during ventricular ejection, causing the atria to expand more rapidly than they fill; a negative wave is therefore inscribed. Following the V wave is the Y descent, representing rapid atrial emptying after the AV valves have opened.[5]

The ventricles generate a systolic pressure that is much greater in magnitude than the atrial pressures; ventricular diastolic pressures are essentially the same as atrial pressures in the normal heart. The greater ventricular systolic pressure is appreciated as compared with atrial pressures, when muscle bulk is considered. Contraction of the muscular ven-

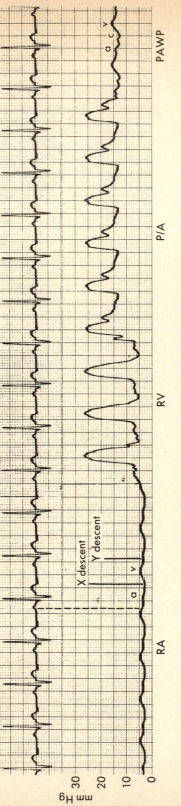
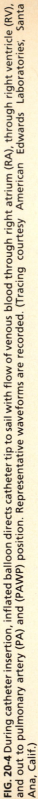

FIG. 20-4 During catheter insertion, inflated balloon directs catheter tip to sail with flow of venous blood through right atrium (RA), through right ventricle (RV), and out to pulmonary artery (PA) and (PAWP) position. Representative waveforms are recorded. (Tracing courtesy American Edwards Laboratories, Santa Ana, Calif.)

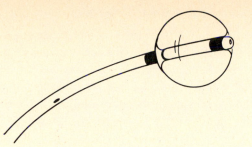

FIG. 20-5 When inflated, balloon actually protrudes over catheter tip, which comes to lie below surface as if withdrawing into "hole in doughnut." Forces that would ordinarily be concentrated at catheter tip are dispersed over wider surface of flotation balloon.

tricular chamber understandably produces a higher pressure than that of the smaller mass atria.

Pressure waveforms monitored from the PA differ from the RV because of the pulmonic valve. Although the PA systolic pressure is normally identical to right ventricular systolic pressure, PAEDP is higher than right ventricular diastolic pressure because the pulmonic valve closes and prevents the diastolic pressure from further decline.[11]

Waveforms during Swan-Ganz catheter insertion

The waveforms are idealized for clarity. As the catheter is advanced under sterile technique, pressures are continuously monitored, and the location of the catheter tip is identified by the characteristic waveform. Increase in respiratory fluctuation confirms that the catheter tip is in the thorax. At this time the balloon is inflated with the recommended volume to encourage "flotation" of the catheter through the right heart circuit. Spurious oscillations are observed with cardiac catheter pressure recordings because of the catheter movement associated with the beating heart. It is desirable to monitor the pressure waveforms from dual-channel recorders when available so that simultaneous Swan-Ganz pressures and the electrocardiogram may be recorded on graph paper. Sources do not agree on absolute pressure values, and therefore the most generally accepted values are presented.

RA: normal mean pressure 1 to 7 mm HG (Fig. 20-6)

Normal right atrial pressure is recorded as a mean value, since the pressure in this chamber is low. Such a low pressure enables the heart to readily receive the deoxygenated blood along a downhill pressure gradient; the vena cava serves only as a passive conduit. The pressure generated during ventricular systole is blocked to the RA by the closed tricuspid valve. Right atrial pressure is therefore equivalent to the right ventricular pressure in diastole when the tricuspid valve is open and the RA and RV are common chambers (Fig. 20-7).

Millimeters of mercury (mm Hg) are the universally used units in measuring Swan-Ganz pressures. The normal CVP when recorded from the proximal port (right atrial) is 1 to 7 mm Hg. Caution is extended when comparing this value to a CVP recorded with a water manometer in centimeters (cm) of water units.[9] To convert centimeters of water to millimeters of mercury divide $\dfrac{\text{cm of H}_2\text{O}}{1.36}$.

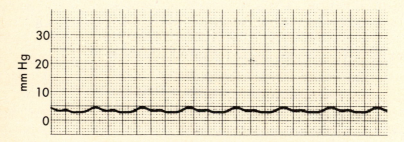

FIG. 20-6 RA pressure waveform. Normal pressure is recorded as mean value, since pressure is so low. (Tracing courtesy American Edwards Laboratories, Santa Ana, Calif.)

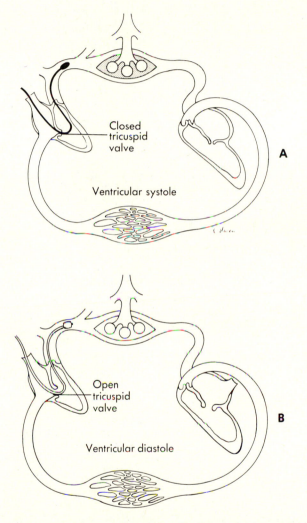

Closed
tricuspid
valve

Ventricular systole

A

Open
tricuspid
valve

Ventricular diastole

B

FIG. 20-7 A, Ventricular systole. Closure of tricuspid valve blocks transmission of right ventricular diastolic pressure. **B,** Ventricular diastole. Right atrial pressure is equal to right ventricular diastolic pressure as RA and RV become common chamber when tricuspid valve is open.

RV: normal pressure $\dfrac{20\text{-}25}{5\text{-}8}$ mm Hg (Fig. 20-8)

After the pressure waveform is documented to represent right atrial positioning of the catheter, the balloon is inflated to the recommended volume. The inflated balloon has a diameter of approximately 13 mm, which is sufficient to guide the soft catheter through the tricuspid valve into the RV and thereafter out into the PA.

As the catheter tip enters the RV, the range of the pressure excursion on the pressure monitor markedly increases, whereas the diastolic pressures remain essentially the same as the right atrial pressure. Catheter location in the RV is easy to affirm because of the large pressure variations in systole and diastole.

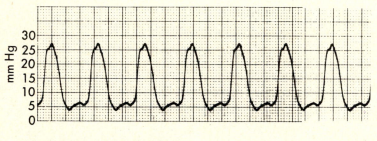

FIG. 20-8 RV pressure waveform.

Normal pressure = $\dfrac{20\text{-}25}{5\text{-}8}$ mm Hg

PA: normal pressure $\dfrac{20\text{-}25}{10\text{-}12}$ **mm Hg** (Fig. 20-9)

As the catheter continues to advance, close observation is made for an increase in diastolic pressure. Systolic pressure does not change. PA catheter location is verified simply by this visible increase in diastolic pressure.

The diastolic phase involves movement of blood from the PA into the capillaries; the systolic component of the PA pressure tracing represents ejection of blood from the RV into the PA.

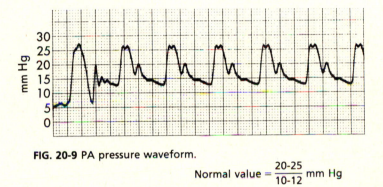

FIG. 20-9 PA pressure waveform.

$$\text{Normal value} = \frac{20\text{-}25}{10\text{-}12}\ \text{mm Hg}$$

PAWP: mean normal $\leq$ 12 mm Hg (Fig. 20-10)

Further progression of the catheter is stopped once it migrates into a branch of a pulmonary vessel slightly smaller in diameter than the inflated balloon. Forward blood flow is terminated in that vessel. Since the catheter tip is just distal to the balloon, the distal lumen records only the downward stream pressure, referred to as PAWP.

The pulmonary vascular bed has a low resistance, and blood flow from the pulmonary capillaries to the left atrium (LA) traverses a valveless course. Normally there is no obstruction between the occluded segment of the distal PA and the LA. Pulmonary capillary wedge pressure (PCWP) is therefore a phase-delayed and amplitude-damped version of left atrial pressure.[38] During diastole the normal nonstenotic mitral valve is open, and the pulmonary venous bed, LA, and LV become a common chamber (Fig. 20-11). Therefore in the absence of mitral valve disease, the PAWP approximates left atrial pressure, LVEDP, and PAEDP. With deflation of the balloon, pulmonary arterial pressure reappears. Reinflation causes the balloon to again float into the "wedge" position.

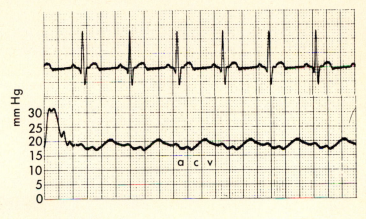

FIG. 20-10 PAWP.

Normal value ≧ 12 mm Hg.

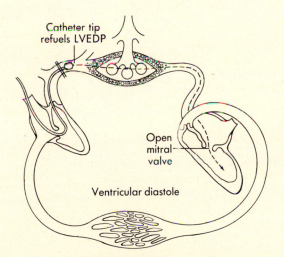

FIG. 20-11 In diastole normal nonstenotic valve is open, and pulmonary venous bed, left atrium (LA), and left ventricle (LV) become common chamber. Therefore in absence of mitral valve disease, distal catheter tip with inflated balloon reflects forward pressure (i.e., pressure recording tip "sees" into LV or reflects left ventricular end-diastolic pressure (LVEDP).

TABLE 20-1 Troubleshooting Swan-Ganz catheters

Problem	Cause	Prevention	Correction
Ventricular arrhythmias	Irritation of RV endocardium by catheter on insertion or after implantation, or catheter floats back to RV after implantation	Suturing of catheter at insertion site; continuous monitoring of electrocardiogram	Ventricular irritability may require lidocaine and/or catheter repositioning
Spontaneous wedging of catheter	Migration of catheter forward, since it is flow directed and catheter material softens at body temperature		Spontaneous wedging leads to pulmonary infarction if not corrected; catheter must be pulled back into larger portion of PA
Right ventricular waveform appears rather than PA pressure waveform	Migration of catheter backwards into RV	Suturing of catheter at insertion site	Turning patient on his left side and having him cough may float catheter out into PA; inflating to facilitate flotation; observing for ventricular ectopy once catheter is documented to be in RV
Unable to withdraw blood from distal port	Ball clot on end of catheter	Continuous slow infusion of catheter; plumbing system with heparin drip	Clot may occasionally dissolve or dislodge, but catheter may have to be removed; no flushing with tuberculin syringe, as this blows clot off catheter and causes embolization to patient
Unable to obtain PA wedge tracing	Insufficient air used to inflate balloon; it may be ruptured; thin latex of balloon absorbs lipoproteins from blood and gradually loses its elasticity, increasing chance of rupture	Inflating balloon gradually and not overinflating; if no resistance is felt, inflation should not be continued	Deflating and trying again; if no resistance is felt, balloon may be ruptured; discontinuing attempts to reinflate; notifying physician

TABLE 20-1 Troubleshooting Swan-Ganz catheters—cont'd

Problem	Cause	Prevention	Correction
Damped tracing as indicated by flush with poor ring; tracing may exhibit decreased amplitude and lower systolic readings	Most common cause is air bubbles in dome; infusion bag may have lost pressure	Flushing all bubbles out of system when assembling line; periodically checking for bubbles in tubing and stopcocks; maintaining 300 mm Hg pressure on infusion bag	Flushing bubbles in dome to outside but not to patient and reevaluating flushing and tracing
Bleeding back from catheter into connecting tubing	Patient's pressure is higher than counterpressure from pressure infusion bag; loose connections in system	Maintaining 300 mm Hg pressure on infusion bag; checking to see that all connections from patient catheter to transducer are secure	Reestablishing counterpressure in infusion bag if pressure was lost; checking all connections and stopcock positions; replacing any fractured components of software system
PAWP waveform drifts upward on scope	Balloon is over-inflated	Observing monitor during inflation; not adding more air to balloon once PA waveform pattern has changed to PAWP	Deflating balloon and observing monitor on reinflation, and adding only amount of air needed to change waveform from PA tracing to PAWP
Unable to obtain pressure readings	Loose connections in system; incorrect stopcock position (transducer open to air); transducer dome is loose; malfunctioning transducer or monitor	Initiating proper system checkout according to unit/hospital biomedical protocols before activating system	Troubleshooting for loose connections; checking calibration of monitor and transducer accoring to unit/hospital biomedical established procedures

Alterations in magnitude and morphology of hemodynamic waveforms
Right atrial pressure

Reduced right atrial pressure is generally secondary to hypovolemia. Elevation of pressure has the following three major causes: right ventricular failure, tricuspid regurgitation, and pericardial tamponade. In patients with acute myocardial failure, elevated right atrial pressure most commonly reflects right ventricular failure.[19]

Clues to the diagnosis of tricuspid insufficiency and pericardial tamponade can be made from the inspection of the pressure waveforms. Fig. 20-12 illustrates a right atrial pressure tracing from a patient with tricuspid regurgitation diagnosed by the presence of a giant V wave. When the tricuspid valve does not close competently in systole, a reflection of ventricular systole is shown by the morphology of a large right atrial pressure V wave.[7]

Pericardial tamponade may be suspected in the presence of an elevated right atrial pressure, and if right atrial pressure equals PAEDP, right ventricular diastolic pressure, and PAWP (Fig. 20-13).[6] The rising intrapericardial pressure interferes with the diastolic filling of the heart so that the usual differences between PAWP and RA pressure practically disappear.

PA pressure

In the absence of pulmonary disease, PA pressure is equal to right ventricular pressure during systole while the pulmonic valve is open. Increased PA pressure occurs with coexistent lung disease, pulmonary embolism, or elevated pulmonary flow as in ventricular septal defect. PAEDP is virtually equal to the PCWP if pulmonary vascular resistance is normal and the patient's lungs are not being mechanically ventilated. Therefore the PAEDP is often substituted for PAWP to reduce the frequency of balloon inflation.[5] An increase in pulmonary vascular resistance elevates PAEDP substantially in comparison to pulmonary capillary pressure. Differentiation of pulmonary embolism from cardiogenic shock can be made by comparison of PAEDP and PAWP. PAEDP usually is elevated secondary to the increased resistance (mechanical obstruction) following vasoconstriction caused by pulmonary embolism, whereas the wedge pressure is normal. Both pressures are comparatively equal in elevation in cardiogenic shock.[13]

PAWP

The PAWP is usually equal to LVEDP. However, the mitral valve begins to close before the onset of ventricular systole, producing an equality between PAWP and LVEDP. When the atrial contribution to ventricular filling is substantial, or if left ventricular compliance (ability to improve the force of contraction with increased stretch on the fibers before contraction) is reduced, LVEDP may exceed PAWP by as much as 20 mm Hg.[16]

Elevated PAWP. Elevation of the PAWP is critical, since it is the hemodynamic cause of pulmonary congestion. The alveoli normally are kept free from fluid entry to provide sufficient space for ventilation by the force of osmotic pressure of the blood proteins,

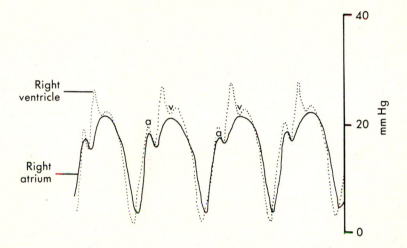

FIG. 20-12 Right atrial pressure tracing of tricuspid regurgitation, illustrating large V waves that are reflection of ventricular systolic pressure, since tricuspid valve does not close competently in systole.

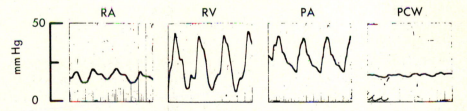

FIG. 20-13 Pressure tracings recorded from patient with cardiac tamponade. Characteristically there is equalization of right atrial pressure, right ventricular end-diastolic pressure, pulmonary artery end-diastolic pressure, and PAWP. (From Buchbinder, N., and Ganz, W.: Anesthesiology **45**:146, 1976.)

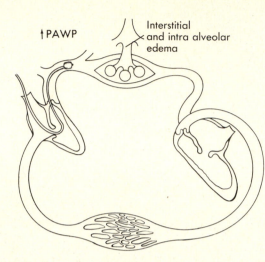

FIG. 20-14 Increased hydrostatic pressure reflected by increased PAWP; fluid is forced out of pulmonary capillaries and into interstitial and intraalveolar spaces.

which pulls fluid into the vessels. Hydrostatic pressure is the force that favors egression of fluid from the capillaries. Whether fluid remains in the capillaries or moves out is dependent on the net difference in these two pressures. An elevation of PAWP causes the hydrostatic pressure to force fluid out of the pulmonary vascular space and into the interstitial and intraalveolar spaces (Fig. 20-14), and pulmonary congestion ensues.[22]

PAWP and preload. Cardiac function is frequently defined by Starling's law of the heart, which states that the strength of cardiac contraction is proportional to myocardial fiber length or left ventricular volume at the onset of contraction. The PAWP is therefore used as an index of left ventricular end-diastolic volume, an elevation of PAWP reflects an increased left ventricular end-diastolic volume or preload [15] (Chapter 2). An increase in PAWP in acute myocardial infarction generally reflects increased left ventricular volume secondary to a diminution of ejected volume.[39] Acute myocardial infarction may precipitate an increase in left ventricular stiffness, which has a role of unknown magnitude in increasing PAWP.[35]

PAWP and mitral insufficiency. Mitral insufficiency alters the normal bifid low magnitude PAWP. The presence of large V waves in the PAWP is commonly interpreted as being diagnostic of significant mitral regurgitation (Fig. 20-15). Some cardiologists appreciate that large V waves are not specific for the detection of significant mitral regurgitation.[21,29] Researchers at Johns Hopkins University[18] studied the usefulness of large V waves in pulmonary capillary wedge tracings for establishing the diagnosis of mitral regurgitation. Data on 1021 cardiac catheterizations were reviewed. Mitral regurgitation was the most common cause of large V waves, which were, however, neither highly sensitive nor specific for severe regurgitation. In this study one third of the patients with

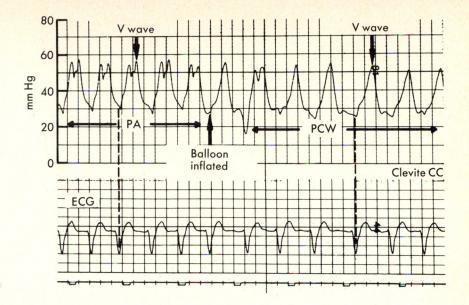

FIG. 20-15 Large V waves are present in PA and PAWP tracing from patient with mitral insufficiency. (From Buchbinder, N., and Ganz, W.: Anesthesiology **45**:146, 1976.)

severe mitral regurgitation displayed only trivial V waves, and one third of those with large V waves had no significant mitral regurgitation.

Major determinants of V-wave amplitude are (1) the volume of blood entering the LA during filling, (2) the position on the left atrial pressure-volume curve at the onset of filling, and (3) the shape of that curve (i.e., atrial compliance). Relative hypovolemia may therefore prevent the development of large V waves in the presence of severe mitral regurgitation. Congestive heart failure, mitral valve obstruction, and ventricular septal defects may also produce large V waves in the absence of significant regurgitation.

Concerns and cautions in measuring waveforms
PAEDP as a substitute for PAWP recording

At the time of right heart catheterization, the PAEDP can be compared to the PAWP. Normally these two measurements are within 4 to 5 mm Hg. The PAEDP can be used as an alternative measure of the PAWP and therefore the LVEDP in most patients.[27] In the presence of left ventricular dysfunction and elevated LVEDP, the PAEDP correlates well with PAWP but fails to represent LVEDP accurately. The PAEDP is consistently lower by 2 to 18 mm Hg than LVEDP when the LV dysfunctions.

Reading PA and PAWP waveforms with respiratory cycle variations

The PAEDP and PAWP signals have a significant cyclic respiratory effect (Fig. 20-16). During inspiration the pressure falls as a result of the negative intrathoracic pressure, whereas during expiration the pressure rises because of the positive intrathoracic

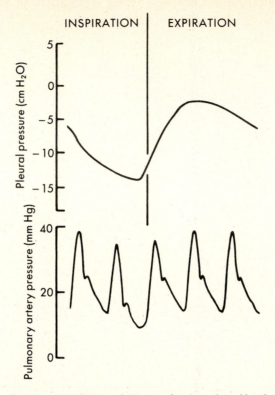

FIG. 20-16 Respiratory variations in PAWP and PA waveform produced by changes in intrathoracic pressure that are necessary to expand and deflate lungs during breathing. (From Riedinger, M.S., et. al.: Heart Lung **10**:675, 1981.)

pressure generated. Further swings in cyclic respiratory pressure waveform alterations are noted in patients with a reduction in lung compliance, which heightens the inspiratory effect.

Reading pressures on and off the ventilator

Ventilator assistance used in the care of the critically ill patient provides intermittent positive pressure ventilation (IPPV). IPPV increases pleural, PAWP, and PA pressure on inspiration when the ventilator is triggered[20] (Fig. 20-17). This effect is in opposition to spontaneous breathing during which pleural pressure decreases on inspiration.

An increase in pleural pressure with IPPV could alter PA pressure and PAWP in several ways. (1) The increased pleural pressure could decrease venous return, thereby decreasing right ventricular filling volume and PA pressure. (2) The increased pleural pressure could increase all intrathoracic vascular pressures as related to pulmonary vascular resistance, thereby elevating right-sided pressures.

For these reasons it has been assumed that to obtain accurate and stable central pressure measurements, patients must be disconnected from the ventilator. Such action disturbs a resting patient, removing him from the ventilator may not provide an accurate account of

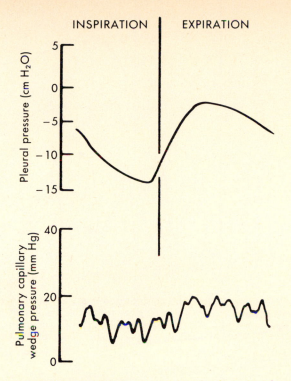

FIG. 20-17 Inspiratory and expiratory pleural pressure changes during mechanical ventilation. PA pressure is increased whenever respirator is triggered during inspiration. (From Riedinger, M.S., et. al.: Heart Lung **10:**675, 1981.)

the pressures to which he is being subjected as a result of the ventilator. Recording the wedge pressure without the ventilator may actually over estimate this hemodynamic measurement, since venous return may be reduced with IPPV.[30]

Shinn and co-workers[32] examined the effect of IPPV on PA pressure and PCWP in patients requiring mechanical ventilatory support. No correlations could be found between tidal volume, PA pressure, and PAWP differences on or off the ventilator. In the hemodynamically stable patient receiving IPPV, the wedge pressure did not change whether it was measured on or off the ventilator. The PA pressures decreased when the patient was breathing spontaneously as compared to these recordings taken during IPPV.

Pressure averaging

Fig. 20-18 illustrates a technique for determining the numerical values of PA systolic and diastolic pressures that account for pressure fluctuation with the respiratory cycle. The systolic and diastolic portions of a representative sampling of morphological waveforms are averaged over two to three respiratory cycles. This technique may not be accurate if used on patients who display grossly inconsistent inspiratory and expiratory pleural pressures (i.e., Cheyne-Stokes respiration).[30]

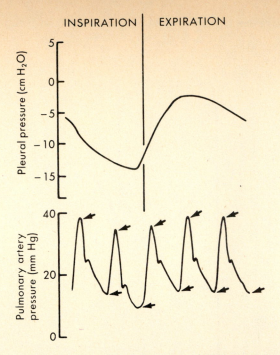

FIG. 20-18 Pressure averaging. Systolic and diastolic points of PA pressure waveform are recorded over two to three respiratory cycles (one respiratory cycle is illustrated), and values are tallied to obtain average measurement. PA measurement in this tracing, by pressure averaging, is approximately 37/13 mm Hg. (From Riedinger, M.S., et. al.: Heart Lung **10**:675, 1981.)

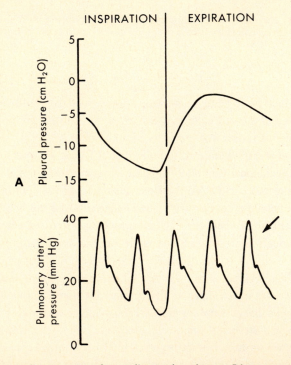

FIG. 20-19 A, Arrow indicates point of recording end-expiratory PA pressure on patient breathing spontaneously. Pressure is 39/15 mm Hg. (From Riedinger, M.S., et al.: Heart Lung **10**:675, 1981.)

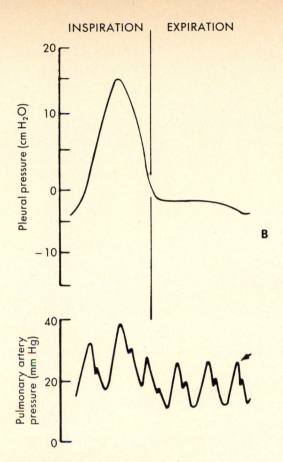

FIG. 20-19, cont'd B, Arrow indicates point of recording end-expiratory PA pressure on ventilated lungs of patient. Pressure is approximately 26/10 mm Hg.

End-expiratory recorded values

A definite fluctuation in intravascular pressure occurs with the respiratory cycle because of the alteration in pleural pressure that is necessary for inspiration-expiration. IPPV produces higher pressures during peak inspiration, but these peaks are not always consistent. Pressure waves may also be altered after an ectopic beat. Wide excursions in pressure waveforms caused by respiration, either spontaneous or mechanical, conflict with pressure recordings at the moment of inspiration. Therefore it is recommended that the PAWP and PA pressure, whether taken on or off the ventilator, be recorded at end-expiration to facilitate easy recording of a more stable pressure waveform (Fig. 20-19). End-expiration is defined as the period of the respiratory cycle preceding the start of inspiration. The pressure in the thoracic cavity is constant at the end of the expiratory cycle; pressures recorded at this point inscribe a usually stable baseline.[9,30]

Confirming PAWP as a good tracing

Any hemodynamic pressure waveform displayed must be evaluated with a critical eye. Deleterious treatment errors can be made by assigning numerical values to waveform morphologies that are technically poor. Suggested criteria are listed to assure that the waveform labeled as the PAWP is a correct measurement.[10]

1. The PAWP must be lower than the mean PA pressure.
2. A visible change in the tracing should be noted in transition from PA pressure to PAWP.
3. A good dynamic response should be present while the balloon is inflated (Chapter 31).
4. The tracing should convert to a PAWP mode when between 1.0 to 1.5 cc of air has been injected into the balloon.
5. Pulmonary capillary gases withdrawn from the distal port (with balloon inflated) confirm a true wedge; P_{CO_2} is lower than usual arterial norms (about 25 mm Hg), and capillary P_{O_2} should be equal to but usually greater than the arterial P_{O_2} sample.

Derived hemodynamic measurements[2,26,34]

As an adjunct to the care of the patient requiring the IABP, several derived measurements must be calculated in addition to the directly gauged values of right atrial pressure, PA pressure, and PAWP.

Body surface area (BSA) is an important denominator in many of the derived parameters. The difference in body size is minimized in establishing an assemblage of an ordered array of normal values that account for the individual's height and weight. Fig. 20-20 reproduces the DuBois body surface chart. By intersecting the patient's height and weight on this scale, the BSA is calculated.

Stroke volume (SV)

Definition: milliliters of blood ejected with each heart beat

Formula: $\dfrac{\text{Cardiac output}}{\text{Heart rate}}$

Normal value: 60 to 100 ml/beat

Stroke volume index (SVI)

Definition: SV adjusted for BSA

Formula: $\dfrac{\text{SV}}{\text{BSA}}$

Normal value: 33 to 47 ml/beat/m^2

Systemic vascular resistance (SVR)

Definition: Resistance against which the LV must eject to force out its SV with each beat (as the peripheral vessels constrict, the systemic vascular resistance or afterload increases)

Formula: $\dfrac{(\overline{\text{MAP}} - \text{RA}) \times 80}{\text{CO}}$

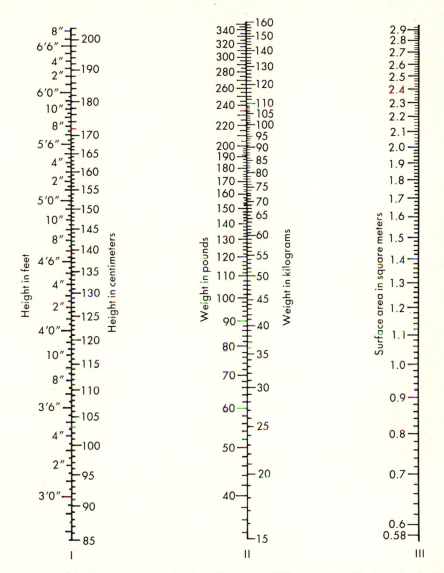

FIG. 20-20 DuBois body surface chart. Body surface area (BSA) is calculated by locating patient's height on scale I and weight on scale II. Straight edge is placed between two points, which intersect on scale III at patient's BSA. (From DuBois, E.F.: Basal metabolism in health and disease, Philadelphia, 1936, Lea & Febiger.)

Normal value: 900 to 1300 dynes/sec/cm^{-5}

$$\overline{MAP}, \text{Mean arterial pressure} = \frac{\text{Systolic pressure} + 2 \text{ diastolic pressures}}{3}$$

RA, Mean right atrial pressure

80, Constant for converting to absolute resistance units

CO, Cardiac output in liters/min

Pulmonary vascular resistance (PVR)

Definition: Impedance in the pulmonary vascular bed against which the RV must eject

Formula: $\dfrac{(\overline{PA} - PAWP) \times 80}{CO}$

Normal value: 155 to 255 dynes/sec/cm^{-5}

$\overline{PA}$, Mean pulmonary artery pressure

PAWP, Pulmonary artery wedge pressure

80, Constant for conversion to absolute units

CO, Cardiac output

NOTE: Although SVR and PVR are presented in absolute resistance units of dynes/sec/cm^{-5}, practical monitoring of these measurements is often done in relative units. The formulas remain the same with the omission of multiplying times 80, which is the conversion factor into absolute units.

$$\text{SVR relative units: SVR} = \frac{\overline{MAP} - RAP}{CO} = 12 \text{ to } 18 \text{ units}$$

$$\text{PVR relative units: PVR} = \frac{\overline{PA} - PAWP}{CO} = 0.5 \text{ to } 1.0 \text{ unit}$$

The PAWP is used as an indicator of preload.[22] However, the PAWP as a singular measurement is very limiting. An individual with healthy ventricular function could be overloaded to a wedge of 30 + mm Hg if volume were infused rapidly. Conversely, a patient with severe myopathy could be phlebotomized to the point of a PAWP reading of 5 mm Hg. Fig. 20-21 represents an attractive healthy Starling curve graphed from the CO and PAWP of patients A and B. Patient A maintains this curve with a heart rate of 60 beats per minute and a mean blood pressure of 90 mm Hg. Patient B, on the other hand, is also maintaining a normal-appearing Starling curve but at the expense of a heart rate of 118 with a mean arterial pressure that has dropped to 60 mm Hg.

Therefore in caring for patients with left ventricular dysfunction, it is important to become familiar with and monitor the additional measurement of stroke work index (SWI).

SWI

Definition: The work involved in moving the volume of blood in the LV with each heart beat against the aortic impedance

Formula: SWI = $(\overline{MAP} - PAWP) \times SVI \times 0.0136$

Normal value: 38 to 80 g/beat/m^2

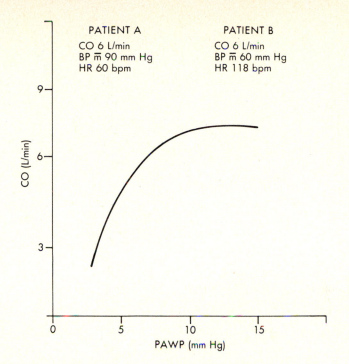

PATIENT A
CO 6 L/min
BP m̄ 90 mm Hg
HR 60 bpm

PATIENT B
CO 6 L/min
BP m̄ 60 mm Hg
HR 118 bpm

CO (L/min)

PAWP (mm Hg)

FIG. 20-21 Normal Starling curve from two patients. Patient B requires heart rate (HR) of 118 beats/min. to maintain curve in contrast to patient A whose HR is 60 beats/min. Blood pressure is correspondingly lower in patient B. Examples illustrate how misleading measurements of cardiac output (CO) and PAWP can be.

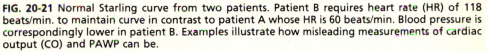

MAP, Mean arterial pressure
PAWP, Pulmonary artery wedge pressure
SVI, Stroke volume index
0.0136, Conversion factor from pressure to work

Plotting the SWI against the PAWP provides a left ventricular function curve (Fig. 20-22) for monitoring ongoing left ventricular performance. A left ventricular function flow sheet can be initiated at the beginning of every 24-hour period. By plotting these two indices with an X, left ventricular performance can be documented as improving or deteriorating. Such tracking of left ventricular function is crucial in monitoring patients who are receiving balloon pump assistance.

Ejection fraction

An index of ventricular function that is often available to the nurse caring for a patient receiving balloon assistance is the ejection fraction. The percentage of total ventricular volume that is ejected during each contraction (i.e., SV divided by end-diastolic volume) equals the ejection fraction.[22] Normally the ejection fraction is about 65%. Opacification of the ventricular cavity with contrast medium during a heart catheterization (ventriculography) enables the end-systolic and end-diastolic volumes to be determined. The ven-

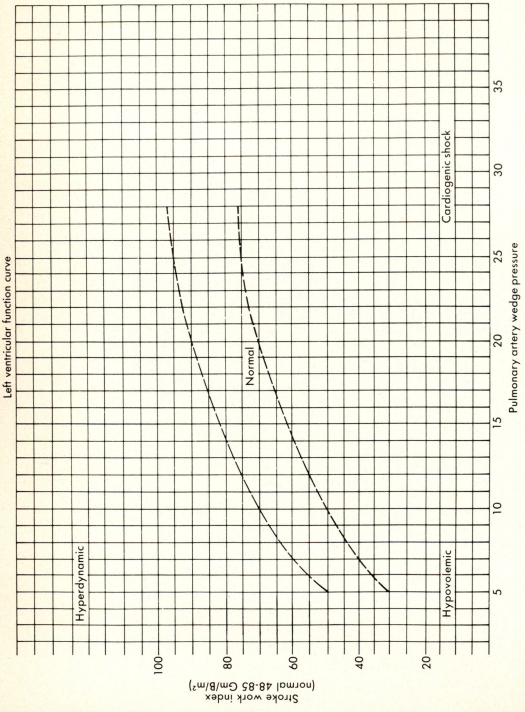

FIG. 20-22 Left ventricular function curve. Stroke work index (SWI) is plotted against PAWP. Low SWI and PAWP represent hypovolemia.

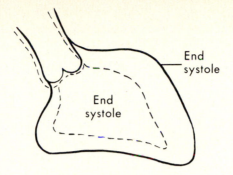

FIG. 20-23 Ejection fraction. Opacification of ventricular cavity with contrast medium during heart catheterization allows ventricular cavity to be outlined at end-systole and end-diastole. Dimensions are obtained that permit calculation of end-systolic and end-diastolic volumes. Stroke volume is end-systolic volume subtracted from end-diastolic volume. Ejection fraction is computed by dividing stroke volume by end-diastolic volume. Normal value is about 65%.

tricular cavity is outlined at end-systole and end-diastole from the ventriculogram, and dimensions are obtained. SV is then calculated by subtracting the end-systolic volume from the end-diastolic volume (Fig. 20-23).

CO

CO is the amount of blood pumped by a ventricle during 1 minute and is determined by SV and heart rate. SV is governed by contractility, afterload, and preload. To standardize the CO to the patient's size, CO is usually expressed as the *cardiac index*, obtained by dividing the CO by the patient's BSA.[34] CO can be measured by the dye-dilution method, the Fick calculation, or the thermal dilution technique.

Dye-dilution method[2]

A dye, such as indiocyanine green, is injected into the venous system. The concentration of dye is measured from a downstream site (usually the femoral or radial artery) by a densitometer. The greater the final concentration, the lesser the flow. Since the blood is in motion, the addition of dye must be rapid, and measurement of the dye concentration at the downstream site must be continuous until all or most of the added dye flows past the sampling site. Disadvantages of this method include (1) recirculation of the dye, which interferes with repeated studies, (2) allergic reaction to the dye, and (3) necessity of frequent blood withdrawal.

Fick method[11]

The Fick concept prescribes that the uptake or release of a substance by an organ is the product of blood flow through that organ multiplied by the arteriovenous concentration of the substance. The organ is the lung, and the substance released is oxygen.

$$CO = \frac{\text{Oxygen consumption in milliliters per minute} \times 100}{\text{Arteriovenous } O_2 \text{ content difference}}$$

Accurate Fick analysis requires simultaneous collection of arterial and mixed venous blood samples and expired gas. However, an estimated Fick analysis is more often performed when oxygen consumption is assessed to be 125 ml/min/m^2 of BSA.

The O_2 content for this formula is determined as follows:

1. Hemoglobin value $\times$ 1.36 ml/O_2/g of hemoglobin = O_2 carrying capacity
2. O_2 carrying capacity $\times$ O_2 saturation = O_2 content
3. Arterial O_2 content $-$ Mixed venous O_2 content = Arteriovenous O_2 difference

EXAMPLE: Patient's BSA = 2 m^2
Hemoglobin = 15 g
Arterial O_2 saturation = 94%
Mixed venous O_2 saturation = 76%

Estimated O_2 consumption = (125 ml/min $\times$ 2m^2) = 250 ml/min/m^2

O_2 carrying capacity = (1.36 $\times$ 15) = 20.40 ml O_2

Arterial O_2 content = 20.40 $\times$ 0.94 = 19.18

Mixed venous O_2 content = 20.40 $\times$ 0.76 = 15.50

Arteriovenous O_2 difference = arteriovenous 3.68

$$CO = \frac{250 \times 100}{3.68} = \frac{25,000}{3.68} = 6790 \text{ ml/min or } 6.79 \text{ liters/min}$$

Thermal dilution[24,37]

As with the dye-dilution method, thermal dilution also uses an indicator technique, but in this case the indicator is temperature. A bolus of a solution (the volume and temperature are known) is added to the bloodstream. The resultant cooling of the blood temperature is sensed by the thermister, located at the tip of the transducer, situated in the PA. The CO is inversely proportional to the change in the blood temperature invoked by instillation of the injectant.

More specifically, 5 to 10 cc of iced or room air with 5% dextrose in water is injected into the right atrial (proximal) lumen of the Swan-Ganz catheter. As the blood carries a portion of the bolus into the RV, the injectant, which is cooler than blood temperature, mixes with the blood. The injection and sampling sites are separated by the RV, tricuspid valve, and pulmonic valves. When the RV contracts, the injectant ejects out into the PA. Thus a reduction in the temperature of the blood in the PA occurs, which is registered by the thermister on the distal tip of the catheter. The temperature change is recorded in the computer attached to the catheter, and a "thermal dilution curve" is constructed from this blood temperature change. Peak thermal dilution curve is reached as the coolest portion of blood flows past the thermister. (Fig. 20-24).

CO is inversely proportional to the area under the curve. A high CO yields a small area under the curve; the injectant is more quickly perfused out to the thermister, producing a lesser drop in blood temperature. Conversely, since CO is inversely proportional to the area under the curve, a larger area under the curve represents a higher CO (Fig. 20-25). A curve that appears distorted (i.e., notched or grossly different in morphology from the norms) should be disregarded. A distorted curve represents faulty injection and an invalid value.

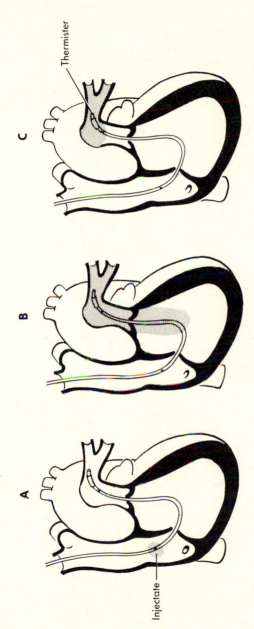

FIG. 20-24 A, Known quantity and temperature of solution is injected into proximal (right atrial) lumen of Swan-Ganz catheter. **B,** As blood carries portion of bolus into RV, injectant mixes with blood. **C,** Injectant, which is cooler than blood temperature, is carried out to PA with right ventricular systole. Ensuing temperature change is recorded by thermister on distal tip of catheter.

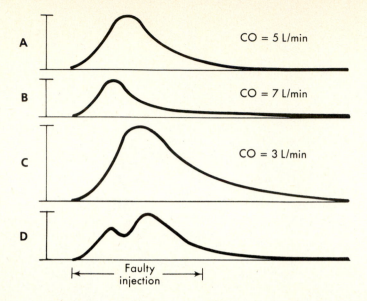

FIG. 20-25 Thermal dilution CO curves. **A,** Area under curve is inversely proportional to CO. This represents normal thermal dilution curve. **B,** Comparatively higher CO (less area under curve.) **C,** Comparatively lower CO (greater area under curve). **D,** Notched thermal dilution curve represents faulty injection technique.

Normal value = 4 to 6 liters/min

$$\text{Cardiac index} = \frac{\text{CO}}{\text{BSA}} = 2 \text{ to } 4 \text{ liters/min/m}^2$$

Conclusion

Hemodynamic monitoring offers a pragmatic approach to the problems at hand in the care of the critically ill. The information obtained from the Swan-Ganz catheter is vital to the management of the patient who is receiving left ventricular assistance in the form of IABP. The addition of hemodynamics to the patient's clinical findings gives a degree of specificity and accuracy in monitoring patient status, making alterations in treatment plans, and rapidly assessing the results of therapy. Hemodynamic monitoring techniques may also be valuable in the diagnosis of mitral regurgitation, pulmonary embolism, and cardiac tamponade. Directly measured and derived hemodynamic monitoring is only a useful adjunct in the management of the patient receiving balloon assist if used judiciously to improve patient care.

REFERENCES
1. Adams, N.R.: Reducing the perils of intra-cardiac monitoring, Nursing **16**:66, April 1976.
2. American Edwards Laboratories: Understanding hemodynamic measurements made with the Swan-Ganz catheter, Santa Ana, Calif., June 1981.
3. Berglund, E.: Balance of left and right ventricular output: relation between left and right atrial pressures, Am. J. Physiol. **178**:381, 1954.
4. Bolognini, V.: The Swan-Ganz pulmonary artery catheter: implications for nursing, Heart Lung **3**:976, 1974.

5. Bouchard, R.J., et al.: Evaluation of pulmonary arterial end-diastolic pressure as an estimate of left ventricular end-diastolic pressure in patients with normal and abnormal left ventricular performance, Circulation **44:**1072, 1971.

6. Braunwald, E.: Heart disease, Philadelphia, 1980, W.B. Saunders Co.

7. Buchbinder, N., and Ganz, W.: Hemodynamic monitoring, Anesthesiology **45:**146, 1976.

8. Buda, A.J., et al.: Effect of intrathoracic pressure on left ventricular function, N. Engl. J. Med. **301:**453, 1979.

9. Burton, A.C.: Physiology of the circulation, ed. 2, Chicago, 1972, Year Book Medical Publishers, Inc.

10. Clemmer, T.S., and Orme, J.F., Jr.: Critical care medicine, Salt Lake City, 1982, Latter Day Saints Hospital Division of Critical Care.

11. Daily, E.K., and Schroeder, J.S.: Techniques in bedside hemodynamic monitoring, ed. 2, St. Louis, 1981, The C.V. Mosby Co.

12. DuBois, E.F.: Basal metabolism in health and disease, Philadelphia, 1936, Lea & Febiger.

13. Elkins, R.C., et al.: Pulmonary vascular response to experimental embolism and reversal leg embolectomy, J. Surg. Res. **25:**135, 1978.

14. Falicov, R.E., and Resnekov, L.: Relationship of the pulmonary artery end-diastolic pressure to the left ventricular end-diastolic and mean filling pressures in patients with and without left ventricular dysfunction, Circulation **42:**65, 1970.

15. Forrester, J.S., and Diamond, G.A.: Clinical application of left ventricular pressure. In Corday, E., and Swan, H.J.C., editors: Myocardial infarction, Baltimore, 1973, The Williams & Wilkins Co.

16. Forrester, J.S., et al.: Filling pressure in the right and left sides of the heart in acute myocardial infarction: a reappraisal of central-venous pressure monitoring, N. Engl. J. Med. **285:**190, 1971.

17. Forrester, J.S., et al.: Medical therapy of acute myocardial infarction by application of hemodynamic subsets, N. Engl. J. Med. **295:**1404, 1976.

18. Fuchs, R.M., et al.: Limitation of pulmonary wedge v-waves in diagnosing mitral regurgitation, Am. J. Cardiol. **49:**849, 1982.

19. Givetta, J.M., and Gabel, J.C.: Flow directed–pulmonary artery catheterization in surgical patients, Ann. Surg. **176:**753, 1972.

20. Grenvik, A.: Respiratory, circulatory and metabolic effects of respirator treatment, Acta Anesthesiol. Scand. Suppl. **14:**7, 1966.

21. Grossman, W., and Dixter, L.: Profiles in valvular heart disease. In Grossman, W., editor: Cardiac catheterization and angiography, Philadelphia, 1980, Lea & Febiger.

22. Guyton, A.C.: Textbook of medical physiology, ed. 6, Philadelphia, 1980, W.B. Saunders Co.

23. Herzlinger, C.A.: Absolute determinations of cardiac output in intra-aortic balloon pumped patients using the radial artery arterial pressure trace, Circulation **53:**417, 1976.

24. Hewlett Packard: A guide to hemodynamic monitoring using the Swan-Ganz catheter, Waltham, Mass., 1979.

25. Hoie, J.: Determination of cardiac output from pulse pressure contour during intra-aortic balloon pumping, Scand. J. Clin. Lab. Invest. **40:**445, 1980.

26. Hurst, J.W., et al.: The heart arteries and great veins, New York, 1982, McGraw-Hill Book Co.

27. Kinney, M.R., et al.: AACN's clinical reference for critical care nursing, New York, 1981, McGraw-Hill Book Co.

28. Lategola, M., and Rahn, H.: A self-guiding catheter for cardiac and pulmonary arterial catheterization and occlusion, Proc. Soc. Exp. Biol. Med. **84:**667, 1953.

29. Meister, S.G., and Helfant, R.H.: Rapid bedside differentiation of ruptured intraventricular septum from acute mitral insufficiency, N. Engl. J. Med. **287:**1024, 1972.

30. Riedinger, M.S., et al.: Reading pulmonary artery and pulmonary capillary wedge pressure waveforms with respiratory variations, Heart Lung **10:**675, 1981.

31. Sammarco, M.E., et al.: Measurement of cardiac output by thermal dilution, Am. J. Cardiol. **28:**54, 1971.

32. Shinn, J.A., et al.: Effect of intermittent positive pressure ventilation upon pulmonary artery and pulmonary capillary wedge pressures in acutely ill patients, Heart Lung **8:**322, 1979.

33. Shubin, H., and Weil, M.H.: Routine central venous catheterization for management of critically ill patients. In Ingelfinger, F.J., editor: Controversy in internal medicine, II, Philadelphia, 1974, W.B. Saunders Co.

34. Siegel, R., and Tresh, D.: Bedside hemodynamic measurements: principles and practical applications, Primary Cardiol. **80:**113, Aug. 1980.
35. Smith, M., et al.: Early consecutive left ventricular compliance changes after acute myocardial infarction, Am. J. Cardiol. **31:**158, 1973.
36. Starling, E.H.: The Linacre Lecture on the law of the heart, London, 1918, Longmans, Green & Co.
37. Swan, H.J.C., and Ganz, W.: Use of balloon flotation catheters in critically ill patients, Surg. Clin. North Am. **55:**501, 1975.
38. Swan, H.J.C., et al.: Catheterization of the heart in man with use of a flow-directed balloon-tipped catheter, N. Engl. J. Med. **283:**447, 1970.
39. Swan, H.J.C., et al.: Hemodynamic spectrum of myocardial infarction and cardiogenic shock: a conceptual model, Circulation **45:**1097, 1972.
40. Visalli, F., and Evans, P.: The Swan-Ganz catheter, Nurs. 81 **11:**37, Jan. 1981.
41. Wade, J.I.: Comprehensive respiratory care: physiology and technique, ed. 3, St. Louis, 1982, The C.V. Mosby Co.
42. Walinsky, P.: Acute hemodynamic monitoring, Heart Lung **6:**838, 1977.
43. Wesseling, K.H.: Pulse contour cardiac output as a clinically valuable tool for intensive patient monitoring, Basic Res. Cardiol. **72:**82, 1977.
44. Wood, S.L.: Monitoring pulmonary artery pressures, Am. J. Nurs. **76:**1765, 1976.

CHAPTER 21 Bioinstrumentation of hemodynamic monitoring

Today's intensive care nurse is ensconced in a milieu of biomedical instrumentation. Nurses frequently assume the responsibility for obtaining physiological pressure recordings from highly specialized equipment, but they have little knowledge of the instrument or the principles by which it operates. The objective of physiological pressure monitoring is to obtain a record that is an exact facsimile and a high quality reproduction (fidelity) of the physiological event. Instrument-determined measurements, however, are not infallible. All measurements must be related to the patient's clinical condition, and these informational instrument slaves require that the nurse understand and assess their function to provide a safe, intelligent operation. Maximum use and accuracy can be achieved from instrument reproduction of the patient's physiological event if the nurse masters a few basic principles of assessing good fidelity reproduction of the recorded waveform. Understanding the components of a hemodynamic monitoring system and correcting the underlying factors that reduce the fidelity are crucial if the clinician is to have confidence in the physiological information that is sensed by the instrument. This chapter prepares the nurse for supportive hemodynamic monitoring of the patient receiving balloon pump assist by examining the following components of the hemodynamic monitoring system: the dynamic response and the technique of balancing and calibrating the system.

Components of the system

The basic invasive hemodynamic monitoring system consists of a catheter inserted into the vessel from which the pressure is to be monitored, a transducer connected to the patient catheter via a plumbing system, a pressurized continuous fluid infusion, stopcocks, and a fast-flush device. A column of fluid carries the mechanical physiological pressure of the patient through the transducer, which converts the physiological pressure to an electrical signal that is processed through an amplifier and displayed on an oscilloscope (Fig. 21-1).

Catheter

A primary determinant of the fidelity of the system is the monitoring catheter. Short but large-diameter catheters record the highest fidelity. However, placement usually requires a long catheter. Thrombosis caused by the catheter requires that the catheter be as

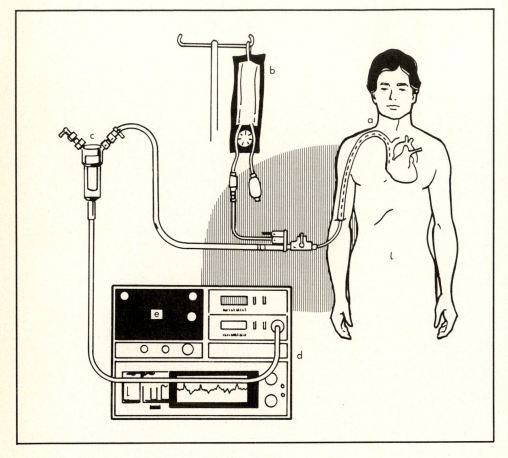

FIG. 21-1 Components of hemodynamic monitoring system. *a*, Catheter; *b*, pressurized continuous fluid infusion; *c*, transducer; *d*, amplifier; *e*, oscilloscope.

small in diameter as possible. Therefore a compromise must be reached in achieving fidelity in catheter usage.[16]

Transducer

The transducer converts the patient's mechanical energy in the form of pressure to an electrical signal that can be amplified and monitored on a display oscilloscope. Virtually all the electrical transducers emit their signals in response to displacements imposed by direct application of mechanical force. Pressure recording therefore involves the displacement of the elastic diaphragm or sensing mechanism of the transducer.[5]

The most commonly used transducer is the unbonded strain gauge (Fig. 21-2). Four strain-resistant wires that support a metal slide are housed in a metal bellows. These strain-sensitive resistant wires measure the displacement of the diaphragm, which is proportional to the pressure transmitted to the diaphragm from the patient catheter through the fluid-filled connecting tubing. The four wires are arranged in what is termed a *Wheatstone bridge* configuration. As the diaphragm of the transducer is displaced by the patient pressure, the bridge becomes unbalanced; there is a change in the length and diameter of the strain wires. Two wires become more strained or stretched, and two become more relaxed. As the diameters of the strain wires increase or decrease, the electrical resistance is concomitantly altered, thereby affecting current flow, which is directly proportional to changes in pressure. Thus pressure applied on the diaphragm from the patient's mechanical energy causes the strain-sensitive wires to move in their Wheatstone bridge arrange-

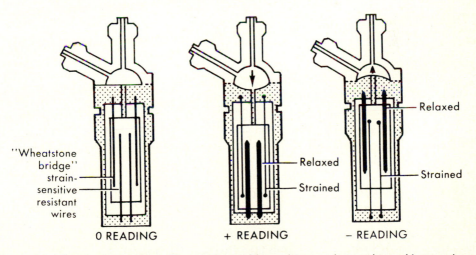

FIG. 21-2 Strain-gauge transducer. Four strain-sensitive resistance wires are housed in transducer and measure displacement of diaphragm, which is proportional to pressure transmitted to diaphragm from patient catheter through fluid-filled connecting tubing. Positive pressure applied to diaphragm causes inner wires to become more relaxed and outer wires to become more strained. Opposite effect occurs with negative pressure reading. (Modified from teaching illustration, courtesy Reed Gardner, Salt Lake City.)

ment, converting the mechanical pulse into an electrical signal that passes through an amplifier to be displayed on the oscilloscope.[8,12]

Most transducers are designed to measure both positive and negative pressures in a range of -50 to $+300$ mm Hg. When 300 mm Hg is applied to the transducer, the center of the diaphragm moves only the distance of a thin human hair. The transducer, however, tolerates pressure from 5000 to 10,000 mm Hg before damage occurs. A common source of overpressurization is the pressure from a tuberculin syringe (25,000 mm Hg) that is directed toward the transducer.[12] When not in use, storage of the transducer is extremely important; the dome must be protected from trauma by a proper covering, such as a plastic cap.

Amplifier

It is necessary to enlarge the mechanical signal transmitted from the patient through the transducer into the displayed electrical signal. This is the function of the amplifier. Amplifiers contain the following components:
1. Analog or digital display reproduces the actual graphic pressure waveform and/or numerical value of the pressure.
2. Zero control allows for adjustment of the monitor to read whatever pressure the transducer is receiving.
3. Gain control allows for adjustment of the amplitude of the waveform signal.
4. Alarm system provides visual and audible alarms, which signal a pressure that has violated preset alarm limits.
5. Selector switch provides options of selecting systolic, diastolic, mean, or a combination of waveforms displayed.

Domes

Both disposable and nondisposable domes are available to cover the transducer membrane. Disposable domes contain a thin membrane that acts as a sterile barrier between the nonsterile transducer and the solution in contact with the patient's blood. Disposable domes are commonly used because they eliminate the need for resterilization. Nondisposable domes require sterilization of the dome and transducer. Linden fittings provide a secure accommodation when there is anticipated frequent movement of the transducer, such as in the catheter laboratory, and Luer-Lok fittings are used in the bedside application of the transducer.[12]

Obtaining excellence in fidelity transmission by understanding frequency and damping

The accurate measurement of hemodynamic pressures depends on the ability of the fluid-filled catheter system to transmit the pressures with good fidelity. Long catheters with small diameters, stiffness of the diaphragm, and entrapped air bubbles distort the pressure signal being transmitted and therefore impede good fidelity. Assessment for these technical errors in the catheter-plumbing system must be undertaken before accepting any pressure waveform as a fidelity representation of the patient's hemodynamic pressures.

The responsiveness of a system can be examined by understanding the concepts of frequency, underdamping, and overdamping, which therefore aid in the recognition of technical problems in the system that prohibit accurate waveform reproduction.

Frequency response of the system

Frequency refers to the number of cycles generated per second from a particular wave. Cycles per second is the definition of the term *Hertz* (Hz), or the units of frequency. The time frame for just one cycle of the waveform is termed a *period*. Any signal or waveform that is periodic and includes pulsatile pressure waveforms can be electronically resolved into a series of signals of various frequencies.[7]

Natural frequency. Natural frequency can be explained as being analogous to the action of a bouncing tennis ball when dropped on a hard, flat surface. The ball oscillates and then comes to rest. With each successive bounce, the ball does not rise as high as it did on the last[5] (Fig. 21-3). Each bounce has a characteristic frequency. The time it takes the ball to come to rest is referred to as the *damping coefficient*. Frequency response of a catheter-plumbing system can be determined by driving the system with a known input signal and observing the oscillatory overshoot or ringing-like effect that occurred with the earlier example of a bouncing tennis ball. Such a response is termed *dynamic response*. Regardless of the technical excellence applied in engineering a hemodynamic monitoring system, not all of the frequency components of the signal are passed through the system. Only a sufficient number are transmitted to generate an adequate but not exact replica of a signal.

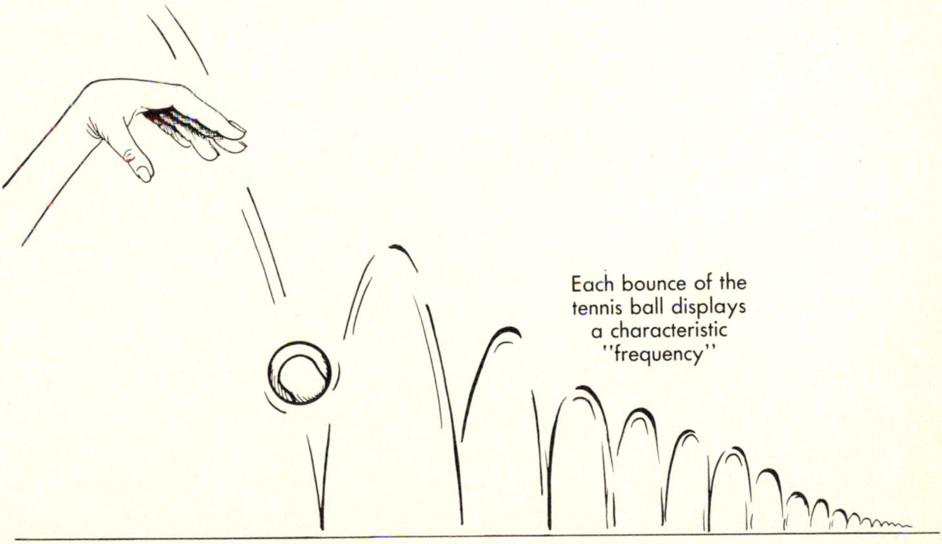

Each bounce of the tennis ball displays a characteristic "frequency"

FIG. 21-3 Tennis ball dropped on hard floor bounces or oscillates and then comes to rest. Each bounce has characteristic frequency. Time it takes ball to come to rest is referred to as damping coefficient.

Dynamic response

The flush device of the plumbing system provides a method for assessing dynamic response. Several flush devices are marketed with various designs (Fig. 21-4); they allow an infusion of a very minimal and predictable flow of a heparinized saline solution through the catheter and into the artery continuously as a preventive method for thrombus formation.[9] Flush devices should also incorporate a fast-flush mechanism that allows opening of the system in a high-pressure flush bag and closing of the system quickly enough to produce an oscillatory square wave, which then permits evaluation of the dynamic response of the system. Specifically, rapid closure of the fast-flush valve excites the system, producing an oscillatory response.[5] Fig. 21-5 illustrates the qualities of a system with good dynamic response. The fast-flush valve is opened and released, producing an oscillating flush.

The following criteria must be present in the flush to assure a good dynamic response:

1. Two or three rapid oscillations occur from top to bottom of the tracing.
2. The tracing does not stick on the bottom after the flush device is released.
3. The pattern goes directly back into the waveform after oscillation.
4. When the flush device is open, the pressure should exceed 200 mm Hg on the graph paper or oscilloscope (provided the pressure infusion bag is pumped up to 200+ mm Hg).[4]

Property of damping

Damping is that property of an oscillatory system that diminishes and eventually arrests the oscillations recorded from the closure of the fast-flush device. Some degree of damping is desirable in the system. The physical characteristics of a catheter-plumbing system with its relatively small-bore catheter, connecting tubing, and stopcocks make it an underdamped system. That is why oscillations are produced when the fast-flush valve closes. If after displacement of the fast-flush device, the system simply returns to the position of rest without oscillatory overshoot, it is said to be "critically damped."[9]

Underdamping. An underdamped plumbing system transmits all frequency components without a reduction in amplitude. Fig. 21-6 illustrates an underdamped system with wide excursions above and below the baseline before the oscillations come to rest. High systolic and low diastolic readings are the consequence of a greatly underdamped system.[13] A device is available, the Accudynamic (Fig. 21-7), which consists of a 0.1 ml sealed air bubble placed on the side port of the transducer dome or somewhere between the flush device and the patient. This small sealed bubble serves to reduce the underdamping of the system and presents more accurate waveform transmission.[5]

Overdamping. An overdamped system is recognized by a square wave that does not fall below the baseline once the fast-flush device is released (Fig. 21-8). The recorded flush rises slowly to return to the morphology of the transmitted waveform without oscillations. Overdamping reduces the amplitude of the components of the waveform being transmitted; the waveform appears sluggish and has a diminished or absent dicrotic notch.

Text continued on p. 228.

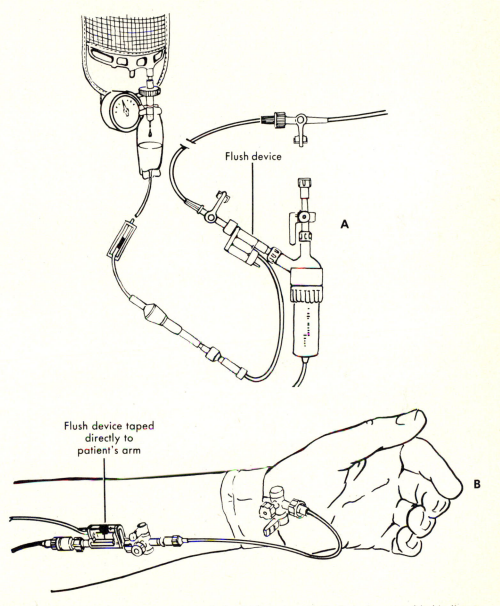

Flush device

A

Flush device taped
directly to
patient's arm

B

FIG. 21-4 A, Flush device in line as part of plumbing system. **B,** Flush device assembled in line to accommodate taping to patient's arm.   *Continued.*

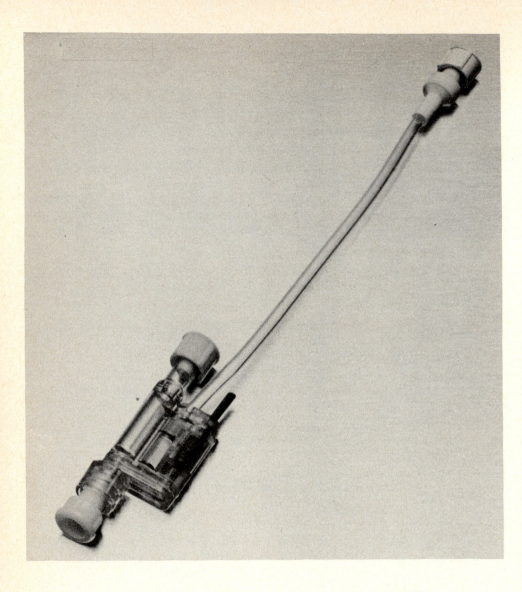

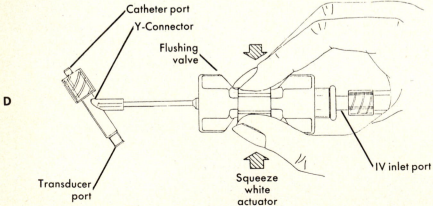

Catheter port
Y-Connector
Flushing valve
Squeeze white actuator
IV inlet port
Transducer port

D

FIG. 21-4, cont'd C, Sorenson Intra-Flo flush device. **D,** Pharmaseal flush device. (C, courtesy Sorenson Research Co.; D, courtesy Pharmaseal Inc.)

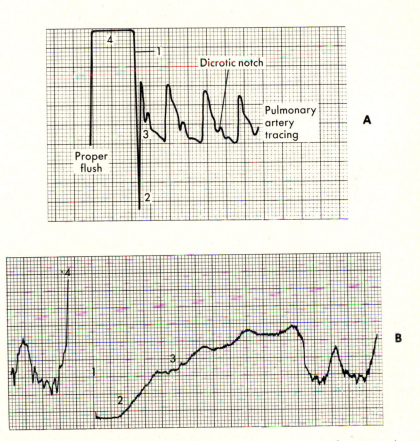

FIG. 21-5 A, Proper flush response. **1,** Two or three rapid oscillations occur from top to bottom; **2,** tracing does not stick on bottom of graph paper after flush device is released; **3,** pattern goes directly back into waveform after oscillating; **4,** when flush device is opened, pressure exceeds 200 mm Hg on graph paper (provided that pressure infusion bag is pumped up to pressure greater than 200 mm Hg). **B,** Bad flush. **1,** No oscillations; **2,** tracing sticks on bottom of graph paper; **3,** pattern does not go directly into waveform; **4,** pressure is not full scale when fast-flush device is opened.

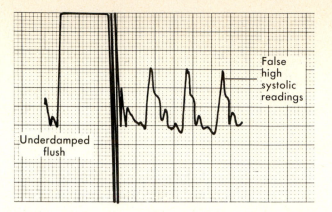

FIG. 21-6 Underdamped flush response. Wide excursions occur above and below baseline before oscillations come to rest.

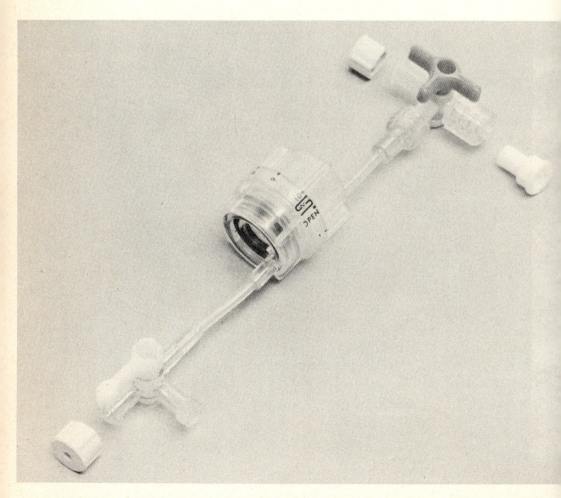

FIG. 21-7 Accudynamic. Sealed air bubble (0.1 ml) is positioned on side port of transducer dome, which serves to reduce underdamping of system.

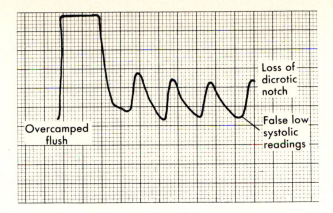

FIG. 21-8 Overdamped flush response. Flush square wave does not fall below baseline once fast-flush device is released.

False low systolic and high diastolic readings occur with an overdamped system. Diastolic pressure is more tolerant of dynamic response inadequacies.

The most common cause of overdamping is the presence of air bubbles in the pressure line, introduced through air leaks in the system. Air bubbles are compressed by the transmitted pressure wave; the pressure component's energy is absorbed, producing a distorted waveform. The greater the pressure waveform energy lost to compression of air bubbles, the greater is the distortion in waveform reproduced on the oscilloscope and strip recorder, and false readings occur.[7]

Soft, compliant catheter and extension tubings are altered in diameter by transmission of the pressure waveform. Energy is imparted from the pressure waveform to compression of the soft, compliant tubing that distorts the waveform. The longer the tubing, the more material available for compression and more of the pressure waveform energy is absorbed, thereby distorting the waveform. The length of the pressure line should not exceed 4 to 5 feet. Catheters with small internal diameters constrict the movement of the fluid medium. In overcoming the frictional resistance to motion, energy of the pressure wave transmitted is again lost, reducing the amplitude of the waveform frequency components.[13]

Optimum dynamic response is required to accurately measure hemodynamic pressures. Simply looking at the waveform does not provide the information necessary to determine dynamic response. Visual observation of the flush waveform can determine if the system is overdamped or underdamped. Highly specific computational techniques can also be performed to quantitatively measure the natural frequency (fn) and damping coefficient (D).[5]

Balancing the transducer

Physiological pressures are relative to atmospheric pressure; therefore the transducer must be balanced or "zeroed," at atmospheric pressure. Before zeroing, the transducer should be fluid filled and attached to the monitor with the power on for whatever warm-up time is recommended by the manufacturer. The zero reference point depends on the catheter tip location, which is considered to be in the midchest position. Windsor and Burch[15] researched a reference level, the phlebostatic axis, which has beome the acceptable standard for localizing the midchest position (heart level) for people of any build.

Phlebostatic axis

The phlebostatic axis (Fig. 21-9) is the point of junction between a frontal and transverse plane on the chest. To locate this reference point, one imaginary line is drawn from the fourth intercostal space at the sternal border and extended around to the right side of the chest. The second imaginary line is drawn vertically from the patient's midaxillary line down to bisect with the transverse line. The junction of these two points is the phlebostatic axis.[16]

Specific points on zeroing

Zeroing the system to atmospheric air is usually accomplished by using a fluid-filled zero stopcock. The most convenient location of this stopcock is between the connection of the software tubing and the external catheter hub (Fig. 21-10). The system could also be zeroed by opening the stopcock to air that is attached to the dome of the transducer, which is mounted on a pole (Fig. 21-11) or directly on the patient (Fig. 21-12). It is the point at which the stopcock is opened to air and *not* the transducer that is leveled to the patient's phlebostatic axis.[1,3,13] Therefore if the stopcock in line between the catheter hub and tubing connection is opened to air, it must be placed at the patient's phlebostatic axis (Fig. 21-10). If the slopcock on top of the transducer dome is opened to air, then it must be leveled to the patient's phlebostatic axis. The longer the connection tubing, the more material is available for compression and more of the pressure waveform energy is absorbed, thereby distorting the waveform. It is therefore recommended that the transducer be mounted directly on the patient (Fig. 21-12). Personal experience with this type of arrangement leads to the conclusion that this is not an uncomfortable or unrealistic restriction for the patient. Once the system is opened to air, the monitor is adjusted to read zero, and the stylus on the strip recorder is adjusted to a zero position on the graph paper. The system must always be zeroed before recording a pressure reading.

Calibrating

The transducer requires calibration or verification that a known millimeter of mercury pressure applied to the transducer is displayed on the monitor (Fig. 21-13). The blood pressure cuff is removed from the sphygmomanometer so that the tubing and pressure pump bulb from the mercury manometer can be attached to one of the Luer-Lok fittings of the transducer dome. The hand bulb is squeezed to elevate the mercury column to 200 mm Hg. The digital readout on the manometer should also read 200 mm Hg. Following release of the hand bulb, the digital readout should return to zero. The transducer should also be checked at lower pressure levels (i.e., pumping the bulb to elevate the pressure to 50 mm Hg). The digital monitor display should also read 50.[1,3,8,13]

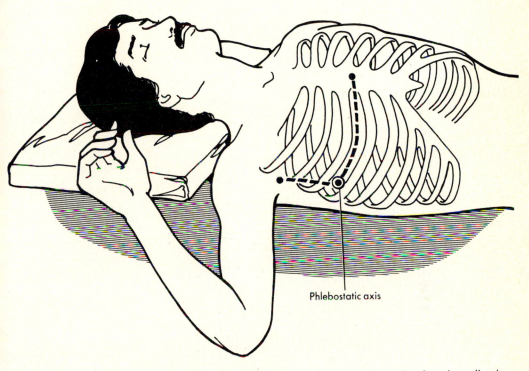

Phlebostatic axis

FIG. 21-9 Phlebostatic axis is point of approximation of level of right atrium. One imaginary line is drawn from fourth intercostal space around right side of chest; a second imaginary line is drawn vertically from patient's midaxillary line down to bisect transverse line. Junction of these two points is phlebostatic axis.

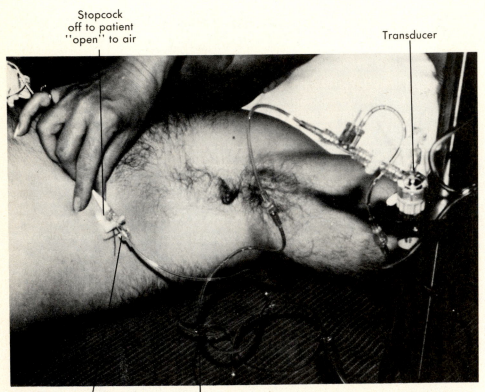

Stopcock
off to patient
"open" to air

Transducer

Phlebostatic
axis

Connecting tubing

FIG. 21-10 Zeroing system to atmospheric air is accomplished by opening stopcock to air at level of phlebostatic axis. This system has excess connection tubing for illustration purposes, but it is recommended that no more than 4 to 5 feet of tubing be used for proper compression and absorption of pressure waveform energy.

If this stopcock is
opened for "zeroing," it must
be adjusted to level of
patient's phlebostatic axis

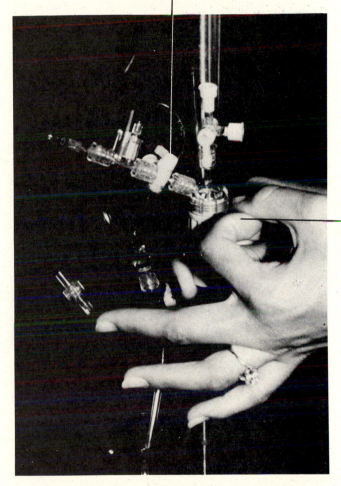

Snapping
finger against
dome to remove
air bubbles

FIG. 21-11 Transducer mounted on pole. It is extremely important to remove all air bubbles from softwear system, and that can often be done with snap of finger. If stopcock on transducer is opened to air, stopcock (and in this case, connecting transducer) is leveled to patient's phlebostatic axis).

Stopcock used to open system
to air for zeroing

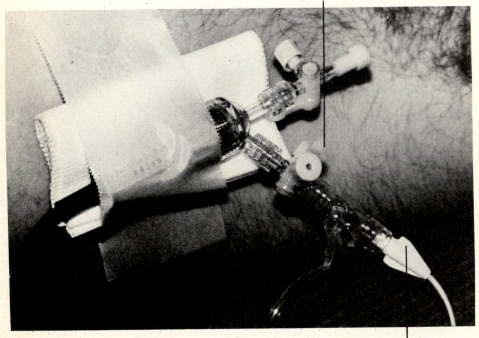

Distal port
of Swan-
Ganz catheter

FIG. 21-12 Transducer can be mounted directly on patient. In example transducer that connects with Swan-Ganz catheter is mounted at phlebostatic axis. Stopcock, opened to air for zeroing, is at phlebostatic axis.

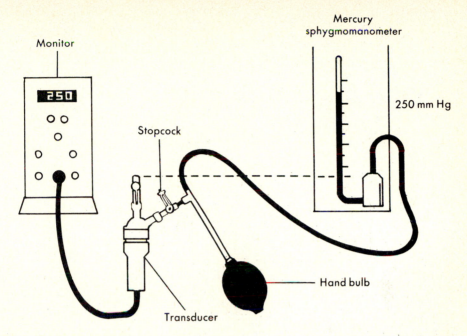

FIG. 21-13 Mercury calibration of transducer. Known value of mercury is applied to transducer, which should in turn register on oscilloscope.

REFERENCES

1. Daily, E.K., and Schroeder, J.S.: Techniques in bedside hemodynamic monitoring, ed. 2, St. Louis, 1981, The C.V. Mosby Co.
2. Fry, D.L.: Physiologic reading by modern instruments with particular reference to pressure readings, Physiol. Rev. **40:**753, 1960.
3. Gardner, R.: Bioinstrumentation and dynamic response lecture presented at Veterans Administration Conference on hemodynamic monitoring, Salt Lake City, March 1982.
4. Gardner, R.: Blood pressure monitoring—a summary of dynamic response consideration. In Latter Day Saints Hospital critical care manual, Salt Lake City, 1982.
5. Gardner, R.: Direct blood pressure measurement—dynamic response requirements, Anesthesiology **54:**227, 1981.
6. Hewlett Packard: Guide to physiological pressure monitoring, Waltham, Mass., 1977.
7. Karselis, T.C.: Descriptive medical electronics and instrumentation, Thorofare, N.J. 1973, Charles B. Slack, Inc.
8. Kinney, M.R., et al.: AACN's clinical reference for critical care nursing, New York, 1981, McGraw-Hill Book Co.
9. Latimer, K.E., and Latimer, R.D.: Continuous flushing systems, Anesthesiology **29:**307, 1974.
10. Rushmer, R.F.: Cardiovascular dynamics, Philadelphia, 1976, W.B. Saunders Co.
11. Shapiro, G., and Krovetz, L.J.: Damped and undamped frequency responses of underdamped catheter manometer systems, Am. Heart J. **80:**226, 1970.
12. Smith, R.N.: Invasive pressure monitoring, Am. J. Nurs. **78:**1514, 1978.
13. Smith, R.N.: Arterial and pulmonary artery pressure monitoring syllabus, Invasive pressure parameters and autotransfusion seminar, Salt Lake City, Jan. 18, 1982, Sorenson Research Co.
14. Underhill, S.L., et al.: Cardiac nursing, Philadelphia, 1982, J.B. Lippincott Co.
15. Windsor, T., and Burch, C.E.: Phlebostatic axis and phlebostatic reference levels for venous pressure measurements in man, Proc. Soc. Exp. Biol. Med. **58:**169, 1945.
16. Woods, L.: Monitoring pulmonary artery pressures, Am. J. Nurs. **76:**1765, 1976.

CHAPTER 22 Nursing care of the patient requiring the balloon pump

Nursing care of the patient requiring the IABP demands the same intense and expert care afforded any critically ill patient. It is imperative that the nurse place into proper perspective the importance of nursing a patient requiring the assistance of an IABP, rather than caring for a pump patient. A plan of care is outlined that includes rationale for the stated measures.

Nursing care plan for the patient requiring the IABP: removal artery insertion

Problem	Rationale	Expected patient outcome	Nursing orders
POTENTIAL FOR INJURY			
Hematological abnormalities: anemia and thrombocytopenia	Mechanical trauma of balloon inflation causes disruption of platelet integrity	Prevention of anemia, thrombocytopenia, and hemorrhaging	Guaiac all stools
			Observe for bleeding of mucous membranes and skin bruising
	Blood loss occurs during insertion of balloon and frequent blood sampling		Attempt to minimize laboratory work drawn
	Patients are often heparinized to reduce threat of thrombus formation at insertion site		Assure that a unit of blood is on hand at all times
			Record all blood losses, including milliliters of blood samples drawn
			Monitor platelet count: hemaglobin, hematocrit, prothrombin time, and partial thromboplastin time
			Replace platelets and red blood cells as laboratory work indicates and per physician's order
Infection	Number of indwelling catheters and high frequency of invasive procedures, combined with patient's debilitated and immunosuppressed condition, predisposes patient to risk of infection	Absence of infection:	Sterile technique with insertion of all lines and subsequent dressing changes
		a. Patient afebrile	Meticulous hand washing by anyone caring for patient
		b. Absence of leukocytosis	Monitor temperature every 2 hours
		c. Invasive catheter sites are free from redness, swelling, tenderness, and drainage	Change IV tubing every 48 hours; clean all catheter insertion sites with betadine, and redress with sterile technique
			Perineal and Foley care every 24 hours
			Sterile technique with endotracheal suctioning
			Culture any drainage; blood cultures per physician's order
			Administer antibiotics per physician's order

Continued.

Nursing care plan for the patient requiring the IABP: femoral artery insertion—cont'd

Problem	Rationale	Expected patient outcome	Nursing orders
POTENTIAL FOR INJURY—cont'd			
Inadequate peripheral circulation caused by: 1. Occlusion of femoral artery by catheter or thrombus 2. Peripheral embolization 3. Transient arterial spasm	Femoral artery balloon insertion in setting of peripheral vascular disease carries increased risk of peripheral embolization and aortic dissection Balloon catheter resting in situ in aortoiliac system can compromise distal blood flow in leg Inadequate perfusion of leg may necessitate balloon removal to preserve limb viability	Good peripheral perfusion to maintain viability of leg in which balloon catheter is inserted	Record quality of peripheral pulses before balloon insertion to establish baseline; record dorsalis pedalis and posterior tibial pulses (Fig. 22-1) Following insertion of balloon, note pulses, color, and temperature of legs every 15 minutes, four times every 30 minutes, every hour four times, then every 2 hours while balloon catheter remains in place
Inadequate perfusion to hand because of compromise from radial artery indwelling catheter for blood pressure monitoring	Radial artery catheter may occlude arterial perfusion; if flow through ulnar artery is also compromised, inadequate perfusion to hand will occur	Good perfusion through radial artery to maintain viability of hand	Perform Allen test[1] at least every 4 hours to assess perfusion through radial artery as follows: 1. Have patient open his hand and palpate ulnar artery (Fig. 22-2, A) 2. Compress ulnar artery, and instruct patient to make closed fist (Fig. 22-2, B) 3. Maintain pressure on artery as patient opens his fist (Fig. 22-2, C); hand should flush and regain pink color if perfusion is adequate through radial artery (around indwelling catheter) 4. If patient is unable to cooperate, nurse can manually close his hand into fist and release while compressing ulnar artery

Decubitus formation and atelectasis	Immobility imposed by balloon catheter in situ; restrictive movement in body because of catheters and invasive lines	Absence of decubitus ulcers, atelectasis, and stiffness of joints	Turn patient from side to back every 2 hours, maintaining straight alignment of leg in which balloon catheter is inserted
			Good skin care; proper cleansing after bowel movement; keep skin dry
			Use alternating pressure mattress
			Encourage coughing and deep breathing once patient is extubated
			Appropriate pulmonary toilet for intubated patient and continued pulmonary toilet with suctioning after extubation if patient is unable to cough
			Passive range-of-motion exercises

POTENTIAL FOR INAPPROPRIATE BALLOON PUMP FUNCTIONING

Loss of signal electrocardiogram [ECG] or arterial waveform necessary for balloon triggering)	Balloon pump is dependent on good quality ECG with tall R wave or arterial waveform tracing; if such signal is lost, balloon pumping ceases	Ongoing quality signals to maintain continued pumping	Proper preparation of electrode site before applying:
			1. Sites must be free of oil film or residue that could affect electrode adhesion
			2. Use a brisk dry rub with gauze to prepare each site; avoid using alcohol or solvents when preparing—solvents trapped beneath electrodes cause skin irritation and adhesion loss
			3. Avoid bone protuberances, joints, and creases or folds in skin; shave excessive hair from site
			4. Limit contact between fingers and adhesive surface
			5. Make sure that gel pad is moist before applying electrode
			6. After applying gel pad, smooth adhesive surface to reduce motion artifact

Continued.

Nursing care plan for the patient requiring the IABP: femoral artery insertion—cont'd

Problem	Rationale	Expected patient outcome	Nursing orders
POTENTIAL FOR INAPPROPRIATE BALLOON PUMPING FUNCTION—cont'd			
			7. Properly flush arterial line after drawing blood samples to maintain patency
			8. Change dressing daily using sterile technique
Damage to balloon catheter	Damage to catheter prevents effective augmentation	Catheter integrity and effective counterpulsation maintained	Instruct patient not to flex involved leg; restrain leg if necessary
	With femoral insertion, marked hip flexion may bend and fracture balloon catheter		Do not raise head of bed above 30°
	Raising head > 30° may crack catheter or force balloon proximally into aortic arch	Catheter integrity and effective counterpulsation maintained	Log roll patient to maintain immobility of leg that has balloon catheter in place
	Pumping efficacy is variable if balloon's position in aorta is changed		Passive range of motion to leg joints without flexing hip
POTENTIAL FOR LACK OF HEMODYNAMIC IMPROVEMENT FOLLOWING INSTITUTION OF BALLOON COUNTERPULSATION			
Continued or worsening left ventricular failure	Afterload is potentially reduced and perfusion potentially increased through coronary circulation and distal arterial tree; improper timing can prevent such improvements and patient's left ventricular dysfunction can be so severely impaired that IABP does not improve hemodynamic functioning	Reduction of afterload and improvement of left ventricular function as measured reduction of systemic vascular resistance, pulmonary artery, and pulmonary artery wedge pressures	Monitor hemodynamic measurements every 30 minutes until patient stabilizes, then every hour, further increasing to every 2 to 3 hours with patient improvement
		Adequate urine output	Measure urine output every hour, check vital signs of hemodynamic
		Improved mixed venous Po_2	
		Skin warm and dry	
		Patient alert and oriented	
		Absence of chest pain	
		Decreased dosage of cardiotonic drugs needed	
		Chest auscultation free of rales	

...els, measure blood gas levels, electrolyte concentrations monitored at least every 8 hours, more often if abnormal	No arrhythmias Patient can be weaned from balloon pump support	
		Check chest x-ray film and ECG daily; measure serial cardiac enzymes for 3 days keep strict record of intake and output
		Monitor heart rhythm and auscultate chest every hour until stable, then every 2 hours

POTENTIAL FOR SENSORY DEPRIVATION

Alteration in sleep pattern and disorientation	Patient is oriented, participating in his care, and understanding treatments and procedures	Organize nursing care to allow for blocks of time for "sleep therapy"
Noise level produced by equipment used, unfamiliar environment, necessity of performing nursing procedures 24 hours per day, immobility and lack of privacy		Orientation of patient to special procedures and treatments before they are done, which includes explaining therapeutic goal of counterpulsation
Lack of good night's sleep contributes to patient becoming disoriented		Facilitate sleep environment at night by turning down bright lights
		If patient is intubated, provide for written communication; reassure patient that opportunity to communicate his needs will be provided for, if patient cannot write, provide flash cards that allow for communication of basic needs
		Provide for comfort measures
		Allow patient to participate in decisions of care whenever possible
		Frequently reorient patient to surroundings, date, and time
		Provide for diversion (e.g., music therapy, favorite tape recordings)

Continued.

Nursing care plan for the patient requiring the IABP: femoral artery insertion—cont'd

Problem	Rationale	Expected patient outcome	Nursing orders
POTENTIAL FOR INEFFECTIVE FAMILY MEMBER COPING			
Family anxiety and distress	Family undergoes great stress because of:	Family acknowledges concerns and anxieties	Afford thorough explanations to family regarding patient's treatments and care
	1. Fear of patient not recovering	Family conveys that they understand meaning and goals of patient's plan of care, which includes balloon counterpulsation	Prepare family before they make first visit to bedside so that they understand tubes and lines that are in place in patient (use of pictures is helpful adjunct); assure family that tubes and lines are normal part of patient's comprehensive critical care
	2. Submersion into frightening environment		
	3. Seeing loved one strapped with tubes and lines	Family is able to effectively cope with patient's illness	
	4. Disruption of family life and schedule		Encourage family to communicate questions or express feelings that they are having at this time of crisis for them
	5. Financial burden imposed by patient's hospitalization; often family members need to stay close to hospital and away from home, which causes added financial burden		Keep family appraised of changes in patient's condition
	6. Feeling of helplessness in aiding patient's recovery		At change of shift, oncoming nurse should introduce herself to family who is often keeping vigil, demonstrate professional mannerism, which helps family to have confidence in care being rendered

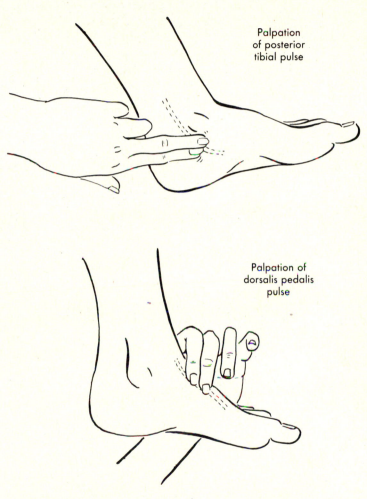

Palpation
of posterior
tibial pulse

Palpation of
dorsalis pedalis
pulse

FIG. 22-1 Location of dorsalis pedalis and posterior tibial pulses.

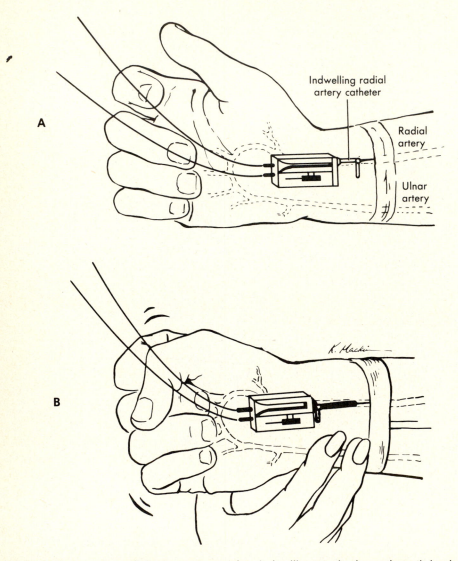

FIG. 22-2 Allen test for radial artery patency when indwelling monitoring catheter is in place in radial artery. **A,** Catheter is in place in radial artery. **B,** Patient makes fist while examiner manually compresses ulnar artery or positions hand in fist if patient is unable to cooperate.

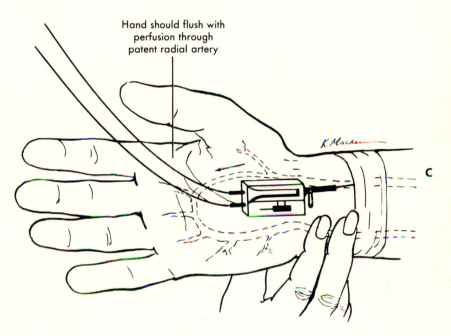

Hand should flush with
perfusion through
patent radial artery

Fig. 22-2, cont'd C, Examiner maintains compression on ulnar artery while patient opens fist. Hand should flush and resume pink color if blood perfusion through radial artery is adequate with catheter in place.

REFERENCES

1. Allen, E.J.: Thromboangitis obliterans: methods of diagnosis of chronic occlusive arterial lesions distal to the wrist with illustrated cases, Am. J. Med. Sci. **177:**237, 1929.
2. Bricker, P.L.: The intense nursing demands of the intra-aortic balloon pump, RN **43:**23, 1980.
3. Collier, P., and Dohas, P.: The intra-aortic balloon pump, Physiotherapy **66:**156, 1980.
4. Purcell, J., et al.: Intra-aortic balloon pump therapy, AJN **83:**775, 1983.
5. Shively, M.: The physiologic principles of intra-aortic balloon counterpulsation. In Pollock-Lathum, C., and Canobbio, M., editors: Current Concepts in Cardiac Care, Rockville, Md., 1982, Aspen Publications.
6. Sturm, J.T., et al.: Treatment of postoperative low output syndrome with intra-aortic balloon pumping: experience with 419 patients, Am. J. Cardiol. **45:**1033, 1980.
7. Whitman, G.: Intra-aortic balloon pumping and cardiac mechanics: a programmed lesson, Heart Lung **7:**1034, 1978.

CHAPTER 23 Cardiac catheterization and balloon pumping

Balloon assistance before and during cardiac catheterization

IABP has been used to provide a period of stabilization for patients who have demonstrated hemodynamic decompensation, before subjecting them to coronary angiography. Before catheterization, balloon pumping has enabled angiograms to be performed with less risk during a usually high-risk state of ischemia. Bardet and co-workers[2] performed coronary angiograms during IABP without complication (arrhythmia or progressive angina) on 21 patients with angina after infarction, thereby confirming severe coronary artery disease. Pumping was begun in the intensive care unit, continued enroute to the cardiac catheter laboratory, and carried out during the angiogram. Counterpulsation continued until the patient was placed on extracorporeal circulation if bypass surgery was indicated.

Leinbach[4] at Massachusetts General Hospital established criteria for cardiac catheterization for patients who receive balloon pump assist following myocardial infarction. The criteria included:
1. Failure to improve significantly after 12 to 24 hours of IABP and catecholamine infusion.
2. Continued high or increasing catecholamine requirements in spite of IABP.
3. Refractory pump failure more than 1 week after myocardial infarction.
4. Balloon dependence after 48 hours of assistance, as diagnosed by abrupt discontinuance of counterpulsation and a drop in arterial pressure to 55 mm Hg, cardiac index to less than 2.0 liters/min/m^2, and a rise of pulmonary wedge pressure above 20 mm Hg in spite of diuretics or development of angina pectoris.

Transfemoral coronary catheterization approach

Selective coronary angiography undertaken with patients on balloon assist may be performed via the brachial or Sones'[8] approach to avoid mechanical interference with the intra-aortic balloon resting in situ in the descending thoracic aorta. Angiographers may, however, favor the use of the femoral approach because of the ease and speed preferable in catheterization of the critically ill patient.

When the patient who already has the balloon pump in situ is transported to the cardiac catheter laboratory for femoral arterial catheterization, the femoral artery not occupied by the balloon is used (Fig. 23-1). Curved-tip guide wires are used for insertion of the catheter

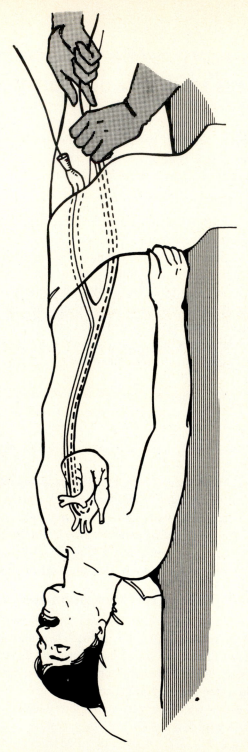
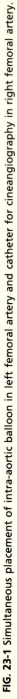
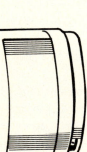

FIG. 23-1 Simultaneous placement of intra-aortic balloon in left femoral artery and catheter for cineangiography in right femoral artery.

to diminish the possibility of balloon damage by inadvertent contact with the end of a guide wire.

Aroesty and associates[1] described the technique for femoral (Judkins) catheterization via the opposite femoral artery from balloon placement. The catheterization is performed under fluoroscopy; the guide wire is advanced retrogradely through the femoral artery to a position 5 cm below the distal end of the intra-aortic balloon. Care is taken not to advance the guide wire to the level of the pulsating balloon. Immediately before advancement of the Judkins' catheter into the thoracic aorta, the balloon pump console is turned off, allowing the catheter to be guided past the deflated balloon. Once the tip of the catheter has passed the distal portion of the balloon, pumping is resumed as the catheter is advanced to the ascending aorta.

Angiography is performed with the balloon pulsing. Following completion of the cineangiographic examination, the catheter is withdrawn to the proximal tip of the balloon. At this point balloon pumping is halted and the intra-aortic balloon remains deflated, as the catheter is withdrawn past the balloon, down to its distal tip. Once the catheter has been withdrawn around the balloon, pumping is resumed.

Good quality angiograms are obtainable, and the mobility of the catheter is not impaired by the operating counterpulsating balloon. Examination of balloons that were pumping in situ during simultaneous catheter manipulation for coronary angiography failed to produce evidence of trauma or thrombosis. Therefore the intra-aortic balloon does not constitute an obstacle to the introduction or manipulation of the transfemorally inserted catheter placed for angiography.

REFERENCES

1. Aroesty, J.M., et al.: Transfemoral selective coronary artery catheterization during intra-aortic balloon by-pass pumping, Radiology **111**:307, 1974.
2. Bardet, M.J., et al.: Treatment of post-myocardial infarction angina by intra-aortic balloon pumping and revascularization, J. Thorac. Cardiovasc. Surg. **78**:445, 1979.
3. DeLaria, G.A., et al.: Delayed evolution of myocardial ischemia injury after intra-aortic balloon counter-pulsation, Circulation **49**(suppl. 2):242, 1974.
4. Leinbach, R.C., et al.: Selective coronary and left ventricular cineangiography during intra-aortic balloon pumping for cardiogenic shock, Circulation **45**:845, 1972.
5. Mundth, E.P., and Austen, W.G.: Surgical measures for coronary artery disease, N. Engl. J. Med. **293**:13, 1975.
6. Petch, M.C.: Safety of coronary arteriography, Br. Heart J. **35**:377, 1973.
7. Proudfit, W.L., et al.: Selective cine coronary arteriography correlation with clinical findings in 1,000 patients, Circulation **33**:901, 1966.
8. Sones, F.M., Jr.: Indications and value of coronary arteriography, Circulation **46**:1161, 1972.

CHAPTER 24 Datascope, Hoek Loos, Kontron, and SMEC balloon pumps

The four models of IABPs available are presented to introduce the reader to options in the selection of a pump. Information presented is not intended to be all inclusive. Each of the four manufacturers of balloon pumps afford expert resource personnel who can provide the reader with a much more in-depth understanding of specific pump features and operation. IABPs should never be used with a patient unless the operator has a thorough understanding of the physiological principles of IABP and of the controls and functions of the instrument. All models have been designed with consideration of safety and ease of operation; however, each manufacturer emphasizes precautionary protocols specific to its pump to ensure proper and effective use and optimum counterpulsation. The pumps are presented in alphabetical order.

Datascope System 82[2,3]

The current generation of IABP manufactured by Datascope Corp. is the System 82; this pneumatic drive instrument may be used for IABP and pulsatile assist with the Datascope pulsatile assist device (PAD). Carbon dioxide (CO_2) and helium may be used with the Datascope pump.

The System 82 has three main components (Fig. 24-1).

1. Datascope Model 870 nonfade monitor and electrosurgical interference suppression (ESIS) module provide monitor viewing for the patient electrocardiogram (ECG) waveform and arterial pressure. The ESIS module eliminates interference from electrocautery during surgery.
2. Model 3520 Cardiac Assist Control accepts the ECG and arterial pressure from the monitor and delivers alternate drive pressure and vacuum to the balloon or PAD. Adjustments are provided for achieving the desired timing and magnitude of the pneumatic output.
3. The System 82 cart houses a compressor-aspirator that develops the necessary pressure and vacuum. Storage tanks of CO_2 are also mounted on the cart and used to develop the required pressure when in portable operation, while an internal Venturi tube develops the required vacuum. A changeover to portable operation occurs whenever the line cord is unplugged or line power is interrupted.

Inflation and deflation of the balloon are accomplished by alternately applying pres-

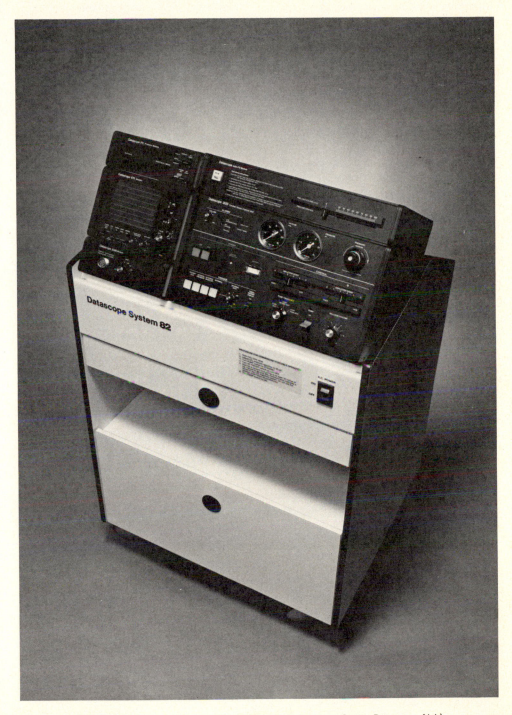

FIG. 24-1 Datascope System 82. (Courtesy Datascope Corp., Paramus, N.J.)

sure and vacuum to a closed circuit, consisting of the intra-aortic balloon and a slave balloon with a safety chamber. This circuit is charged before use with a fixed amount of CO_2 or helium.

Specifications

System components
Model 82C mobile cart
Model 3520 cardiac assist control unit
Model 3500 safety chamber
Model 3520B battery pack
Model 870 dual-trace, nonfade physiological monitor
ESIS module
Positive and negative pressure pump
Blood pressure transducer

Control system
Power switch: Two-station interlock push-button switch
Battery indicator: Amber LED indicates battery operation
Battery meter: Monitors battery condition
Trigger input selector: Four selectable inputs on interlocked push-button switch; push-button flashes on each trigger pulse
Positions: Patient ECG—triggers from 870 monitor, ECG display, or other ECG monitor
  Arterial pressure—triggers from 870 monitor or other monitor pressure waveform display
  External monitor—triggers from output of most electronic pulse generators
  Internal—triggers from internal rate generator; adjustable from 60 to 120 beats per minute
Timing marker display: Three-level signal indicates pump sequence in relation to the pressure waveform display
Inflation control: Slide control adjusts balloon inflation from 125 to 625 msec after trigger pulse; with Arterial Pressure Trigger or Internal switches on, adjustment is from 3 to 540 msec
Inflation indicator: Red LED illuminated during inflation
Deflation control: Slide control adjusts balloon deflation from 3 to 625 msec after start of inflation
Deflation indicator: Amber LED illuminated during deflation
Balloon volume: Rotary selector adjusts safety chamber filling time from 2 to 200 msec, allowing adjustment of balloon volume
Pump frequency: Selects triggering on every beat, every second beat, or every third beat
Pump switch: Two-position switch—Pump On and Standby. In the Standby position balloon is deflated
Pump indicator: Red LED indicates pump operation

Pacer timing switch: Rear panel switch permits later balloon deflation when pump triggers on pacer spike; front panel LED flashes when pacer timing is selected

Minimum inflation Point switch: Rear panel switch permits adjustable inflation delay of 3 to 540 msec for special clinical applications; front panel LED flashes when engaged

Front panel controls (Fig. 24-2)

1. **OFF**

   Push-button switch that is used to turn off power to the Model 3520. Internal batteries continue to charge if line cord is plugged into AC outlet.

2. **ON**

   Push-button switch that is used to supply power to the Model 3520. Before depressing this push button, verification that the Pump Switch is in the Standby position should be made.

3. **PATIENT ECG**

   Push-button switch that is used to select the ECG signal as the trigger source for cardiac assist.

4. **ARTERIAL PRESSURE**

   Push-button switch that is used to select the arterial pressure as the trigger source for cardiac assist.

5. **EXTERNAL MONITOR**

   Push-button switch that is used to select the ECG from a compatible external monitor or synchronization pulse as the trigger source for cardiac assist.

6. **INTERNAL RATE**

   Push-button switch that is used to select the internal pacing generator as the trigger

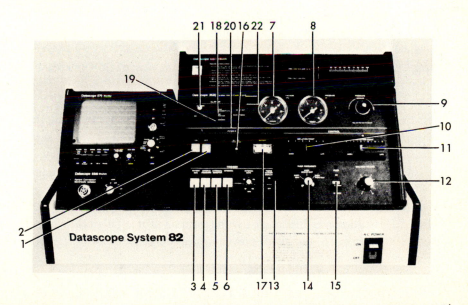

FIG. 24-2 Front panel controls of System 82. (Courtesy Datascope Corp., Paramus, N.J.)

source for cardiac assist. The pacing rate is determined by the setting of the Internal Rate Control.

7. VACUUM

Gauge that indicates the vacuum generated by an internal pump.

8. PRESSURE

Gauge that indicates a controlled pressure generated by an internal pump and regulator.

9. PRESSURE INCREASE

Rotary control with locking ring that permits adjustment of the pressure.

10. INFLATION POINT

Slide control that is used to set the point of inflation by adjusting the time period from the trigger event to the beginning of assist.

11. DEFLATION POINT

Slide control that is used to set the point of deflation by adjusting the end of assist.

12. BALLOON VOLUME

Rotary control that is used to adjust the pumping volume by varying the duration that pressure is applied to the cardiac assist device (intra-aortic balloon, PAD).

13. TIMING MARKER DISPLAY

Switch that is used to turn the Timing Marker on or off.

14. PUMP FREQUENCY

Three-position switch that is used to determine whether assist will occur on every beat, every other beat, or every third beat.

15. PUMP

Switch that is used to initiate cardiac assist. This switch should be turned to on only after all preliminary control settings have been made. LED indicator becomes illuminated whenever the switch is in the On position.

16. BATTERY OPERATION

Amber LED that indicates the operating power is being derived from internal batteries and not from an external power source.

17. BATTERY

Meter that indicates the approximate charge condition of the internal batteries.

18. LOW AUGMENTATION

Alarm LED that becomes illuminated if the assisted pressure falls below a level established by the setting of the Ref Pressure Control. When tripped, an audible tone is sounded.

19. NO VACUUM

Alarm LED that becomes illuminated if the vacuum source falls below 3 inches of mercury. When tripped, the alarm prevents pressure delivery to the cardiac assist device, and an audible tone is sounded.

20. TRIGGER

Alarm LED that becomes illuminated as a result of a loss of a trigger or in the event of an extremely high trigger rate (generally indicative of an open electrode lead, noise, artifact). When tripped, an audible tone is sounded.

21. **VOLUME**

Rotary control that is used to set the volume of the audible tone produced by low augmentation, no vacuum, or trigger alarms.

22. **DELAY OUT, PACER**

Alarm LED indicators that operate in conjunction with two rear panel switches. These switches are for specialized applications.

Abbreviated operator's manual

A. Establish AC power

1. Plug power cord into AC power receptacle.

CAUTION: Power cord should only be connected to a three-wire AC power system containing a separate ground line. Do not remove the ground (round) prong off the plug; do not use adaptors to defeat the ground prong, or a potentially dangerous shock hazard may result.

2. Set AC power switch on cart front at On.
3. Turn on Datascope 3520 control unit by depressing the On push button.
4. Turn on Datascope 870 monitor by rotating main selector to 25 mm Hg/Div position.

B. Establish gas pressure

1. Turn on either one of the CO_2 tanks at the rear of the cart by using a gas cylinder wrench. Open the corresponding shut-off valve on the pressure manifold. The right-hand gauge of the pressure regulator should indicate at least 500 pounds per square inch.
2. Rotate the pressure regulator/manifold's black control knob (clockwise) until the left-hand gauge reads 50 pounds per square inch.

C. Verify proper operation of safety chamber (Fig. 24-3)

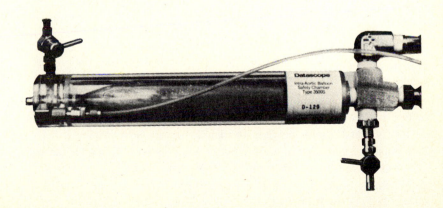

FIG. 24-3 Safety chamber. (Courtesy Datascope Corp., Paramus, N.J.)

CAUTION: The safety chamber should be replaced after 1000 hours of cycling or 2 years from date of delivery. Safety chambers that exceed these limits should be regarded as suspect.

WARNING: This procedure should not be performed when the system is connected to the patient.

1. Set front-panel controls on Model 3520 as follows:

Control	Setting
Balloon Volume	5
Pump	On
Internal Rate	80
Internal	Depress
On/Off	Depress On
Inflation Point	2
Deflation Point	2

2. Attach a stopcock or syringe to the Balloon Connector on the safety chamber.
3. Check the Run/Fill push button on the autofill module. If Run is illuminated and system is already pumping, proceed to step 4. If Fill is illuminated, press Run/Fill push button to illuminate Run, begin pumping, and then proceed to step 4.
4. Depress the Run/Fill push-button switch. Pumping stops, and the Run light extinguishes. Verify that both the safety chamber balloon and patient balloon are fully deflated.
5. The Preload slide control on the autofill module (front panel) will be at "0" position. Press the Run/Fill push-button switch again. The system will begin to pump. The safety chamber and the patient balloon were intentionally not preloaded (remain deflated); thus introduction of pressure to the safety chamber should not inflate either balloon. If either balloon inflates during this test, a pneumatic leak exists in the patient balloon/safety chamber drive system. Check all fittings and connection for tightness.
6. If no initial leak is evident, continue the procedure with these settings for a minimum of 5 minutes, and verify that both balloons remain deflated.
7. If in doubt about the integrity of the safety chamber, replace it. (Installation instructions are supplied with the replacement safety chamber.)
D. Establish initial setup
   1. Set Inflation Point control at 2.5.
   2. Set Deflation Point control at 2.5.
   3. Set Balloon Volume control at 0.
   4. Set Pump switch to Standby.
   5. Set Timing Marker Display switch at Off.
   6. Verify that Vacuum gauge is 16 inches mercury or more.
   7. Adjust Pressure control until Pressure gauge is set at 8 pounds per square inch. Press red ring in to lock setting.
   8. Set Pump Frequency switch at Every Beat.
   9. Set Trigger for Patient ECG.
   10. Set 870 monitor's Beep switch at ECG.
   11. Set 870 monitor's ECG size control at 1.

E. Establish ECG
1. Connect the patient cable to the ESIS module. See ECG Acquisition for details on setup.
F. Establish arterial pressure trace
1. Connect a Datascope compatible pressure transducer to the Pressure Transducer connector on the 870 monitor's rear. See arterial pressure monitoring for details on setup.
G. Initiate timing
1. Set initial timing by using Timing Marker Display, and adjust Inflation Point. See triggering and timing for details.
H. Preload the safety chamber balloon
See instruction on autofill module for details.
I. Initiate counterpulsation
1. Initiate counterpulsation, and verify diastolic augmentation by adjusting Balloon Volume to "8" and setting Deflation Point control to achieve a 5 to 15 mm Hg diastolic unloading.

Timing sequence. When activated, a Timing Marker Display switch changes the ECG tracing to a square wave (Fig. 24-4). To set inflation, rotate the Reference Pressure control until the reference trace line intersects the dicrotic notch of the arterial line. Next rotate ECG Size control until the square wave superimposes on the arterial pressure waveform (Fig. 24-5). Using Inflation Point control, set inflation at the dicrotic notch (indicated by the reference trace line). Verify that deflation occurs before onset of the next cardiac cycle. Then set Timing Marker Display at Off, and observe return of ECG signal on top half of monitor screen. This is a preliminary timing setup.

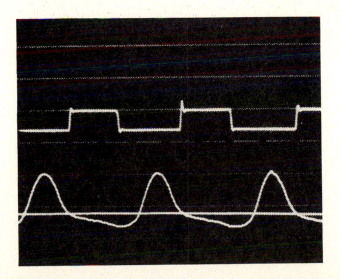

FIG. 24-4 Electrocardiogram waveform is changed to square wave when Timing Marker Display switch is activated. (Courtesy Datascope Corp., Paramus, N.J.)

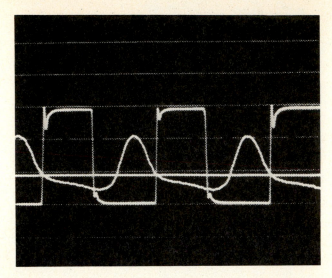

FIG. 24-5 Reference trace line is adjusted to intersect dicrotic notch of arterial line. Square wave is set to superimpose on arterial waveform and inflation (square wave) is set to occur at dicrotic notch, indicated by reference line. (Courtesy Datascope Corp., Paramus, N.J.)

Routine checks

1. Recharging of the safety chamber balloon is required every 2 to 3 hours.
2. If the heart rate deviates more than 10 beats per minute, timing adjustments may be necessary to achieve optimum diastolic augmentation and reduction of end-diastolic pressure.

System alarms

1. Low augmentation: A lamp lights, and an audible tone sounds whenever the assisted diastolic pressure falls below the setting established by the Reference Pressure Marker. The horizontal linear Reference Pressure Marker should be set 5 mm Hg below the peak level of diastolic augmentation. Decreased augmentation indicates loss of CO_2 in the safety chamber or decreased arterial pressure.
2. No vacuum: A lamp lights, and an audible tone sounds whenever the vacuum pressure falls below 3 inches of mercury. Balloon pumping automatically ceases on activation of this alarm, with the balloon deflated until the situation is corrected.
3. Trigger: A lamp lights, and an audible tone sounds whenever the ECG or trigger signal is disrupted. Balloon pumping automatically ceases until an adequate trigger is established.

Troubleshooting guidelines

ECG: There are several methods to correct conditions that alter or hamper the acquisition of a reliable ECG. Repositioning or replacing the ECG electrodes, choosing an alternate lead selection, and verifying that the patient cable is properly connected are the most common solutions.

Pressure: Adequate flushing to maintain pressure line patency and alignment of stopcocks in the proper position eliminate the majority of pressure trace problems that are encountered.

Arrhythmias—atrial: Constant atrial arrhythmias are a source of problems in obtaining maximum benefit for the patient. By timing inflation and deflation to the majority of the beats, the maximum augmentation and unloading should be produced in these patients.

Arrhythmias—tachycardia: Tachycardia compromises ventricular ejection by a reduction in ventricular filling time. The ejected systolic blood volume is reduced, thereby lessening the amount of diastolic augmentation. It is recommended that a pump frequency of every other beat be used to obtain the maximum benefit for the patient.

Arrhythmias—ventricular premature contractions (PVCs): This arrhythmia simply causes the balloon to deflate. No special adjustment is needed.

Cardiac assist—ventricular fibrillation: In the event of this arrhythmia, all that is necessary is to treat the patient with defibrillation. The System 82 is completely isolated from the patient so that there is no danger of damaging the unit during defibrillation.

Ventricular standstill: In this situation you may leave the unit alone using ECG triggering or time the unit using arterial triggering with the cardiopulmonary resuscitation compression as your pressure signal.

● ● ●

For further information on the Datascope pump contact:

Datascope Corp.
580 Winters Ave.
Paramus, N.J. 07652
(Telephone [201] 265-8800)

or

Datascope B.V.
P.O. Box 3870 CA
Hoevelaken, Holland
(Telephone 03495-34514)

Hoek Loos IABP[6,7]

In cooperation with the Universities of Amsterdam and Nijmegen, the firm of Hoogstraat developed the Hoek Loos system that features simplified operation and greater dependability. The complete unit consists of two separate modules: (1) a control unit and (2) a bedside unit (Fig. 24-6). The unit can be supplied with a trolley and an emergency power pack. It uses CO_2 as the gas of inflation with automatic blood leak detector, automatic QR-wave tracking with average beat inflation-deflation correction, and no skipped function with detection of an extrasystolic complex.

Control module (Fig. 24-7)

The control module consists of two sections. The top section is an intensive care unit that embraces four modular elements, as follows:

1. A module containing a two-channel nonfading memory scope with hold. The scope

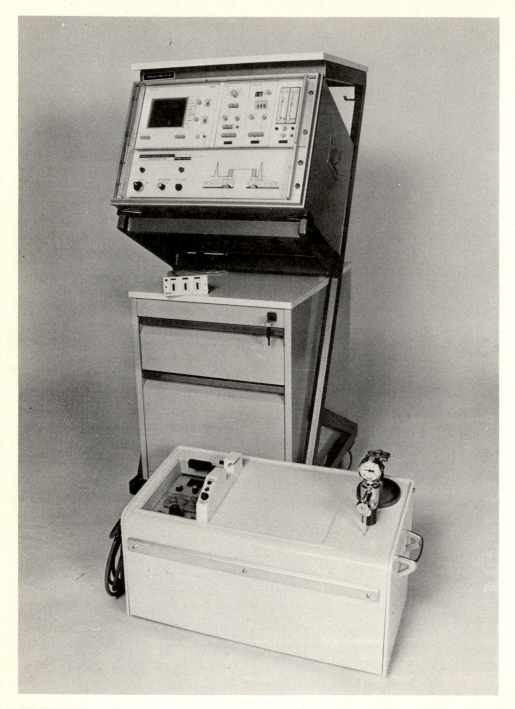

FIG. 24-6 Hoek Loos pump consisting of control and bedside unit. (Courtesy Hoek Loos Medical Group, The Netherlands.)

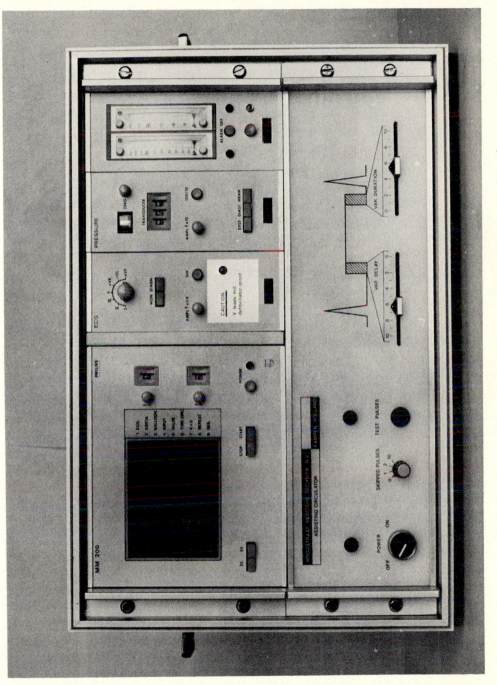

FIG. 24-7 Control model regulators of Hoek Loos pump. (Courtesy Hoek Loos)

has two standard (25 and 50 mm/sec) speeds for display of the ECG and the arterial pressure curve.

2. An ECG module that triggers the pump system with a control pulse derived from the lead showing the most adequate QRS complex.
3. A module that houses the arterial blood pressure amplifier and displays the systolic, diastolic, or average blood pressure as required.
4. A module designed to contain the meters for heart rate and arterial blood pressure. Both instruments have adjustable upper and lower limit controls that set off a visual alarm and deactivate the pump is either limit is exceeded.

Bottom section is the circulation assistance unit, triggered on the R wave, equipped with built-in electronic circuitry that makes pump inflation and deflation adapt automatically to a change in heart rate. Inflation and deflation are timed with two slide potentiometers. Selector switch provides assistance on 1:1, 1:2, 1:3, and 1:11 ratios.

Use of the trolley pack is recommended for patient transport without interrupting balloon pumping. The power pack can provide 1 hour of assistance and activates whenever the main power supply is unavailable. The control unit is positioned on top, and the power pack, which is kept charging when not in use, is on the bottom.

Bedside module (Fig. 24-8)

The gas system is housed in the bedside module, which should be mounted as close to the patient as possible, preferably by means of sturdy brackets at the foot of the bed. The bedside module is linked to the control module by a single cable, 4.5 m in length.

The system includes two gauges that record the positive and negative pressure applied. If the gas pressure falls below the minimum level, a visual and acoustic alarm is activated; the system is protected from excessive pressure by relief valves. Since the balloon is inflated by pressure, it can keep pace with higher heart rates. The system allows any available type of balloon catheter to be adopted, regardless of capacity.

Specifications

Control module two-channel memory scope (12-lead floating input circuit [insulated])

Display unit: Electrostatic deflection; diameter 5 inches, useful screen dimensions 100 × 80 mm

Memory: Digital; 4-second sampling rate, 256 Hz per channel

Amplitude: Maximum 5 cm per channel

Speed: 25 and 50 mm per second

ECG selector: I, II, III, AVR, AVL, AVF, and V

Frequency range: 0.05 to 100 Hz (−3 db) 0.5 to 27 Hz (−3 db)

Input impedance: Minimum 150 m ohms measured at the electrodes; protected from defibrillator shock

Pressure amplifier range: 0 to 30 and 0 to 300 mm Hg floating input (insulated)

Pressure transducers: Philips AE 840; Statham P23 db and P37; Bell & Howell 4-327; Transtec 800; Biotec BT70; etc.

Requisite transducer sensitivity: 42.5 to 500.0 uV per V10 mm Hg

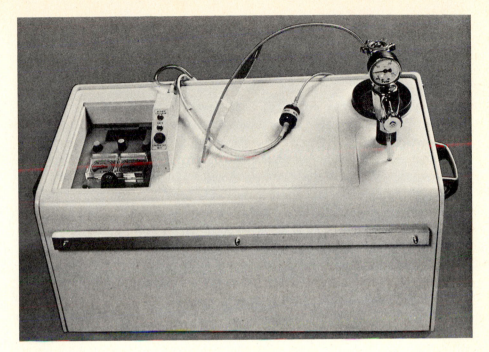

FIG. 24-8 Bedside unit of Hoek Loos pump. (Courtesy Hoek Loos Medical Group, The Netherlands.)

Bridge supply: 5V; DC

Meters: Moving-coil meters, dial length approximately 60 mm, class 1.5, with emergency setting

Electronic IABP control circuit with automatic adaptation to heart rate, including trimming potentiometers

Supply voltage: 110-, 120-, 220-, and 240 V; 50 and 60 Hz

Dimensions: Length 510 mm, width 520 mm, height 350 mm

Weight: 34 kg

Bedside module

Blood leak detector

Pump function blocked during extrasystoles

Balloon catheter: All available IABP types with Luer-Lok

Balloon inflation time: 100 msec

Balloon deflation time: 80 msec

Cable to control module: Length 4500 mm

Driving gas (closed circuit): CO_2

Gas cylinder capacity: 1.3 liters

Maximum gas pressure: 450 mm Hg

Dimensions: Length 310 mm, width 710 mm, and height 475 mm

Weight: 27.5 kg

Trolley with emergency power pack for automatic standby duty

Supply voltage: 110-,120-, 220, and 240 V; 50 and 60 Hz

Maximum standby capability: 1 hour

Abbreviated operation

Standard setup requires an artifact-free ECG signal and an arterial trace.

A. Check the pressure in the CO_2 tank, which needs to be replaced if the pressure is below 4 kg/cm^2.

B. With the console pressure switch off, open the main gas valve on the CO_2 tank and the reducing valve. Slightly open the overpressure knob on the bedside unit. When the CO_2 filling button is depressed, gas can be heard escaping through the overpressure valve, if the system is functioning properly. The gas pressure needle on the bedside alarm must be in the green zone.

C. Connect the balloon catheter from the patient to the Luer-Lok blood leak detector on the bedside manual. The pump is ready to be turned on.

D. A digital readout of the chamber pressure is displayed on the bedside module. Generally optimum balloon function occurs at chamber pressures of +260 and −100 mm Hg. If a pressure of ±400 mm Hg or more is displayed at the digital outlet, open the overpressure valve until the correct pressure is achieved. The digital readout of the gas pressure varies during balloon operation.

Timing sequence. Inflate and deflate slides allow for adjustment of inflation to occur immediately after the dicrotic notch with deflation adjusted to obtain as low as possible an end-diastolic pressure. A good arterial blood pressure is essential for timing. It is recommended that the skipped-pulse switch be turned to position 1 for timing adjustment for every other beat inflation. With heart frequency changes, the pump is fitted with an automatic correction for onset and duration of inflation; however, this can be done by hand with adjustment of the slide potentiometers.

Alarms

1. Alarms that stop the pumping action: Alarm triggering valves for heart rate and blood pressure can be preset. If these limits are violated, alarm lights are activated.

2. An alarm may be acoustically signaled if balloon pressure is too low, which can be caused by a leaking connection, a leaking balloon, or a rapidly increasing heart frequency.

3. Blood leak detection system: This system prevents blood from entering the pump system in case of a leaking balloon. As soon as traces of blood pass by the blood leak detector, a blocking system closes off the rest of the unit, and balloon pumping ceases. An alarm sounds, and the red CO_2 leak light illuminates.

● ● ●

For further information on the Hoek Loos pump contact:

Hoek Loos Export Department
1, Havenstraat, 3115 HC Schiedam
P.O. Box 78, 3100 AB Schiedam
The Netherlands
(Telephone 010-731122)

Kontron Model 10 (Fig. 24-9)

The Model 10 features waveform monitoring of the ECG; arterial or pulmonary artery and balloon pressures; fully automated triggering from the patient's ECG, arterial pressure, or internal 80 beats per minute simulator; variable balloon pump control; switch selection of the ECG lead configuration; fail-safe computerized diagnostics that inform the operator of specific conditions or pump malfunctions that require immediate staff action; alphanumerical displays of derived physiological data; and a self-contained battery system. A built-in automatic cardiac output computer and a single-channel strip recorder are available as options.

Specifications

ECG Input/Processor

Patient safety: Designed to meet UL specification 544

Bandwidth: .05 to 500 Hz

Leakage current: 10 uA maximum

Common mode rejection rate: 115 db at 60 Hz with 5 kilohm lead unbalance

Defibrillator protection: Input is protected against defibrillator voltages up to 5 kilovolts

R-wave trigger: Proper ECG triggering is assured by computer

   Pattern mode—the shape of the wave must conform to a defined pattern that includes rise and fall times, complex width, and amplitude.

   Peak mode—a positive wave is examined for scope and amplitude.

Pacer rejection: Computer rejects pulses less than 20 msec wide to prevent triggering on pacer spikes in pattern ECG recognition mode

Inflation-deflation timing: Balloon inflation is from 20% to 70% of R-R interval; balloon deflation is from 70% to 100% of R-R interval

High level input: Accepts ECG signals from a remote monitor; high level ECG input is ±1.1 volts maximum; connection is facilitated by the ECG Mon In jack.

High level output: Provides ECG signals for display on a remote monitor; high level ECG output depends on the setting of the ECG Gain control; maximum output is ±3.5 volts; connection is facilitated by the ECG Out jack; impedance of this output is typically 1000 ohms resistive

Lead selection: Thumbwheel switch allows selection of leads I, II, III, AVR, AVL, AVF, and all V leads

Polarity: Computer processes positive or negative R waves in pattern ECG mode and in peak triggering mode

General input power: Factory configured for any one of the following operating ranges: 100 V, $\pm10\%$; 110 V, $\pm10\%$ or 120 V, -10 V $+5$ V (user selectable); 220 V, $\pm5\%$, 230 V, $\pm5\%$ or 240 V, $\pm5\%$ (user selectable); line frequency range is 50 to 63 Hz. Average power consumption is approximately 400 volts

Battery power: An internal battery system allows operation for more than 1 hour during patient transport; external supplementary battery system can be connected for additional battery operation

Dimensions (shroud in): Height 10 inches, width 26⅛ inches, and depth 29 inches

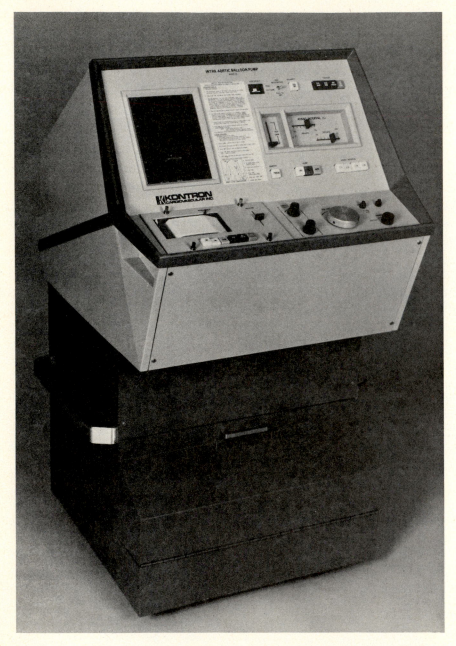

FIG. 24-9 Kontron Model 10. (Courtesy Kontron Cardiovascular Inc., Everett, Mass.)

Weight: 375 pounds (170.5 kg)

Diagnostics: A series of coded messages is available for display to inform the operator of conditions relating to improper IABP timing, noisy arterial pressure signals, poor balloon gas pressure signals, poor balloon drive signals, or improper balloon operation

Balloon gas system

Operating gas: Helium (recycled)

Water vapor trap: Thermoelectric system cools helium and removes moisture

Displays type: Nonfade, memory type display with approximately 40 mm per second apparent sweep speed

ECG: Green trace with red trace on assisted portion

Blood pressure: Red trace—display screen calibrated for direct reading of arterial and pulmonary pressures; any external pressure amplifier may be fed into the Aux In jack; input is calibrated for 100 mm per volt when the front panel Arterial Pressure Sensitivity control is in the fully counterclockwise position

Balloon pressure: Blue trace—sensed through internal solid state pressure transducer; display screen calibrated for direct pressure measurement in millimeters of mercury

Derived data: Heart rate—derived from ECG or arterial pressure triggering signals and automatically updated every eight beats

Arterial pressure—absolute peak diastolic and computed mean pressures are derived by beat-to-beat analysis; each beat is sampled, and pressure is averaged over eight beats of the heart rate; display is automatically updated every eight beats

Cardiac output (optional)—derived from the radial artery pressure wave and is calculated and automatically updated approximately every 10 seconds

Trigger—an asterisk next to the heart rate display flashes red with each recognized trigger

Controls (Fig. 24-10)

1. DISPLAY

    Monitor that presents waveform displays of ECG, arterial pressure, and balloon pressure; continuously updated physiological data in alphanumerical form; system diagnostics.

2. ECG GAIN

    Continuously variable control by which the operator sets the ECG amplitude for proper triggering (normally two divisions peak-to-peak). Control must be at the minimum position when using internal 80 BPM oscillator.

3. LEAD SELECT

    Thumbwheel switch that allows the operator to select the ECG lead configuration (I, II, III, AVR, AVL, AVF, or any one of the V leads).

4. POLARITY

    Push-button switch that allows the operator to invert the ECG and display a positive-going R wave.

5. ECG RECOGNITION

    Peak and pattern modes are used.

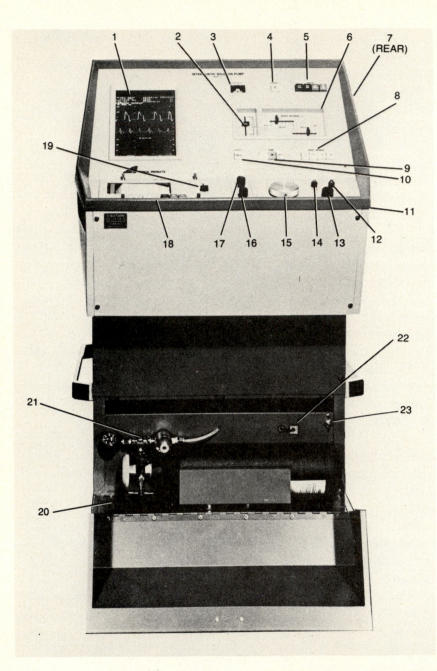

FIG. 24-10 Controls of Model 10. (Courtesy Kontron Cardiovascular, Inc., Everett, Mass.)

6. **TRIGGER SELECT**

Push-button switches that allow the operator to select the trigger signal for balloon inflation-deflation from one of the following:

ECG SKIN: ECG derived from skin electrodes and processed by the Model 3010's ECG front end.

ECG MON: ECG monitored by remote equipment and brought to the Model 3010 for display via the ECG Mon In connector.

ART PRESS: Arterial pressure waveform is monitored at any radial artery.

80 BEATS/MIN: An internal 80 beats/min R-wave simulator.

7. **ASSIST INTERVAL**

Continuously variable controls that allow the operator to set the time of balloon inflation and deflation. Timing is related to a percentage of the R-R interval and is displayed as a red segment on the normally green ECG waveform to aid the operator in making the initial setting.

8. **INPUT/OUTPUT CONNECTIONS**

Recessed connector fittings and controls that facilitate proper balloon use, display, and recording.

ALARM VOLUME: Control is continuously variable and allows the operator to adjust the volume of the system shutdown alarm.

ECG MON IN: Phone jack allows single-ended ECG signals from a remote monitor to be displayed. The ECG signals can be a minimum of 0.3 volts and a maximum of 1.8 volts peak-to-peak.

AUX IN: Phone jack allows any auxiliary waveform of the operator's selection to be recorded via the strip-chart recorder (optional) and displayed as a red trace on channel 3. The gain of this input is adjusted via the Arterial Pressure Sensitivity control. With this control adjusted fully counterclockwise, the input is calibrated for 100 mm Hg per volt.

CARDIAC OUPUT: Phone jack allows signals representative of cardiac output measurements to be brought to an external recorder. This output provides 1.0 volt per liter per minute.

ECG OUT: Phone jack allows monitoring of the patient's ECG via an external monitor. The ECG output is ±3 volts maximum, depending on the setting of the ECG Gain control. (System's maximum overall gain is 5000.)

BALLOON PRESS: Phone jack allows signals representative of balloon pressure to be externally monitored or recorded. This output is calibrated at 100 mm Hg per volt, and it may be connected to the Aux In phone jack for recording on the Model 3010 recorder. For proper calibration, the Arterial Pressure Sensitivity control should be fully counterclockwise.

ART PRESS Out: Phone jack allows signals representative of the monitored arterial pressure to be externally monitored or recorded. This output is normally calibrated at 100 mm Hg per volt.

ART PRESS TRANS: Connector facilitates hookup between Model 3010 and the external arterial pressure transducer. Statham P231a, P23Db, P23AA, or any other transducers with equivalent electrical characteristics may be used.

ECG IN: Connector facilitates hookup of the patient cable (Roche no. 8329). The use of pregelled disposable electrodes are recommended.

BALLOON INPUT: Connector accepts the balloon line and facilitates the helium connection. Electrical connections provide a reference for the nominal balloon volume to prevent overinflation of the balloon.

9. ASSIST/INTERVAL

Push-button switches used to select ratio of assisted to unassisted cardiac cycles. In the 1:1 setting, every cardiac cycle is assisted. In the 1:2 setting, every other cardiac cycle is assisted. In the 1:4 setting, every fourth cardiac cycle is assisted. In the 1:8 setting,, every eighth cardiac cycle is assisted.

10. PUMP

Push-button switches that control operation of the balloon pumping action.

OFF: Stops operation of the pump, and clears any diagnostic messages.

ON: Automatically fills pneumatic system to +5 mm Hg pressure, and starts pumping in the manual mode.

AUTO: Activates automatic gas surveillance and maintenance functions.

11. DISPLAY

Push-button switch that allows operator to "freeze" the waveform portions of the display. Pushing the switch again clears the frozen waveforms and returns the display to real time.

12. TILT ADJUST

Recessed handle mechanism that allows operator to change the viewing angle of the display and controls for maximum visibility and to minimize the height of Model 3010 when transporting the patient in an ambulance.

13. AC

Indicator lamp lights when Model 3010 is powered from the AC power line.

14. POWER

Three-position switch that allows the operator to select AC or battery operation.

15. BATTERY/FLASH LOW

Indicator lamp lights steadily when Model 3010 is powered from the internal battery supply. Indicator flashes to alert operator that the reserve capacity of the battery is low.

16. VOLUME ADJUST

Continuously variable control by which the operator regulates the volume of helium gas displaced into the balloon. An electrical interlock prevents the operator from setting the volume above the allowable limits for each size balloon.

17. ARTERIAL PRESSURE SENSITIVITY

Continuously variable control that allows operator to adjust amplifier's output to agree with externally applied manometer pressure. This control normally does not require readjustment as long as the pressure system is in use; therefore a locking mechanism is provided to prevent inadvertent changes in the control's setting. This control also adjusts the Aux In gain (automatically calibrated to 100 mm Hg per volt when set fully counterclockwise).

18. ARTERIAL PRESSURE ZERO ADJUST

Continuously variable control that allows operator to adjust the zero baseline of the external pressure transducer with no pressure applied. This control normally does not require readjustment as long as the pressure system is in use; therefore a locking mechanism is provided to prevent inadvertent changes in the control's setting.

19. RECORDER MODE SELECT

A set of six push-button switches that allow the operator to select the chart drive speed (25 or 50 mm per second) when recording ECG or arterial pressure; the chart drive automatically operates at 100 mm per hour when recording cardiac output. Any auxiliary signal connected to the Aux In jack (see Input/output connections) is recorded when the Art Press switch is depressed. A marker pen records the assist interval when in the ECG or arterial pressure triggering modes.

20. POSITION

A continuously variable control that allows the operator to set the recording stylus position when recording ECG. For arterial pressure and cardiac output recording, the stylus is automatically calibrated. (Position of the marker stylus is fixed.)

21. HELIUM TANK COMPARTMENT

Hinged cover provides access to interior compartment where helium tank, regulator, cold trap drain, and external battery connection are located.

22. HELIUM TANK REGULATOR

Pressure reduction system that converts the high-pressure output from the helium tank to a regulated 5 pounds per square inch. A pressure gauge provides the operator with an accurate reading of the pressure in the tank; a low pressure alarm provides a diagnostic display if the regulated tank pressure depletes to 3 pounds per square inch.

23. BATTERY WIRING

Connections are made to the internal battery supply.

24. COLD TRAP DRAIN

A push-button actuated drain that allows easy removal of condensed water from the helium system.

Abbreviated operation

A. Start before pumping
   1. Wall power connected.
   2. Front panel power switch on (allow 5-minute warm-up, but continue start-up and check out). (Turn Alarm Volume control down.)
   3. Helium tank on (minimum 200 pounds per square inch); *have spare tank available*.
   4. Electrode placement. Five-lead cable is required. Leads I, II, III, AVR, AVF, AVL, and V must be operative. Suggested lead placement for use with the Avco Model 10 is point of shoulders for arm leads or point of hips for legs. V is appro-

priate for the V lead. These are suggested positions. It is very important to note that electrode position should be such that muscle artifact or surgical team interference is minimized. Prophylactic preoperative placement of the electrodes and cable is beneficial.

5. Plug ECG cable into back of Model 10 console; depress ECG Skin button.
6. Set height of QR segment between 2.0 and 2.5 divisions on display; observe red band on ECG and flashing heart rate asterisk. Observe and ensure regular flashing. The asterisk and red band confirm that the computer is processing the signal. If the red asterisk is flashing irregularly, adjustments should be made to the gain or lead selection.

B. Purging procedure
   1. Set balloon on half volume:
      a. Press Assist Interval control (weaning control) to 1 to 2.
      b. Place beginning of red band on peak of T wave (inflate), and place end of red band before R wave (deflate).
   2. Connect balloon hookup plug to back of console.
   3. Have surgeon open purge vent hole by pulling back on rubber sleeve (Fig. 24-11).
   4. Press Off button to clear any diagnostic messages.
   5. Press On button and release; system is purging (allow 1 minute).
   6. Close purge valve hole by sliding back rubber sleeve over hole.
   7. Adjust timing based on arterial pressure waveform.
   8. Press Off button.
   9. Set balloon to full volume.
   10. Return Assist Interval to 1:1.
   11. Press Off.
   12. Press On (confirm balloon filling).
   13. Press Auto, check when necessary.

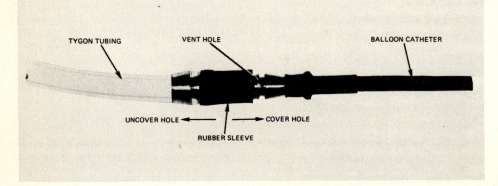

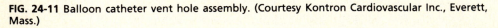

FIG. 24-11 Balloon catheter vent hole assembly. (Courtesy Kontron Cardiovascular Inc., Everett, Mass.)

Timing. Timing is achieved by monitoring the patient's arterial waveform and following the criteria for proper timing as described in Chapter 15.

Routine checks. Emptying the water trap is a necessary routine check. The water vapor trap is a thermoelectric system that cools the helium and removes moisture. Condensate is brought to the helium tank compartment via a plastic line. A push-button operated valve (Fig. 24-1, helium tank compartment) allows easy removal of the moisture.

NOTE: To reduce nonessential power drains, the water vapor trap is nonoperative during battery operation.

When the trap requires emptying, a diagnostic message flashes in yellow on the display screen. To empty the trap, perform the following:

1. Turn the pump off by depressing the Pump Off switch.
2. Open the helium tank compartment; place a paper cup under the drain; depress the push button.
3. Close the compartment's door.
4. Restart pumping by depressing On to fill the pneumatic system and initiate manual mode pumping; depress Auto to initiate automatic mode pumping.

Manual mode pumping requires regular monitoring of the balloon pressure at least every 30 minutes. Reload balloon line pressure; it should not drop more than 20 mm Hg in 5 minutes. This rate is equivalent to a gas loss of 0.5 cc per minute, which is the alarm level for a leak in the automatic mode. Reload the pneumatic system by momentarily depressing the Pump Off switch and then the Pump On switch whenever the pressure reaches −20 mm Hg.

To check for a leak, measure the drop in balloon pressure from the 0 mm Hg reference for a 5-minute period. If balloon pressure falls more than 20 mm Hg in 5 minutes, assume a leak has developed in either the IABP console or the balloon line.

Alarms. If a system malfunction develops, the Model 10 IABP shuts down. Deflate the balloon in the patient's aorta; open the console vent valves; alert the operator. A system shutdown produces an audible, interrupted alarm tone to alert the operator; the Off indicator lights, and a diagnostic statement informs the operator of possible causes for the shutdown. The system shuts down if any of the following conditions occur:

1. Insufficient balloon pressure. The inflation pressure must be above 50 mm Hg at least once each 30 seconds.
2. Excessively high volume setting of the Volume Adjust control. The volume setting exceeds the nominal design volume for the balloon.
3. Helium pressure loss. There is a possible leak in the pneumatic system or the balloon.
4. Gas loading failure. System does not start up because of a possible leak in the pneumatic system or the balloon.
5. Loss of trigger signal. The ECG (or arterial pressure) is not available, too noisy, or erratic.
6. Improper balloon deflation. Balloon does not deflate properly.

7. High peak pressure. Pressure in the pneumatic system exceeds +300 mm Hg at peak, or +20 mm Hg steady state.
8. Changing from ECG to arterial pressure triggering (or arterial pressure to ECG triggering) provides a reminder to readjust the timing settings.

Brief troubleshooting

Insufficient helium pressure

PROBABLE CAUSE. The balloon pressure does not exceed +50 mm Hg in the 30 seconds before shutdown. This is indicative of a volume setting at 00 cc (a depleted helium supply), a leak in the pneumatic system, or a leak in the balloon.

RECOMMENDED ACTION. Examine the volume setting on the screen and the helium supply for adequate reserve. Reload the gas system, and initiate manual mode pumping. Observe the balloon pressure waveform's zero plateau, and determine the time it takes for pressure to decrease from +5 to −5 mm Hg. If −5 mm Hg is reached in 60 seconds or less, a leak exists. Observe the balloon waveform, and verify that the pressure exceeds +50 mm Hg once each assisted cycle.

Improper balloon deflation

PROBABLE CAUSE. Patient sneezes or coughs, end-expiratory pressure is positive, balloon in aorta is too tight, percutaneous balloon is not totally unwrapped, there is a kink in the catheter, balloon is a false lumen (Fig. 24-12).

RECOMMENDED ACTION.
1. Reduce volume if balloon is too tight in the aorta, and observe a normal balloon pressure waveform.
2. Make sure the percutaneous balloon is unwrapped.
3. Check fluoroscopy or chest x-ray film for balloon position in the aorta.
4. Check for kinks in the catheter or connecting tubing.

High volume setting

PROBABLE CAUSE. The Volume Meter setting exceeds the nominal volume for the balloon connected to the console, or the balloon's connector end is not hooked up properly to the console.

RECOMMENDED ACTION. Check the balloon's connection with the receptacle on the console. Check the setting of the Volume Meter; decrease the setting to coincide with the volume of the balloon. If the catheter or balloon is broken, replace it.

Pressure loss

PROBABLE CAUSE. Probable causes include low gas pressure, helium loss at a high rate, or a severe arrhythmia. Gas pressure does not refill in the automatic mode when −5 mm Hg pressure is reached. A low helium reserve or high rate of loss may prevent the pressure from reaching a proper loaded condition. A high rate of loss may cause the pressure to decrease to −20 mm Hg. In the automatic mode, pumping action shuts down. If the pump requires two refills within 1 minute in the automatic mode, pumping action will shut down. Noisy ECG or severe arrhythmias cause low pressures to be measured. In the automatic mode, pumping action shuts down.

RECOMMENDED ACTION. To locate the cause of this alarm:
1. Check for a depleted helium supply. Lack of pressure reserve may prevent filling of the system.

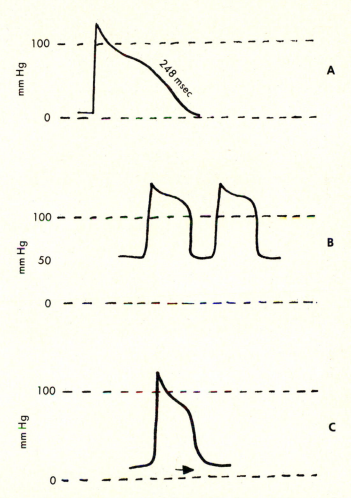

FIG. 24-12 A, From activation of command to deflate until balloon pressure waveform crosses zero baseline, time lapse exceeds 248 msec. **B,** Balloon pressure exceeds +50 msec for longer than 2 seconds. **C,** Deflation waveform never crosses zero baseline in particular clinical event.

2. Check the pneumatic system's connections and tubing for kinks and leaks. If blood is present in the balloon line, the surgical unit must be called for removal and replacement of the balloon. Reload the gas system, and initiate manual pumping.
3. Make sure O ring has been removed from the balloon connector. Observe the balloon pressure waveform's zero plateau, and determine the time it takes for the pressure to decrease from $+5$ to -5 mm Hg. If 5 mm Hg is reached in 60 seconds or less, a leak still exists. If there is no leak in the system, check the ECG waveform for proper triggering. If severe arrhythmias are present, the patient may have to receive pump assist in the manual mode to prevent shutdown.

Loading failure

PROBABLE CAUSE. Manual mode pumping could not be initiated because of an inability to load the pneumatic system. This is defined as the system not reaching $+5$ mm Hg pressure within 70 seconds.

RECOMMENDED ACTION. Check helium bottle pressure, pneumatic system's connections and tubing for leaks, bleed purge valves for leaks, and balloon's connection to the console.

Loss of triggering

PROBABLE CAUSE. The ECG signal is not available, too noisy, or erratic. The triggering logic cannot identify the QRS complex reliably, and 10 seconds has elapsed from the last trigger signal.

RECOMMENDED ACTION FOR ECG TRIGGERING. Check the display for an ECG waveform. If none is present, check the patient's state, electrode placement, patient cable connections, and console connections. If an external monitor is processing the ECG, check the waveform on the monitor and the connections from the monitor to the ECG Mon In connector. If the waveform amplitude is substantially greater or less than two divisions, readjust the ECG Gain control. If the waveform is erratic or noisy, reapply electrode paste, or replace disposable electrodes. If the R-wave width exceeds 130, select another configuration using the Lead Select switch.

NOTE: If an external monitor is being used, the console's Lead Select switch is inoperative. The lead configuration must be changed at the external monitor.

RECOMMENDED ACTION FOR ARTERIAL PRESSURE TRIGGERING. Check and adjust the transducer calibration for 100 mm Hg per volt. If the trigger signal is present but there is no red overtrace on the assisted interval, there is an internal failure. The failure may be in the timing circuitry or the display. The pump should be used on the patient in an attempt to isolate the failure.

If an ECG waveform cannot be obtained for triggering the pump, select arterial pressure triggering. The R-wave simulator should only be used with the physician's knowledge and orders.

NOTE: When switching to arterial pressure triggering, readjust the timing intervals.

High pressure

PROBABLE CAUSE. There is a possible kink in a pneumatic line, which is evidenced by the pressure being above +20 mm Hg during the zero plateau in automatic mode and the pressure exceeding +300 mm Hg at any point in manual or automatic mode.

RECOMMENDED ACTION. Check the pneumatic lines, catheter, and plastic tubing for kinks. Restart the pumping.

• • •

For further information on the Kontron Pump contact:

Kontron Cardiovascular, Inc.
9 Plymouth Street
Everett, Mass. 02149
(Telephone 800-343-3297 or [617] 389-6400)

SMEC Model 1300i[12, 13] (Fig. 24-13)

The SMEC Model 1300i affords a very lightweight, portable system, especially crafted for ambulance and aircraft transport. The patented monitor screen rotates through 360°, providing visibility from any part of the room, without turning the entire system. In displays control arterial pressure (balloon off) and augmented arterial pressure (balloon on) are simultaneously superimposed. A unique balloon deflation signal indicates the actual balloon deflation and inflation, the pneumatic delay in the balloon catheter, and possible misplacement of the balloon without the use of fluoroscopy. A photocell brightness control automatically adjusts the intensity of the screen for varying room lighting.

A telewire telemetry system permits patient isolation and a good quality R wave for precise triggering. Two light pens afford easy timing setup. The arterial pressure trace is intensified to illustrate exactly where the deflate and inflate light pens are positioned before the balloon is turned on. With the balloon on, the console intensifies the arterial pressure trace where the balloon is deflated.

The top panel allows various types of assist for versatility. Controls not used in one mode are automatically disabled for simplicity. The balloon isolation chamber is charged automatically to the exact balloon volume selected. The changeover to portable power is automatic whenever the console is unplugged. Gas bottles are not required with this 100% electric system.

Specifications

Depth (elevator): 17.75 inches
Height × width: 28.5+ tube × 35.8 inches
Weight: 169 pounds per 3 weeks helium
Cabinet: Aluminum
Portable power: 100% battery or aircraft type power
Portable time: 25 minutes, for 80 minutes add 19 pounds
Batteries and cost: 24 VDC, $70 to $112
Maximum pump performance: 200 beats per minute
Rate: 60 cc with full vacuum and pressure
Gas: Helium or air

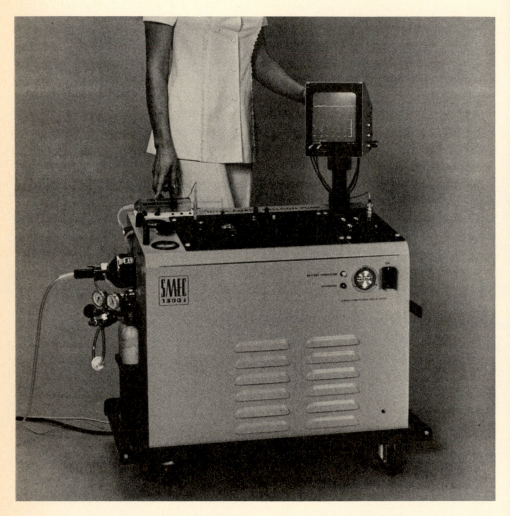

FIG. 24-13 SMEC Model 1300i. (Courtesy SMEC, Inc., Cookeville, Tenn.)

Balloon charging: Automatic
Balloon size, conv[0]1 and average cost: 6 to 60 cc, $220 to $250
Percutaneous sizes and cost: 30, 40, 50 cc per $420/with introducer set
Safety: System type—Closed
    Leak detector—Yes
    Sensitivity—12% per hour
    Slave chamber replacement—$38
Timing of balloon: ECG pickup—Telemetry
    Predetermined—Systole
    Beat by beat—Yes
    Atrial fibrillation—Yes
    Premature ventricular contractions—Yes
    Change in rate—No factor
    Pressure triggering—Yes
    Timing controls—Light pens
Monitor: Viewing angle—any direction
    Balloon off arterial pressure—Yes
    Balloon signal—Balloon volume
PAD versatility: Yes
Pacemaker versatility: Built-in
Training Aids: User instruments—Free videotape
    Servicing—Videotapes and manual
    Simulator—Pneumatic available for sale

Abbreviated operator's manual

A. Position equipment for use
    1. Plug into suitable outlet.
    2. Turn on console (switch at front of console).
    3. Turn balloon adapter off as necessary.
B. Establish ECG trigger
    1. Using Telewire transmitter for direct patient connection:
        a. Place electrodes for best Q or R wave (not an S-wave trigger).
        b. Connect Telewire extension; turn on (temporary light indicates working battery).
    2. As alternative, slave balloon system off wall monitor, using phone jack on console (this disables Telewire). Make sure ECG signal is not delayed.
    3. Select fast-response trigger mode; use "filter artifact" to eliminate mistriggering, as necessary.
    4. Adjust ECG Trigger Sensitivity for reliable trigger.
C. Establish pressure tracing
    With transducer (Size set greater than 0) vented to air, balance as follows, using pressure line controls:
        a. Turn balance control until pressure line trace is exactly on the threshold of

moving upward from the 0 pressure line on the screen (clockwise moves it up; counterclockwise moves it down).

   b. The Size calibration should be checked periodically with a manometer, using the reference pressure readout on the center panel.

 2. Slave pressure (channel 2) to hospital monitor requires no balancing. Calibrate using reference pressure readout.

D. Before connecting console to patient

 1. Select.

   a. Set 200 mm Hg pressure.

   b. ECG triggered, every beat.

   c. Pacemaker off.

 2. Set light pens. For an R-wave trigger, the left Deflate light pen is usually at the extreme left; the right Inflate light pen is a thumb's width to the right.

 3. Store Balloon Off arterial pressure.

 4. Set balloon adapter displacement *only with the patient balloon disconnected* with the balloon adapter correctly charged with water.

E. Connect patient balloon extension to console

 1. Purge adapter twice (helium on); reset alarms; turn balloon on.

   a. In case of leak alarm, purge 1×; reset; turn balloon on.

 2. Check augmentation, and readjust light pens.

Timing. Since the console pneumatic response is exceptionally fast, the balloon is timed to deflate for a predetermined interval with systole and simply remains inflated for the rest of the time, corresponding to diastole. Thereby the balloon is inflated at all times and is simply triggered to deflation by an R wave. Since an R wave exists for a ventricular contraction, the balloon timing is unaffected by changes in rate.

Routine checks

Pressure adjustment

1. Never exceed 250 mm Hg console pressure or peak augmented arterial pressure +100 mm Hg.

2. If the bright portion of the pressure trace is wider than the light pen spacing, the balloon may not be inflating completely because:

   a. Console pressure may be too low.

   b. Balloon adapter displacement setting is too high.

   c. Adapter is not fully charged with water.

   d. Balloon is occlusive or twisted.

3. For augmentation with aortic insufficiency, reduce inflate pressure for less diastolic augmentation while maintaining systolic pressure reduction. In case of poor triggering, adjust ECG trigger sensitivity, reposition electrodes, or select filter artifact trigger mode (delays deflate).

4. At least every 4 hours purge balloon adapter twice (turn balloon off and stopcock to purge until light extinguishes).

5. Store balloon off arterial pressure; reset alarms; turn balloon on; check augmentation.

Diaphragm
1. Change after 250 hours of pumping.
   a. Disconnect balloon; turn console off; set displacement to 60 cc.
   b. Open all three clasps; remove only blue diaphragm, not clear diaphragm.
   c. Clean inside of front dome with a moist cloth; replace diaphragm, convex side facing OUT, red gasket on outside.
   e. Engage all clasps; and *only then* close clasps; reset balloon displacement.

Leak alarms during patient use
1. For the first alarm that cannot be reset without repurging:
   a. If there is blood in the catheter, the balloon is defective.
   b. Otherwise check all balloon connections; purge and turn balloon back on.
2. For the second leak alarm (within 1 hour) that cannot be reset without repurging:
   a. If there is blood in the catheter, the balloon is defective.
   b. Reduce Syringe Setting by 5 to 11 cc; reset alarm and continue to augment if possible, *without* repurging. (This also eliminates erratic leak alarms for competitive balloons that do not unwind.)
   c. For purging at the regular interval, set to original volume for purging and reduce by 5 cc to resume pumping.
3. For the third leak alarm (within 1 hour) that cannot be reset without repurging, change the diaphragm per Supplement no. 1, item 5.
4. Any subsequent leak alarm within 1 hour indicates that the balloon may have a leak and should be changed, unless the leak alarm can be identified to be in other than the balloon. Heparinize if augmentation is discontinued for more than 5 minutes.

● ● ●

For additional information on the SMEC Pump contact:

Vitol/Med Systems Corporation
Box 3553
Englewood, Colo., 80155
(Telephone [303] 841-3199)

SMEC
Rt. 7, Box 354
Cookeville, Tenn., 38501
(Telephone [615] 537-6505)

Intra-aortic balloon designs

Each manufacturer provides a variety of intra-aortic balloons. Clinical studies have established balloon sizes and capabilities for individual needs. Single-, double-, and triple-chambered designs afford segmented balloon inflation, optimizing nonocclusive, nonthrombogenic properties.

Another newer innovation is the balloon mounted on a double-lumen catheter. Through the central lumen of this balloon arterial pressure can be monitored, a guide wire can be passed to aid in difficult insertions, and a contrast medium can be injected to define obstructions or to ensure proper balloon positioning. The percutaneous balloon can be inserted in less than 10 minutes, using the Seldinger technique, as compared with the 30 to 45 minutes necessary for surgical insertion of conventional balloons.

Emergency guidelines for Kontron/Datascope IABP console substitution

Balloon pumps, like other instrumentation, are subject to occasional malfunction. Console failure could further compromise a hemodynamically pump-dependent patient; an implanted balloon that remains deflated in situ in the thoracic aorta could cause clots to develop on its surface. Replacing the inoperable pump with another console of the same type is the most desirable alternative. However, if the only replacement console available is one made by another manufacturer, the implanted balloon can be driven by adopting the in situ balloon to the alternate console. Such improvisation saves time and rescues the patient from further operative intervention.

The University of Washington School of Medicine in Seattle has established guidelines for the emergency driving of a Datascope pump console with a Kontron (formerly Avco) balloon and a Kontron pump console, using a Datascope balloon catheter.[1] The following is a summary of their publication. The authors recommend four factors:

1. An adequate electrogram should be obtained.
2. Arterial pressure output must be maintained.
3. A simple, gas-tight connection is necessary to join the balloon catheter with the pump console.
4. Optimal balloon fill volumes must be determined.

Kontron (Avco) balloon with Datascope console

The Kontron balloon catheter is joined to the Datascope balloon chamber by a standard tapered male to male Luer fitting (4.0 to 4.2 mm) (Fig. 24-14). After purging the system with CO_2, the rubber exhaust sleeve is closed, and the system is evacuated with a large syringe in the usual manner. The safety chamber is filled with a volume of 50 to 52 cc for a 40 cc Kontron balloon. The Datascope console is operated according to the manufacturer's instructions.

Datascope balloon with Kontron console

The Datascope balloon is attached to the Kontron console by interposing a section of salvaged Kontron tigon tubing and a 40 cc pin connector. The Kontron tubing is severed between the rubber exhaust sleeve and the hard fiber catheter. The Datascope catheter is inserted into the end of the Kontron tubing (Fig. 24-15). The system is purged with helium in the usual manner through the rubber sleeve. A fill volume of 30 cc is recommended for a 30 cc dual-chamber Datascope balloon and 33 to 34 cc for a 35 cc dual-chamber Datascope balloon. The vent sleeve is closed, and the Kontron pump is operated according to the manufacturer's instructions.

The most difficult problem encountered with the exchange is that of determining proper fill volumes. Overfill can delay deflation and risk balloon rupture. Underinflation prohibits full expansion, increasing risk of thrombus formation on the balloon surface.

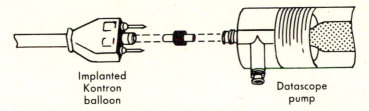

FIG. 24-14 Connection of implanted Kontron balloon catheter to Datascope pump console. Tapered (4.0 to 4.2 mm) metal connector is inserted into Kontron balloon connector and Datascope console safety chamber. (Courtesy Kontron Cardiovascular Inc., Everett, Mass. and Datascope Corp., Paramus, N.J.)

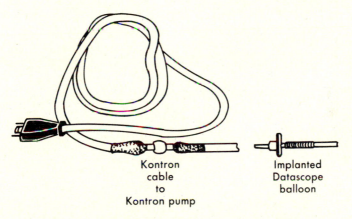

FIG. 24-15 Connection of implanted Datascope balloon catheter to Kontron pump. Datascope balloon is joined to Kontron pump console by means of salvaged Kontron balloon tubing. (Courtesy Datascope Corp., Paramus, N.J., and Kontron Cardiovascular Inc., Everett, Mass.)

Optimal fill volumes were determined by the authors by in vitro pressure-volume curves and by in vivo pressure augmentation.

Use of CO_2 versus helium in IABP

Theoretically differences exist between helium and CO_2 but the practical significance of these differences has not been clinically demonstrated. The shuttle gas moves in and out of the balloon; the driving gas operates the pneumatics of the system. Kontron and SMEC pumps employ helium, Hoek Loos uses CO_2, and Datascope can use either gas.

Inflate-deflate duration

Helium is less dense than CO_2; density is the primary determinant of resistance to turbulent flow. Therefore helium affords faster inflation and deflation of a balloon. *Health Devices*[4] confirmed the efficacy of rapid gas movement in and out of a balloon by using CO_2 in the SMEC and Kontron units and helium in the Datascope unit. Inflation and deflation times of the SMEC and Kontron units almost doubled; Datascope's inflation-deflation cycle was reduced by 40 to 600 msec with the use of helium.

Kayser and associates[8] confirmed that helium could inflate and deflate a balloon in two thirds the time required by CO_2 in the same driving system. Three different driving gases (CO_2, helium, and air) were tested in the Hoek Loos, Datascope System 80, and Avco-7 pumps. The response time was shortest with helium in all three pumps.[14]

Theoretically it seems feasible that a more rapid inflate-deflate cycle and a longer inflation duration would benefit the patient hemodynamically, but no published study investigates and confirms this hypothesis.

Safety comparison of helium and CO_2

CO_2 is 80 times more soluble than helium in water,[5] and it presumably would be absorbed into the blood more rapidly in the event of balloon rupture or leakage. Because of the difference in solubility, CO_2 bubbles more quickly dissipate into smaller bubbles when absorbed into blood than do helium bubbles; neither gas disappears from the bloodstream. Furman and associates[5] confirmed that a bubble as small as 0.25 cc can occlude a coronary artery.

The ratio of a bubble's surface area to exposed blood volume reflects a bubble's ability to shrink. Large bubbles do not shrink as quickly as small bubbles. Dogs have been demonstrated to survive injections of less than 3 cc per kilogram of CO_2 into the left ventricle, but injections of 4.5 cc per kilogram or greater were lethal.[10] Helium (7 cc per kilogram) injected into dogs' left ventricles was definitely lethal.[5] The gas dissipated into the blood from the thoracic aorta was also demonstrated to travel retrogradely to the aortic arch, cerebral vessels, and heart and distally to the abdominal aorta. These studies suggested that injected volumes of either helium or CO_2 greater than 30 cc may be life threatening, and the differences between CO_2 and helium may be less significant in vivo than in theory. Also, patients have been reported to survive both CO_2 and helium-containing balloon rupture with no apparent consequences.

Gas losses from the balloon can occur through diffusional losses, small balloon leaks, or balloon rupture.[4] The primary concern with gas diffusion out of the balloon or pneumatic system continues to be with loss of augmentation over time.

Theoretical performance advantages have been documented with use of helium gas. However, the safety advantage of CO_2 is questionable based on animal studies. Further in vivo human studies are required, however, to affirm the safety superiority of one gas over another.

Acknowledgments

Appreciation is extended to the following:

Datascope Corp., Hoek Loos, Kontron, and SMEC Corp. for permission to reproduce illustrations and to present information from their marketing literature.

Donna Goebel, RN, Datascope Corp.; Berenice Watring, RN, Kontron; and Peter Schiff, SMEC Corp. for their reviews of this chapter.

REFERENCES

1. Binford, J., and Hessel, E.: Emergency guidelines for AVCO/Datascope intra-aortic balloon pump console substitution, Ann. Thorac. Surg. **29:**381, 1980.
2. Datascope Corp.: Abbreviated operator's instructions for Datascope System 82 intra-aortic balloon pump, Paramus, N.J.
3. Datascope Corp.: Datascope System 82 intra-aortic balloon pump operating manual, Paramus, N.J.
4. ECRI: Evaluation: intra-aortic balloon pumps, Health Devices **11:**1, 1981.
5. Furman, S., et al.: Lethal sequelae of intra-aortic balloon rupture, Surgery **69:**121, 1971.
6. Hoek Loos Medical Group: Hoek Loos intra-aortic balloon pump: an advanced Netherlands product, The Netherlands.
7. Hoek Loos Medical Group: Hoek Loos intra-aortic balloon pump operator's manual, The Netherlands.
8. Kayser, K.L., et al.: Comparison of driving gases for IABPs, Med. Instru. **15:**51, 1981.
9. Kontron Medical Instruments: Avco intra-aortic balloon pump Model 10 operator's manual, Everett, Mass., 1976.
10. Kunkler, A., and King, H.: Comparison of air, oxygen and carbon dioxide embolization, Ann. Surg. **149:**95, 1959.
11. Rajani, R., et al.: Rupture of an intra-aortic balloon: a case report, J. Thorac. Cardiovasc. Surg. **79:**30, 1980.
12. Smec Inc.: The SMEC system for balloon assist, Cookeville, Tenn.
13. SMEC Newsletter **19,** Jan. 1982.
14. Tipler, D.R., and Ghadiali, P.E.: A comparative study of some technical aspects of three intra-aortic balloon pump systems, Intensive Care Med. **7:**91, 1981.

CHAPTER 25 **Complications**

Potential complications associated with IABP can be divided into four stages: (1) insertion, (2) counterpulsation, (3) balloon removal, and (4) following balloon removal.[33]

Stage 1: during balloon insertion

1. Dissection of the aorta
2. Dislodgement of plaque producing obstruction
3. Obstruction of femoral artery with severely compromised circulation to lower extremity
4. Inability to pass the balloon catheter

Stage 2: during pumping

1. Emboli to
   a. Head
   b. Upper or lower extremities
   c. Kidneys
   d. Gastrointestinal tract
   e. Spinal column
2. Thrombosis associated with prolonged immobilization
3. Thrombocytopenia
4. Infection
5. Rupture of the aorta
6. Compromised circulation to the leg
7. Compromised circulation because of improper balloon placement
   a. Too high
   b. Too low
8. Intensive care unit psychosis
9. Gas emboli
10. Bleeding
    a. Balloon insertion site
    b. Intravenous and invasive monitoring sites
    c. Stress ulcers
    d. Excessive laboratory work

11. Inability to wean
12. Air emboli through central lumen of catheter
13. Harmfully continued improper balloon timing

Stage 3: during removal

1. Dislodgement of plaque or emboli producing obstruction
2. Bleeding at site

Stage 4: following removal

1. Reversal or relapses of condition
2. Thrombosis
3. Emboli

Further elaboration of selected complications is presented to afford a more in-depth understanding of the cause from which the complication arises and to expand on the clinical course proceeding from the complication.

Complications related to duration of intra-aortic balloon assist

Complications observed do not appear to be related to the length of time that the intra-aortic balloon support is rendered. Two patients have been reported to have been maintained for periods of 34 and 35 days with an intra-aortic balloon counterpulsating in situ without complications.[15] Alpert's series of retrospective analysis of complications associated with balloon pumping did not associate length of pumping with incidence of complications.[1] This retrospective study suggested that patients who developed limb ischemia did so shortly after balloon insertion; there was no evidence that thrombotic complications increased with length of continued pumping.

The record duration of IABP via a femoral artery inserted balloon is 327 days. A patient at Mercy Hospital in Sacramento, California, survived this duration with a single balloon implant; he could not be weaned from the intra-aortic balloon before a suitable heart transplant donor was found. The balloon was fabricated from Cardiothane 51 polymer. Testing of the balloon following removal revealed a highly satisfactory performance of this material. Changes in chemical composition did not affect its blood compatibility. There was a minimum of thrombus formation, very little protein deposit and lipid uptake, and no calcification. Decrease in mechanical properties was not significant enough to affect the balloon's physical performance.[3]

Rupture of a balloon

In the laboratory, rupture of an intra-aortic balloon has been demonstrated as a result of intrinsic weakness of the balloon itself so that it cannot accept repeated inflation and deflation; poor design of the scam, which is infrequently present at one end of the balloon; and overinflation of the balloon with a pressure beyond its capacity.[11]

Rupture in the clinical setting is extremely rare. In three reported cases of rupture,[21,27,28] one patient died of a massive gas embolism, and the other two recovered without complications. Analysis of one balloon removed following rupture[27] revealed a

2×2 mm perforation in the proximal segment. Electron microscopic analysis verified that the leak was caused by a sharp protruding plaque. Other abraded areas had not been perforated. Therefore even though rupture is rare, such a complication has been documented and has verified the need for continuous observation.

Balloon rupture is documented by appearance of blood inside the catheter. Communication between the balloon chamber and aortic lumen occurs with rupture. The diastolic arterial waveform augmented pressure may markedly decrease or disappear all together. Once blood is detected in the balloon catheter, the console must be shut off and the balloon immediately removed. Sensitive leaking devices shut down the pumping action and sound an alarm on consoles that have gas leak detection incorporated into the alarm system.

Effects of intravascular air dispersement following balloon rupture. As early as 1769, Morgagni[22] reported the catastrophic sequelae of air embolism. Arterial pressure has been documented to be high enough to drive air emboli from the arterial to the venous system, thus guaranteeing the presence of air in virtually all body tissues.[9] Arterial gas emboli are essentially nonexistent when air is introduced on the venous side of the circulation[24] where the pressures are inadequate to force the air retrogradely into the arterial side, unless a right-to-left intracardiac communication is present.

Cineangiographic studies have demonstrated that gas in the left ventricle tends to dissipate ventricular force, not so much by compression of a gaseous mass, but by the expenditure of energy moving the gas in and out of the left ventricle and atrium.[11]

Laboratory research performed on the effect of helium release after balloon rupture yielded the following results[11]:

1. Small volumes of helium as low as 30 cc were adequate to kill some dogs within 3 minutes.
2. In other trials, increments of 30 cc up to 300 cc were tolerated before cessation of cardiac activity occurred.
3. The smallest volume of injected helium is widely distributed throughout all of the major arteries and veins and can be visualized within 3 minutes in the cerebral and coronary arteries and veins, the right ventricle, and the coronary sinus, which forms an effective barrier against blood flow.
4. With release of helium in the descending thoracic aorta, the gas immediately traveled retrogradely to the aortic arch, cerebral vessels, and heart and antegradely to the vessels of the abdominal viscera.
5. Helium gas forms a readily compressible, space-occupying mass in the left ventricle, which evolves to a cessation of blood ejection. Both mitral and aortic valves are incompetent to helium.

In the presence of balloon rupture with release of helium, serious embolic consequences would likely occur if enough helium escapes into the arterial tree. Lethal embolization may be avoided if the patient can be treated with hyperbaric decompression.

Air embolism secondary to pulsatile assist device (PAD) rupture treated with the hyperbaric chamber

Air embolism has been documented secondary to rupture of the PAD, which is described in Chapter 29. This disposable device consists of a thin, polyurethane balloon or "skin" inside a rigid chamber that is connected to the balloon pump console. The PAD is operated with compressed air at 9 pounds per square inch of pressure. The PAD is positioned in the arterial line of the heart-lung by-pass setup, about 30 cm from the entrance of the arterial cannula into the ascending aorta. Augmentation of diastolic coronary artery flow is effected as the pulsatile assist chamber rapidly collapses in diastole and inflates in systole. A case of PAD rupture and air embolism that was treated by hyperbaric decompression has been described by Tomatis[33] at Grand Rapids, Michigan.

> A 60-year-old man was placed on PAD at the initiation of an aortic valve replacement and a double vein bypass grafting procedure. After 5 minutes of pumping, the skin of the PAD device ruptured, and a massive amount of air was injected into the ascending aorta. The patient was placed in Trendelenburg position and cooled in deep hypothermia with cardiopulmonary bypass. He was given 16 mg of methylprednisolone intravenously; the valve replacement and revascularization were then carried out. Hypothermia lowered brain metabolism, and steroid administration possibly caused a reduction of the endothelial chemical inflammation in the bubble-capillary interface. Trendelenburg position directed the thrust of air away from the carotid arteries, and possibly by increasing venous return, improved laminar flow and reduced the size of bubbles. Following completion of the operation, the patient was partially rewarmed and placed in a hyperbaric chamber, compressed to 6 atmospheres absolute. He recovered completely with no residual deficits.

Vascular complications

Vascular complications of intra-aortic balloon counterpulsation occur predominately in patients with sclerotic peripheral arteries, whose borderline circulation is further compromised by catheter encroachment on the arterial lumen. Limb ischemia secondary to balloon pumping has been reported as a complication in 16% to 35% in one series of assisted patients who survived long enough for operative balloon removal.[1,21]

In a University of Cincinnati series[32] of 109 patients who received balloon pump assist, three suffered limb loss as a complication. All of them had atherosclerotic disease of the femoral vessels. Pain, pallor, limb cyanosis, mottling, and pulse loss was noted in each case. Thrombectomy was performed to reestablish circulation. Diagnostic angiography revealed arterial occlusion at the bifurcation of the popliteal artery.

Two of the three patients developed the onset of clinical evidence of vascular insufficiency in the lower extremities after counterpulsation had been discontinued. Sutorius[32] suggested that delayed peripheral vascular compromise following balloon removal may be the result of technical problems associated with balloon removal or that the cumulative effects of counterpulsation lead to a set of circumstances that favor the development of acute vascular insufficiency.

Vascular complications have not been reported in patients under 40 years of age.[19] After balloon pump support, however, serious peripheral vascular complications have been reported in as high as 36% of patients at risk (i.e., with evidence of compromised peripheral circulation before balloon insertion).[2]

If the dorsalis pedalis and posterior tibial pulses are easily palpable before and after femoral artery balloon insertion, Doppler examination is not necessary. In the event that these peripheral pulses are weakly palpated either before or after balloon insertion, ongoing Doppler arterial examination is recommended. Doppler ultrasound enables a more precise evaluation of these peripheral pulses. Further deterioration in the arterial supply to the extremity may require reconstructive procedures to preserve the viability of the extremity in which the intra-aortic balloon is inserted.

In view of documented arterial insufficiency after catheter removal, it seems appropriate to continue such peripheral pulse Doppler examinations on a daily basis for 4 to 5 days after balloon removal. Continued anticoagulation after balloon removal has also been suggested for patients with severe distal arterial disease.[32] Prophylactic anticoagulation may not prevent vascular insufficiency, but it may reduce the rate of clot propagation, thereby making reconstructive efforts feasible.

Distortion of hematological and biochemical values influenced by balloon counterpulsation

Objections to the use of balloon therapy are: (1) chronic contact with the aortic wall by balloon overinflation may lead to stripping of endothelium to precipitate mural thrombus formation; (2) nonphysiological eddy currents and turbulence created by the presence of a foreign object in the high velocity blood flow may cause trauma to aortic endothelium, leading to platelet thrombosis. Documented hematological changes reported include leukocytosis, reduction in serum albumin/globulin fraction ratio, and elevation in blood fibrinogen; all of these hematological disturbances have been noted as soon as 24 hours after pumping.[29] Examination of the stained aortic surface after 3 days of pumping in calves showed unequivocal stripping of the endothelium along with adhesion of mural thrombus to the luminal face of the aorta. Episodes of renal infarction occurred as well, probably arising from embolization of denuded endothelium. Stripping of the aortic endothelium resulted in spite of the careful fitting of the balloon to assure that the maximally inflated balloon occupied no more than 85% of the calf aortic lumen.[28]

Intimal tear

Myhre[23] and Durkman[10] have each reported two cases of intimal tear on insertion, which seemed to have no deleterious effect, either anatomically or physiologically, during balloon pumping. Decreased urine output and a fall in blood pressure were the only clues of less than optimum assist following initial clinical improvement after insertion. Although intimal tear occurred, resistance was not always encountered with femoral artery insertion. A postmortem segment of the aorta is illustrated in Fig. 25-1. The balloon catheter in this example entered the intima at the aortic bifurcation and reentered below the renal arteries.[23] In the absence of hypertension and secondary aortic dissection, Myhre speculated that an unknown number of patients who underwent balloon implantation may have survived aortic lesions, occurring with insertion, without apparent sequelae.

Paraplegia

Two case reports have been published on abdominal and lower limb paralysis developing 38 hours after balloon placement.[8] Postmortem examination on one patient disclosed the existence of a subadventitial aortic hematoma with an intact intima. The hematoma compromised the ostia of six intercostal arteries; vascular deficit at the thoracic level led to subsequent spinal medullar ischemia and paraplegia. There is little possibility of

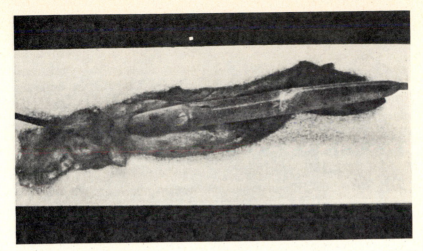

FIG. 25-1 Postmortem segment of aorta. Balloon catheter enters intima at aortic bifurcation and reenters below renal arteries. (From Myhre, J.A., et al.: Int. Surg. **64**:57, 1979.)

collateral circulation at the midthoracic aortic level, which increases the possibility of paraplegia from compromised segmental arteries at that level.[12] Therefore, it is possible for an intra-aortic balloon to cause a subadventitial aortic hematoma with resulting lower limb paralysis. Formation of subadventitial aortic hematoma and dissection on insertion have, however, been described by other surgeons without ensuing neurological symptoms.[4,5]

Complications following ascending aorta insertion

Since cannulation of the ascending aorta for balloon insertion is rarely performed, complications reported are few. Kaiser[14] reported a left hemiparesis after ascending aortic balloon insertion, presumably the result of cerebral emboli as the catheter passed the great vessels. McCabe[20] documented one case of fatal exsanguination from an infected ascending aortic arteriotomy site. Surgeons who have used the ascending aorta have described the tendency for the catheter to enter the abdominal branches. The intended position of the balloon catheter is just distal to the left subclavian artery, which with antegrade insertion, would place the tip in the abdominal aorta.[25] Therefore the potential does exist for inadvertent catheterization of the superior mesenteric artery during antegrade insertion (Fig. 25-2). Mesenteric thrombosis as a complication from ascending aorta insertion has been reported.[13] This potential complication verifies the need for fluoroscopic monitoring or intraoperative films to assure proper antegrade balloon placement.

Catheter fracture

Following satisfactory femoral artery balloon insertion (via percutaneous or cut-down approach), the balloon catheter may be sutured in place, and adhesive tape may be used for

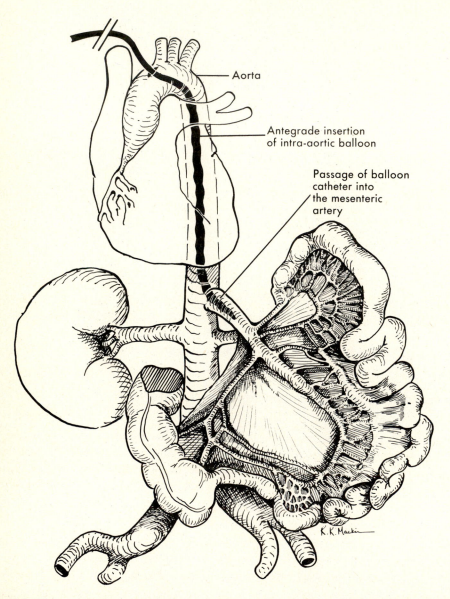

FIG. 25-2 With proper antegrade balloon placement, tip of balloon rests in abdominal aorta. Potential exists for inadvertent catheterization of mesenteric artery during insertion.

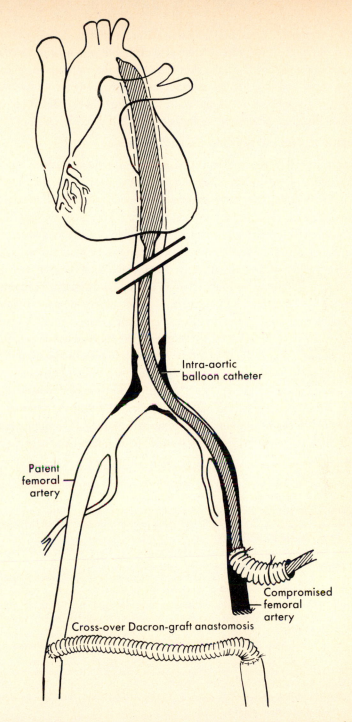

FIG. 25-3 Placement of femoral-to-femoral artery graft to allow for restoration of ischemic limb with balloon catheter remaining in situ. To minimize graft infection, proximal femoral artery is divided and oversewn just below balloon. Crossover Dacron graft anastomosis is completed to establish blood flow to affected leg.

greater security. Removal of residual adhesive during a routine dressing change or preparation of a sterile field before balloon removal is desirable. Acetone is commonly used to facilitate removal of adhesive from the skin and around the catheter. Application of acetone Vi-Drape spray and ether to the catheter causes the catheter to swell and become brittle so that a slight amount of torque causes fracture. Cidex, Betadine, alcohol, and benzoin produce no acute change in stiffness or durability of the catheter.[16]

Surgical femoral-to-femoral grafting for limb ischemia

Alpert and associates[2] reported a 16.5% rate of significant catheter-associated limb ischemia secondary to femoral artery balloon placement. It was also their observation that virtually all intra-aortic balloon catheters are enveloped by a thrombus as a result of (1) catheter thrombogenicity, (2) varying degrees of luminal compromise, and (3) the vascular stasis of diminishing left ventricular function. A buildup of thrombus around the catheter was always noted on removal. Since pericatheter thrombus formation is as prevalent in one femoroiliac artery as the other, Alpert advised against balloon removal and reinsertion in the opposite limb as a remedy for limb ischemia following insertion. Furthermore balloon removal from the ischemic limb with reinsertion on the other side necessitates a period of cessation of counterpulsation. Therefore because of the reasons cited, a femoral-to-femoral graft placement is recommended in the event that limb ischemia is a problem.

Placement of a femoral-to-femoral artery graft to allow for restoration of an ischemic limb while the balloon catheter rests in situ has been described by Parsonnet.[26] In an effort to minimize graft infection, the proximal compromised femoral vessel is divided and oversewn (Fig. 25-3) just below the balloon catheter. A crossover Dacron graft anastomosis is completed to establish blood flow to the affected leg. The implanted graft is not disturbed with balloon removal and is only removed if infection arises.

REFERENCES

1. Alpert, J., et al.: Limb ischemia during intra-aortic balloon pumping: indications for femorofemoral crossover graft, J. Thorac. Cardiovasc. Surg. **79:**729, 1980.
2. Alpert, J., et al.: Vascular complications of intra-aortic balloon pumping, Arch. Surg. **111:**1990, 1976.
3. Ashar, B., and Turcohg, L.R.: Analysis of longest IAB implant in human patient (327 days), Trans. Am. Soc. Artif. Intern. Organs **27:**372, 1981.
4. Beckman, D., et al.: Intra-operative unidirectional intra-aortic balloon pumping in the management of left ventricular power failure, J. Thorac. Cardiovasc. Surg. **70:**1010, 1975.
5. Biddle, T.L., et al.: Dissection of the aorta complication intra-aortic balloon counterpulsation, Am. Heart J. **92:**781, 1976.
6. Bierman, H.R., et al.: Intra-arterial catheterization of viscera in man, A.J.R. **66:**555, 1951.
7. Bron, K.M.: Selective visceral and total abdominal arteriography via the left axillary artery in the older age group, AJR **97:**432, 1966.
8. Criado, A., et al.: Paraplegia following balloon assistance, Scand. J. Thorac. Cardiovasc. Surg. **15:**103, 1981.
9. Durant, T.M., et al.: Body position in relation to venous air embolism: a roentgenologic study, Am. J. Med. Sci. **227:**509, 1954.
10. Durkman, W.B., et al.: Clinical and hemodynamic results of intra-aortic balloon pumping and surgery for cardiogenic shock, Circulation **46:**465, 1972.
11. Furman, S., et al.: Lethal sequelae of intra-aortic balloon rupture, Surgery **69:**121, 1971.
12. Gillilan, A.L.: The arterial blood supply of the human spinal cord, J. Comp. Neurol. **110:**75, 1958.
13. Jurmolowski, C.R., and Poirier, R.L.: Small bowel infarction complicating intra-aortic balloon counterpulsation via the ascending aorta, J. Thorac. Cardiovasc. Surg. **79:**735, 1980.

14. Kaiser, G.C., et al.: Intra-aortic balloon assistance, Ann, Thorac. Surg. **21**:487, 1976.
15. Kantrowitz, A.S., et al.: Initial clinical experience with intra-aortic balloon pumping in cardiogenic shock, JAMA **203**:113, 1968.
16. Karayannacos, P.E., et al.: Counterpulsation catheter fracture: an unexpected hazard, Ann. Thorac. Surg. **23**:276, 1977.
17. Kay, J.N., et al.: Retrograde ilioaortic dissection: a complication of common femoral artery perfusion during open heart surgery, Am. J. Surg. **111**:464, 1966.
18. Kindwall, E.P.: Massive surgical air embolism treated with brief recompression to six atmospheres followed by hyperbaric oxygen, Aerosp. Med. **44**:663, 1973.
19. Kozloff, L., et al.: Vascular trauma secondary to diagnostic and therapeutic procedures: cardiopulmonary bypass and intra-aortic balloon assist, Am. J. Surg. **140**:302, 1980.
20. McCabe, J.C., et al.: Complications of intra-aortic balloon insertion and counterpulsation, Circulation **57**:769, 1978.
21. McEnany, M.T., et al.: Clinical experience with intra-aortic balloon pump support in 728 patients, Circulation **58**(suppl.):124, 1978.
22. Morgagni, G.: The seats and causes of disease, London, 1769. (Translated by B. Alexander.)
23. Myhre, J.A., et al.: Mechanical problems in the use of the intra-aortic balloon, Int. Surg. **64**:57, 1979.
24. Nicks, R.: Arterial air embolism, Thorax **22**:320, 1967.
25. O'Rourke, M.F., et al.: Protection of the aortic arch and subclavian artery during intra-aortic balloon pumping, J. Thorac, Cardiovasc. Surg. **65**:543, 1973.
26. Parsonnet, V., et al.: Femorofemoral axillofemoral grafts: compromise or preference, Surgery **67**:26, 1970.
27. Rajani, R., et al.: Rupture of an intra-aorta balloon, J. Thorac. Cardiovasc. Surg. **79**:301, 1980.
28. Scheidt, S., et al.: Intra-aortic balloon counterpulsation in cardiogenic shock: report of a cooperative clinical trial, N. Engl. J. Med. **288**:979, 1973.
29. Schneider, M.D., et al.: Safety of intra-aortic balloon pumping part I, Throm. Res. **4**:387, 1974.
30. Stewart, D., et al.: Hypothermia in conjunction with hyperbaric oxygenation in the treatment of massive air embolism during cardiopulmonary bypass, Ann. Thorac. Surg. **24**:591, 1977.
31. Stoney, W.S., et al.: Air embolism and other accidents using pump oxygenators, Ann. Thorac. Surg. **29**:336, 1980.
32. Sutorius, D.J., et al.: Vascular complications as a result of intra-aortic balloon pumping, Am. Surg. **79**:512, 1979.
33. Tomatis, J., et al.: Massive arterial air embolism due to rupture of pulsatile assist device: successful treatment in the hyperbaric chamber, Ann. Thorac. Surg. **32**:604, 1981.
34. Watring, B.: Complications associated with intra-aortic balloon pumping, Inservice syllabus, Kontron Cardiovascular Inc., Everett, Mass., 1980.

CHAPTER 26 Weaning from the balloon pump

Protocol

A plan for weaning the patient from balloon assist begins at the onset of implementation. Twenty-five percent to thirty percent of patients with cardiogenic shock caused by myocardial infarction have been reported to have been weaned from balloon assist.[4] Weaning is governed by the hemodynamic status of the patient and is accomplished by decreasing the frequency of assistance from one balloon inflation per cardiac cycle to 1:2 and 1:3, etc., depending on the options of assist ratios available on the particular console in use. Usually each decreasing mode of assist is continued for 1 to 2 hours while the patient is carefully monitored.[6]

Observations essential to patients undergoing weaning include:
1. Presence or absence of chest pain
2. Urine output
3. Skin temperature
4. Cardiac and pulmonary auscultation
5. Sensorium
6. Vital signs
7. Hemodynamic measurements

If the patient remains stable, he is progressed through the less frequent ratios of assist. Finally the patient is advanced to the "flutter mode" on some pumps, in which a minute amount of gas enters the balloon and partially inflates it. Other pumps offer a 1:8 assist ratio. Flutter and/or 1:8 ratio assist provides no hemodynamic augmentation; this infrequent inflation is intended solely to prevent clot formation on the folds of a dormant balloon. Bolooki[2] suggested that the intra-aortic balloon may be discontinued if the following clinical findings prevail:

1. The clinical appearance of the patient is satisfactory, and peripheral evidence of low-output syndrome no longer persists.
2. Urinary output is more than 30 ml/hour with little need for diuretics.
3. Clinical evidence of congestive heart failure has disappeared with or without digitalis therapy.
4. The need for pressor agents is minimal (dopamine $\leq$ 5 mcg/kg/min).
5. Pulse rate has declined to 90 to 100 per minute without multifocal tandem or more than one premature ventricular complex per 10 seconds.

6. Emergency cardiac surgery is not planned.
7. Clinical improvement has persisted during the 1 to 4 hours of the weaning period.

Balloon dependence

Bolooki[2] defined the following criteria for balloon dependence:
1. Inability to wean from balloon assist with two attempts 24 hours apart
2. During the weaning process any of the following develop:
   a. Malignant arrhythmias
   b. Dopamine required in a dosage > 15 mcg/kg/min to maintain the systolic blood pressure > 90 mm Hg
   c. Clinical shock syndrome
   d. Cardiac index decreases > 20% or < 2 liters/min/m^2
   e. Pulmonary artery wedge pressure increases 20% or to 18 to 20 mm Hg
   f. Chest pain or new electrocardiogram changes develop

Austen and others[1] recommended that balloon-dependent patients be studied angiographically. Some patients demonstrate inoperable lesions. Balloon counterpulsation is therefore discontinued when it is proven to be ineffective, and death usually ensues. With the emergence of clinical use of the left ventricular assist device and the artificial heart, another avenue may be available to these patients. The criteria for coronary bypass in patients requiring balloon pump assist include the absence of preexisting debilitating cardiac disease and the angiographic demonstration of stenotic vessels that can be bypassed without major myocardial segments that are angiographically underperfused. Patients are accepted for surgery with large akinetic areas, but success is higher when there is some evidence of persistent motion in the area of ischemia or infarction. Surgical treatment of coronary artery disease, combined with balloon pumping, usually results in a 50% survival rate[1] (Fig. 26-1).

Quantitative indices of balloon dependence

The Cardiovascular Surgical Research Laboratories of the Texas Heart Institute[9] have attempted to quantitate patients who are balloon-pump dependent and to differentiate this group from retrievable patients who receive balloon pump assist following cardiogenic shock.[6] Balloon dependence was recognized by time-course trajectory plots of cardiac

TABLE 26-1 Quantitation of balloon-dependent patients after cardiogenic shock

Class	CI*	SVR†	Outcome
A	> 2.1	< 2100	All survivors
B	< 2.1	> 2100	7 to 14 days; patients finally died
C	< 2.1	> 2100	Died

Data summarized from Sturm, J.T., et al.: Artif. Organs 4:8, 1980.
*CI, = Cardiac index in liters/min/m^2.
†SVR, Systemic vascular resistance in dynes/sec/cm^{-5}.

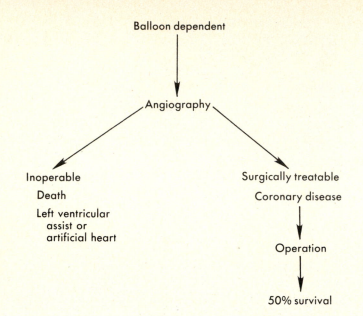

FIG. 26-1 Protocol for management of balloon-dependent patients.

index versus systemic vascular resistance. Class A patients (Cardiac index [CI] > 2.1 liters/min/m^2 with systemic vascular resistance [SVR] < 2100 dynes/sec/cm^{-5}) survived. Class B patients (CI < 2.1 liters/min/m^2 with SVR < 2100 dynes/sec/cm^{-5}) were balloon dependent for 7 to 14 days and eventually died. Patients whose conditions deteriorated to or remained in Class C (CI < 1.2 liters/min/m^2 and SVR > 2100 dynes/sec/cm^{-5}) died despite early balloon support, and they were considered irretrievable.

Antemortem guidelines were developed for identification of salvageable patients early in the course of treatment.

1. Patients receiving balloon support for cardiogenic shock after infarction, who achieve Class A status within 50 hours, appear stable enough to continue balloon pumping with the likelihood that further improvement will occur.

2. Patients receiving balloon support for cardiogenic shock after infarction, who deteriorate to or remain in Class C for more than 12 to 50 hours, appear irretrievable.

3. Patients receiving balloon support for cardiogenic shock after infarction, who maintain Class A for 50 hours, can undergo cardiac catheterization with coronary arteriography with continued balloon support to determine the presence of surgically amenable lesions.

4. Importantly there is a small group of patients receiving balloon support for cardiogenic shock after infarction, who tend to stabilize in Class B for greater than 50 hours. These patients are balloon dependent; they do not improve or deteriorate

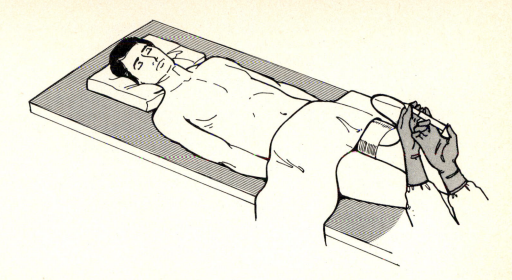

FIG. 26-2 If console must be removed from patient and balloon left in situ temporarily, it must be manually inflated and deflated with syringe one to two times every 5 to 10 minutes to prevent blood stasis and thrombis formation in balloon folds.

rapidly. They should undergo cardiac catheterization. If surgically amenable lesions are not found, such patients could possibly be considered as candidates for left ventricular assist device implantation, such as a bridge to cardiac allografting.

Manual balloon inflation

The rare situation may arise when the pump console may need to be detached from the patient for urgent use on another patient before a physician is available to remove the balloon. The console would only be disconnected if the patient had demonstrated his readiness to be removed from counterpulsation assist. It is recommended that an intra-aortic balloon not be left immobile in the aorta for more than a period of 20 to 30 minutes because of the risk of clot formation on the folds of the dormant balloon.[3,5]

If balloon removal during the time frame of 20 to 30 minutes is impossible, some movement of the balloon membrane must be imposed to prevent thrombus formation. Balloon membrane movement is accomplished by disconnecting the external balloon catheter connection from the pump console and manually injecting into and withdrawing air from this catheter with a Leur-Lok syringe (Fig. 26-2). Manual inflation of the balloon should be done once every 5 to 15 minutes to provide some movement of the balloon membrane.[8] Manual inflation and deflation most likely do not occur in counterpulsation with the cardiac cycle (inflation in diastole). Inflation may occur during peak systole. However, such balloon inflation is mandatory to prevent clot formation. If clots were allowed to form on the balloon, they could be sheared off during balloon removal and embolize to branches of the arterial tree.

The hemodynamic effects of balloon inflation can be observed on the arterial waveform. Inflation during peak systole may produce slight aortic regurgitation, which would manifest on the arterial pressure as a widened pulse pressure. Aortic regurgitation, however, is not usually a problem if the aortic valve is competent. Increased left ventricular work load and systolic pressure are more likely to result from manual inflation during systole. These hemodynamic effects can be minimized by manual inflation of 10 to 15 cc less than full capacity or with some pumps 50% to 60% of preload volume, which allows for dead space of the balloon catheter.[8]

Immediate balloon removal once counterpulsation has ceased is the much preferred and safer approach. Only when it is impossible to retain the console in continued pumping and the time lapse before the balloon is removed is longer than 20 minutes, should manual balloon inflation take place. Such manual inflation then becomes mandatory to prevent potential clot formation on the stagnant balloon.

REFERENCES

1. Austen, W.G., et al.: Intra-aortic balloon counterpulsation: current application, Cardiovasc. Clin. **7**:285, 1975.
2. Bolooki, H.: Clinical application of intra-aortic balloon pumping, Mount Kisco, N.Y., 1977, Futura Publishing Co.
3. Datascope Corp.: Datascope System 82 operator's manual, Paramus, N.J.
4. Igo, S.R., et al.: Intra-aortic balloon pumping: theory and practice. Experience with 325 patients, Artif. Organs **2**:249, 1978.
5. Kontron Cardiovascular Inc.: Model 10 operator's manual, Everett, Mass.
6. Okada, M.: Experimental and clinical studies on the effect of intra-aortic balloon pumping for cardiogenic shock following acute myocardial infarction, Artif. Organs **3**:271, 1979.
7. Rushmer, R.F.: Cardiovascular dynamics, Philadelphia, 1976, W.B. Saunders Co.
8. Self, M.: Manager, Clinical Educational Services Dept., Datascope Corp., Paramus, N.J., Personal communication, Nov. 1982.
9. Sturm, J.T., et al.: Quantitative indices of intra-aortic balloon pump (IABP) dependence during postinfarction cardiogenic shock, Artif. Organs **4**:492, 1980.

CHAPTER 27 **Balloon removal**

Removal of femoral artery balloon that was inserted with a Dacron side-arm graft

Local anesthetic is infiltrated following the preparation of the catheter insertion site. The Dacron graft is exposed, and occluding tapes are placed around the femoral artery proximally and distally to the balloon insertion site. Following heparinization of the patient, the Dacron graft is cut about 1 cm above the suture line. The balloon is aspirated with a syringe to assure maximum deflation. Relaxing the proximal occluding tape around the femoral artery allows for removal of the deflated balloon.

The Dacron graft usually contains some clots that are evacuated at the time of balloon removal. Saini and Berger's[5] technique of inserting a Fogarty catheter proximally and distally to extract any remaining clots from the femoral artery is now standard procedure (Fig. 27-1). The artery is flushed with a heparinized saline solution, and the Dacron graft is

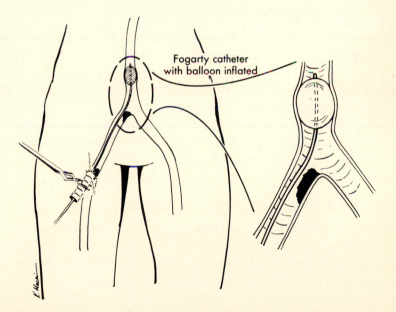

FIG. 27-1 Fogarty catheter is inserted after balloon removal to extract any possible clots from femoral artery.

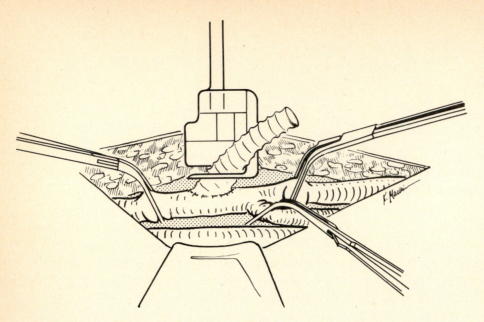

FIG. 27-2 Use of staple device placed over graft, flush with artery, to staple graft shut.

oversewn on the femoral arteriotomy. The occluding tapes are removed, restoring blood flow to the leg, followed by skin and subcutaneous tissue closure.

Staple graft closure as an alternative method

Peake and others[3] described a femoral artery balloon removal procedure like the one just explained with the following alteration: after balloon removal and Fogerty artery catheterization proximally and distally, a staple device with vascular staples is placed over the graft, flush with the artery. The graft is stapled shut (Fig. 27-2). Excess graft material is resected, and the wound is closed (Fig. 27-3).

Removing all of the Dacron graft, when possible, prevents infection that may occur when a larger portion of the graft has been left in situ. Peake's[3] technique affords an effective and rapid means of balloon extraction when the vessel is too small or is invaded with atherosclerosis and therefore is not amenable to primary closure.

Removal of the antegradely inserted balloon

Removal of the antegradely inserted balloon could be accomplished without reopening of the chest.[2,4] However, Bonchek and Olinger[1] and Shirkey and others[6] highly recommended opening the sternotomy incision for balloon removal. Once the balloon catheter is removed from the aorta, the anastomosis site is explored to evacuate any clots. The graft that was sutured over the aorta is cut short, and the remaining stub is oversewn tightly to avoid leaving a pouch of the graft over the intima of the aorta, which could serve as a source of clot formation.

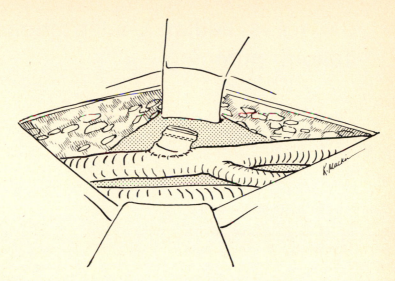

FIG. 27-3 Excess graft material is resected, and wound is ready to be closed.

REFERENCES

1. Bonchek, L., and Olinger, G.: Direct ascending aortic insertion of the ''percutaneous'' intra-aortic balloon catheter in the open chest: advantages and disadvantages, Ann. Thorac. Surg. **32:**512, 1981.
2. Krause, A.H., et al.: Transthoracic intra-aortic balloon cannulation to avoid repeat sternotomy for removal, Ann. Thorac. Surg. **21:**562, 1976.
3. Peake, J.B., et al.: A simple method of intra-aortic balloon removal after open heart surgery, Ann. Thorac. Surg. **32:**510, 1981.
4. Roe, B.B., and Chatterjee, K.: Transaortic cannulation for balloon pumping; report of a patient undergoing closed chest decannulation, Ann. Thorac. Surg. **21:**568, 1976.
5. Saini, V.K., and Berger, R.L.: Techniques of aortic balloon catheter deployment with the use of a Fogarty catheter, Ann. Thorac. Surg. **14:**440, 1972.
6. Shirkey, A.L., et al.: Insertion of the intra-aortic balloon through the aortic arch, Ann. Thorac. Surg. **21:**560, 1976.

CHAPTER 28 Pediatric adaptation in balloon pumping

Modifications in instrumentation

Limited use of the intra-aortic balloon in children under 5 years of age has been reported.[2-4] Modifications in existing balloon pumping instrumentation, appropriate to pediatric patient size, are essential to successful application of counterpulsation. Balloon catheters with much smaller diameters and gas capacities are substituted for the adult balloon catheters. The very small lumen of pediatric patient vessels requires that a correspondingly small balloon catheter be designed for insertion. Pediatric balloons still need to accommodate sufficient gas volume to augment aortic diastolic pressure during inflation, and yet aortic wall intima injury must not be inflicted with inflation. Attention to balloon catheter length is important. The positioned balloon cannot extend below the diaphragm when in situ in the descending thoracic aorta, as mesenteric and renal blood flow might be compromised. Finally the inflation-deflation cycle must occur at a rate compatible with the rapid heart rates of pediatric patients.

Successful miniaturization of equipment is the first step in pediatric application of IABP for use in patients who cannot be weaned from cardiopulmonary bypass and in reducing cardiac work when the left ventricle has failed secondary to a ventricular septal defect, aortic stenosis, or cardiomyopathy.

In vivo testing of balloons and catheters

Dr. George Veasy, Director of Cardiology at Primary Children's Hospital in Salt Lake City, has undertaken extensive research in conjunction with the Division of Artificial Organs at the University of Utah in the fabrication of existing adult intra-aortic balloons for pediatric adaptation.[4] The balloons used in vivo testing were fabricated by dipping stainless steel molds into blood-compatible polyurethanes. Volume capacities of 0.75 to 15.00 ml were fabricated and attached to catheters ranging from 2.5 to 5.0 F.

Trials of intra-aortic balloon augmentation were instituted in cats and dogs following iatrogenically produced mitral regurgitation. Hemodynamics recorded before and after balloon pumping during one such experiment are recorded in Fig. 28-1. Impressive diastolic augmentation was observed. Pulmonary artery pressure decreased from 22/11 mm Hg to 22/9 mm Hg. The mean left atrial pressure decreased by 5 mm Hg with a noticeable

IABP experiment 5-23-80
Dog—4.2 kg   Balloon—2.4 ml   Inflation—3.2 ml
Time—1231   Status—Post MR

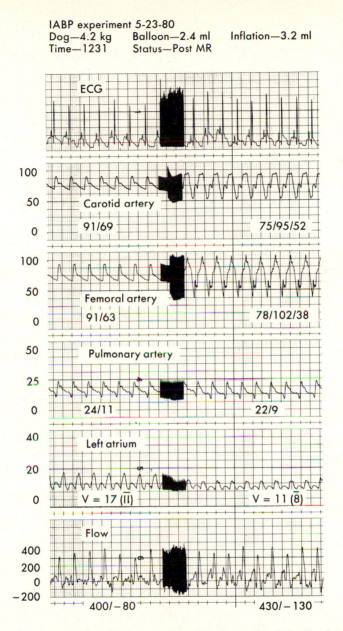

FIG. 28-1 Hemodynamic pressures before and after balloon pumping following iatrogenic mitral regurgitation in experiment with cats. Pressures are in millimeters of mercury. Diastolic augmentation and afterload reduction are observed in carotid and femoral artery tracings. Pulmonary artery and left atrial pressures are impressively reduced with balloon pumping. Flows represent aortic flows. Improvement in forward aortic flow was demonstrated by increase from 400 to 430 ml/min following balloon assist. Increase in negative aortic flow from −80 to −130 ml/min represents coronary artery perfusion. (Photo courtesy L.G. Veasy, Salt Lake City.)

decrease in the V wave produced by mitral regurgitation. Diastolic augmentation was achieved through driving by a Datascope System 80 console.

Clinical IABP in children

The Hospital for Sick Children in Toronto reports relatively little success with balloon pumping in its pediatric series, especially in children under 5 years of age. The conclusion of these researchers was that the aortic elasticity of smaller children prevented hemodynamic improvement following institution of balloon pumping. The smallest of balloons available extended below the diaphragm in these pediatric patients. The mean age of the surviving patients following balloon pump assist was 11.8 years. Better augmentation was confirmed in children over 5 years. Since the human aorta does not reach its adult pattern until age 25, children exhibit greater compliance of the aortic wall compared to the more rigid adult aorta. The Toronto study concluded that the elasticity of pediatric aorta diminished the effect of raising aortic pressure by balloon inflation in diastole and reduced the afterload reduction effect.

Primary Children's Medical Center in conjunction with the University of Utah Medical Center has more recently achieved successful balloon pumping in the pediatric patient.

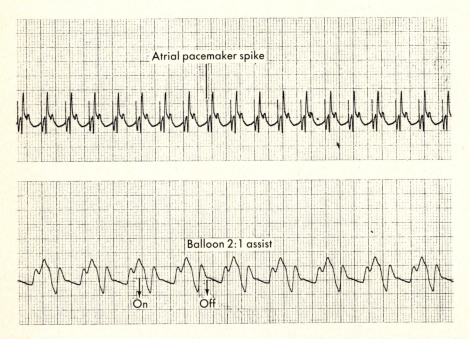

FIG. 28-2 Balloon inflation on every other beat on 4 kg patient with atrioventricular communication and mitral insufficiency. Effective diastolic augmentation and afterload reduction can be noted. Patient is paced atrially with good balloon trigger off pacer spike. (Tracing courtesy L.G. Veasy, Salt Lake City.)

Veasy's experience now consists of seven pediatric patients receiving pump assist and ranging in age from newborn to 1 year.[5] Weight range extended from 4.0 to 16.2 kg. The balloon performed effectively in six out of the seven patients. Balloon catheters employed were from 2.5 to 10.0 F with a 4 to 14 cc gas capacity and were 11 cm in length. Successful diastolic augmentation with afterload reduction was observed in six of the seven patients who were counterpulsated for AV communication and valvular deformity. Two patients were stabilized and weaned from the balloon pump, which allowed elective valvular replacement at a later date. An example of the counterpulsation achieved is illustrated in Fig. 28-2.

Pediatric balloon pumping does seem to be a viable modality with proven clinical effectiveness in the infant patient. A balloon design now exists that provides for appropriate modifications in catheter size, balloon length, and gas capacity to afford diastolic augmentation of aortic pressure with afterload reduction without insult to the aortic intima or compromise to the mesenteric or renal circulation.

REFERENCES

1. Agnagnostopoulos, C.E.: Acute aortic dissections, Baltimore, 1975, University Park Press.
2. Fukumasu, H., et al.: Intra-aortic balloon pumping device for infants, Clin. Cardiol. 2:348, 1979.
3. Pollock, J.C., et al.: Intra-aortic balloon pumping in children, Ann. Thorac. Surg. 29:522, 1980.
4. Veasy, L.G., et al.: Preclinical evaluation of intra-aortic balloon pumping for pediatric use, Trans. Am. Soc. Artif. Intern. Organs 27:490, 1981.
5. Veasy, L.G.: Personal communication, 1983.

CHAPTER 29 Pulsatile flow

Another application of the physiological principles of balloon pumping lies in the use of a pulsatile assist device (PAD). The PAD is a plastic disposable device designed for external application of counterpulsation in the cardiopulmonary bypass circuit. The device is inserted in the arterial line during cardiopulmonary bypass and simulates the action of balloon counterpulsation in the aorta. Thus the usual continuous flow of the cardiopulmonary bypass roller pump is converted to a pulsatile flow. The PAD can provide counterpulsation before and after cardiopulmonary bypass, and its implementation does not require invasive surgery.

Extracorporeal circulation and continuous flow

The usual extracorporeal circulation is illustrated in Fig. 29-1. Returning venous blood is diverted to the cardiopulmonary bypass pump oxygenator via a cannula usually placed in the right atrial appendage to the vena cava. Oxygenated blood is returned from the roller pump to the body through a cannula positioned in the aorta or femoral artery. Continuous, nonpulsating flow is maintained throughout the course of the perfusion circuitry. Physiological changes may potentially occur that may not remain innocuous during prolonged episodes of bypass perfusion.[3]

Pulsatile perfusion has not previously gained wide acceptance because of the mechanical complexity of marketed systems, high pressure gradients across the arterial line when smaller-sized cannulas are used, and increased blood hemolysis, possibly caused by increased turbulence of flow created by the pulsatile device.[8]

Techniques for achieving pulsatile flow

An inline PAD and a roller head modification have been used to convert nonpulsatile bypass flow to pulsatile flow.

PAD

Designed to convert roller pump flow of cardiopulmonary bypass, the PAD is a flexible, valveless balloon conduit through which the arterial return flows. The balloon is inserted in the arterial line close to the aortic root. Contained within a rigid plastic cylinder, the device is connected to a standard IABP by a pneumatic hose (Fig. 29-2).

In addition the PAD can be used as an arterial counterpulsator before and after cardiopulmonary bypass. The counterpulsation mechanism is triggered by the R wave of the electrocardiogram (ECG).[4,18]

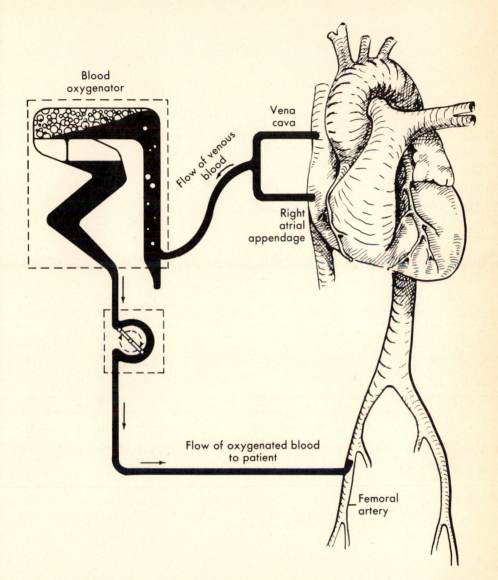

FIG. 29-1 Extracorporeal circulation. Blood flow bypasses heart and lungs. Returning venous blood is diverted to cardiopulmonary bypass pump oxygenator via cannulas usually placed in vena cava and/or right atrial appendage. Oxygenated blood returns from roller pump to body through femoral artery cannula.

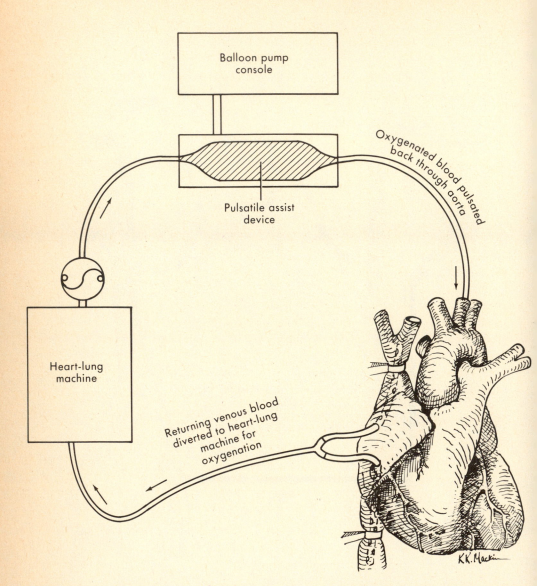

FIG. 29-2 Pulsatile flow during cardiopulmonary bypass. Pulsatile assist device (PAD) is placed in descending thoracic aorta or in arterial line in close proximity to its site of origin in aorta. Counterpulsation is triggered by patient's electrocardiogram (ECG), providing pulsatile flow during cardiopulmonary bypass.

Roller pump modification to produce pulsatile flow

Desjardins and others[7] have described a simple modification of the traditional roller pump, which achieves a pulsatile flow during extracorporeal circulation. A standard roller pump with one roller removed is added to the console and fitted with a length of Silastic tubing. Counterclockwise revolution of the one-roller pump displaces 27 ml of fluid toward the clamped end of the tube, which dilates under the pressure generated; this volume stored in the Silastic tubing is reinjected into the circuit as the single roller ends its half turn of contact with the tube (Fig. 29-3).

Sarns pulsatile flow system

Standard extracorporeal circulation roller pumps provide a continuous blood flow rate because the roller assembly on the pump turns the pump head at a set speed. A roller pump becomes pulsatile when the roller assembly intermittently stops and starts or changes speed. Such changes in roller pump activity return the oxygenated blood from the extracorporeal circuit back to the body at changing rates and pressures.

The 7400 MDX Sarns pulsatile flow pump (Fig. 29-4) synchronizes single pulses with the ECG R-wave signal. Synchronization prevents subjecting the heart to high pressure during contraction. The unit is designed for pulsatile perfusion that might be implemented at the end of the pump run to assist reestablishment of biological circulation or possibly as the heart is recovering from intraoperative cardioplegia. The internally triggered mode provides pulsatile flow during the course of total heart-lung bypass. Flow rates and pressures are intermittently changed by the pump to support metabolic activity. Bypass should begin with continuous rather than pulsatile flow; nonpulsatile flow at the onset of the bypass run allows the operator to adjust venous return and to check the integrity of tubing connections and safety systems before introducing pulsation.[22]

Pulsatile versus nonpulsatile flow
Hematological comparison

Zumbro and colleagues[27] evaluated clinical advantages of the PAD in a prospective randomized study of 100 consecutive coronary artery bypass operations. Serial ECGs, creatine phosphokinase isoenzyme studies, and myocardial scans with technetium-labeled pyrophosphate failed to demonstrate any significant difference between patients with PAD and those receiving nonpulsatile flow. Plasma hemoglobins were significantly higher in the PAD group, indicating increased blood trauma. These researchers concluded that few advantages existed with the use of PAD in routine coronary artery bypass operations. No advantages were offered with the use of PAD in myocardial preservation after coronary bypass grafting in patients with normal left ventricles in the study performed at Massachusetts General Hospital.[11]

In a later study Salerna and others[21] compared hematological studies in patients receiving pulsatile and nonpulsatile cardiopulmonary bypass. A significant drop in platelet count after perfusion was demonstrated in both groups. Similarly, elevations in lactic dehydrogenase and plasma hemoglobin, occurring at the end of bypass, was comparable in both

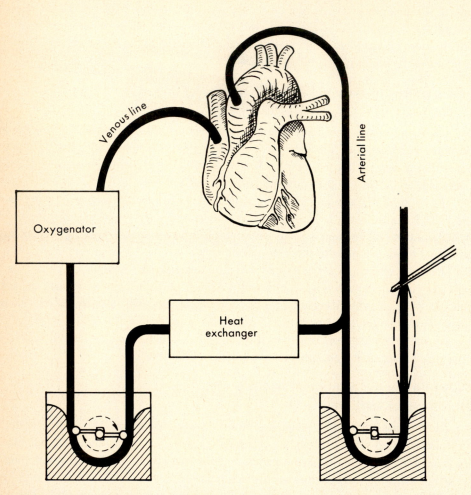

FIG. 29-3 Modification of standard cardiopulmonary perfusion system for achieving pulsatile flow. One-roller pump has been added, turning counterclockwise on Silastic tubing. Proximal extremity of Silastic tubing is connected to arterial line with Y connector. The extremity of distal tube end is clamped. Counterclockwise revolution of single-roller pump displaces 27 ml of fluid toward clamped end of tube, which distends tube. This volume is reinjected into circuit as single roller completes its half rotation of contact with Silastic tube. (Reproduced from Desjardins, J., et al.: Ann. Thorac. Surg. **27**:1979.)

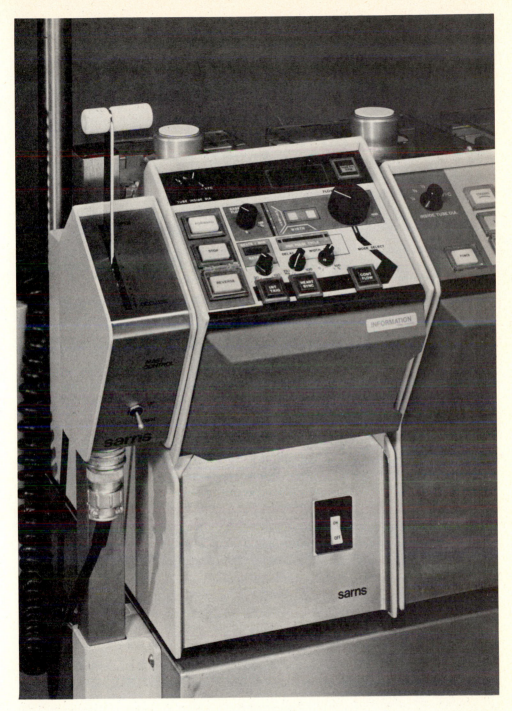

FIG. 29-4 Sarns Model 7400 pulsatile pump. Controls allow continuous roller pump and two pulsatile modes. Internal trigger is provided for use when patient's heart is stilled, and synchronous mode is available when patient's ECG R wave is stable. (Photo courtesy Sarns, Inc., Ann Arbor, Mich.)

groups. There was no significant difference in hemolysis during bypass between the pulsatile and nonpulsatile flow groups.

Effect of restoration of blood flow to the myocardium following ventricular fibrillation

The myocardium of the fibrillating heart is underperfused. Myocardial blood flow occurs primarily in diastole, but systolic flow has also been noted and appears to be directed to the epicardial zones. Loss of this phasic flow during ventricular fibrillation induces ischemia to the subendocardium.[6,10] Salerno[20] studied pulsatile flow as a possible means of restoring blood flow across the ischemic myocardium during ventricular fibrillation. At low flow rates pulsatile perfusion did not restore the abnormal flow distribution in the fibrillating heart. At flow rates considered adequate (70 ml/kg/min) there was no advantage in the use of pulsatile perfusion in terms of blood flow distribution across the myocardium.[20]

Effect on renal perfusion

Bregman[2] described virtual elimination of postoperative renal failure with use of pulsatile flow. Sink and associates[23] at Duke University compared renal cortical blood flow with pulsatile and nonpulsatile extracorporeal circulation in dogs. No difference was found in total renal cortical blood flow or in flow distribution when mean perfusion pressure was held constant at a high (80 mm Hg) or low (50 mm Hg) level. This study did not resolve the question of whether pulsatile perfusion has advantages over nonpulsatile perfusion in maintaining renal function. Rather the data suggested that any differences between the two techniques must be explained by a mechanism other than increased total cortical blood flow or by redistribution of cortical flow.

Pulsatile cardiopulmonary bypass and hypothermia in cardiac surgery

Profound hypothermia with core cooling has been considered unsafe compared with surface heart cooling because of the induced metabolic acidosis. Comparison of pulsatile and nonpulsatile flow has been made during cardiopulmonary bypass with core cooling. Throughout the hypothermia, cerebral excess lactate and metabolic studies on carbohydrates and lipids were made. With pulsatile flow the mean value of excess lactate was significantly lower, and hyperglycemia was reduced. This suggested the higher use of glucose. Thus aerobic metabolism in the brain appears to be reduced by pulsatile cardiopulmonary bypass during the hypothermic period.[24]

Bregman[2] summarized that the best myocardial protection for a patient with a depressed or impaired left ventricle undergoing open-heart surgery is to employ hypothermia and cold potassium cardioplegia and to reperfuse with synchronous pulsatile perfusion in an empty beating heart.

Pulsatile flow and postoperative hypertension

Transient hypertension is recognized as a complication following coronary artery bypass surgery. The incidence has been reported to range from 33% to 58%.[6,19] The sequelae of postoperative hypertension can cause marked subendocardial ischemia and increased afterload.[6]

The actual cause of this transient postoperative hypertension has yet to be elucidated. Patients in whom notable hypertension develops consistently demonstrate elevated peripheral vascular resistance.[19] Taylor and co-workers[25] demonstrated that angiotensin is elevated following aortocoronary bypass surgery. They implicated the induction of the renin-angiotensin system in the production of postoperative hypertension. Renin, which may be secreted through the kidneys, secondary to hypertension, reacts with a plasma globulin to produce angiotensin I. In passage through the lungs, angiotensin I encounters the enzyme that converts it to angiotensin II, the most potent endogenous vasoconstrictor known.[15]

Many[17] and Goodman[9] demonstrated that with a constant perfusion pressure, nonpulsatile flow activated the renin-angiotensin system, resulting in elevations of renin concentrations in the peripheral blood.

Landymore and co-workers[15] evaluated the outcome of pulsatile flow on postoperative hypertension. Hypertension, defined as a pressure of 160/100 mm Hg or higher, was observed in 80% of the patients receiving nonpulsatile flow but in only 20% of the patients perfused during surgery with pulsatile extracorporeal circulation. Patients receiving pulsatile bypass did not demonstrate notable postoperative renin levels. Postoperative catecholamine levels were unchanged in the two groups. This factor may account for hypertension observed in 20% of the pulsatile flow patients, in the absence of significant renin production.

Whether or not to use PAD

Bregman[2] has consistently demonstrated the following effects of pulsatile flow in his series of over 600 patients:

1. An increase in urinary output and virtual elimination of postoperative renal failure occur.
2. Stroke and other neurological complications of cardiopulmonary bypass are minimized.
3. Peripheral vascular resistance is decreased.
4. Subendocardial ischemia is minimal.
5. Perioperative myocardial infarction is reduced to 1.8%.
6. The postoperative period for inotropic support is decreased.
7. There is a decreased time for cooling and rewarming during cardiopulmonary bypass.
8. A decreased time in weaning patients with left ventricular dysfunction after cardiopulmonary bypass is also observed.

Advantages seem to be offered in myocardial preservation in patients with impaired left ventricular function but not in those with normal left ventricles. Blood hemolysis has been demonstrated with pulsatile flow.[27] Bregman[2] cautioned that use of cannulas less than 24 F increases hemolysis, and it is much more difficult to achieve physiological pulsatile flow pressures with the smaller cannulas. Another study showed no difference in hemolysis between the two modes.[21] Therefore except for cannula size, hemolysis is not a definitive argument. Renal flow is improved,[3] but no improvement in total renal cortical blood flow or in flow distribution has been documented.[23]

The former complexity of the systems and the turbulence of flow created by the PAD had limited its acceptance.[8] A pulsatile extracorporeal flow pump is available which synchronizes single pulses with the ECG R-wave signal.[22] Synchronization prevents subjecting the heart to high pressure during contraction. Such an improvement in heart-lung pump design may afford the benefits outlined without the objectionable flow turbulence and potential hemolysis encountered with modification of the standard roller pump to provide pulsatile flow through the inline PAD.

Advantages do seem to exist with pulsatile flow, especially in extracorporeal perfusion of the patient with left ventricular dysfunction. Benefits to the patient with normal ventricular function do not appear to be as dramatic. PAD does not seem to offer the patient with healthy ventricular function any gains beyond the benefits of cold cardioplegia and pharmacological myocardial preservation techniques.

REFERENCES

1. Bolooki, H., et al.: Clinical and hemodynamic criteria for use of the intra-aortic balloon pump in patients requiring cardiac surgery, J. Thorac. Cardiovasc. Surg. **72:**756, 1976.
2. Bregman, D.: Response to paper presented on pulsatile flow, Presented at fifth annual meeting of the Society of Thoracic Surgeons, Phoenix, Ariz., Jan. 15-17, 1979, Ann. Thorac. Surg. **28:**272, 1979.
3. Bregman, D., et al.: Counterpulsation with a new pulsatile assist device (PAD) in open heart surgery, Med. Instrum. **10:**232, 1976.
4. Bregman, D., et al.: A pulsatile assist device for use during cardiopulmonary bypass, Ann. Thorac. Surg. **24:**574, 1977.
5. Bregman, D., et al.: An improved method of myocardial protection with pulsation during cardiopulmonary bypass, Circulation **56**(Suppl. 2):157, 1977.
6. Buckberg, G.D., et al.: Subendocardial ischemia after cardiopulmonary bypass, J. Thorac. Cardiovasc. Surg. **64:**669, 1972.
7. Desjardins, J., et al.: A simple device for achieving pulsatile flow during cardiopulmonary bypass, Ann. Thorac. Surg. **27:**178, 1979.
8. Dunn, J., et al.: Hemodynamic, metabolic and hematologic effects of pulsatile cardiopulmonary bypass, J. Thorac. Cardiovasc. Surg. **68:**138, 1974.
9. Goodman, T.A., et al.: The effects of pulseless perfusion on the distribution of renal cortical blood flow and on renin release, Surgery **80:**311, 1976.
10. Gregg, D.E., and Green, H.D.: Registration and interpretation of normal phasic inflow into a left coronary artery by an improved differential manometric method, Am. J. Physiol. **130:**114, 1940.
11. Hoar, P.F., et al.: Systemic hypertension following myocardial revascularization: a method of treatment using epidural anesthesia, J. Thorac. Cardiovasc. Surg. **71:**859, 1976.
12. Hottenrott, C., et al.: Studies of the effects of ventricular fibrillation on the adequacy of regional myocardial flow. I. Electrical vs. spontaneous fibrillation, J. Thorac. Cardiovasc. Surg. **68:**615, 1974.
13. Hottenrott, C., et al.: Studies of the effects of ventricular fibrillation on the adequacy of regional myocardial flow. II. Effects of ventricular distention, J. Thorac. Cardiovasc. Surg. **68:**626, 1974.
14. Hottenrott, C., et al.: Studies of the effects of ventricular fibrillation on the adequacy of regional myocardial flow. III. Mechanisms of ischemia, J. Thorac. Cardiovasc. Surg. **68:**634, 1974.
15. Landymore, R.W., et al.: Does pulsatile flow influence the incidence of postoperative hypertension? Ann. Thorac. Surg. **28:**261, 1979.
16. Levine, J.H., et al.: The effect of pulsatile perfusion on preservation of left ventricular function after aortocoronary bypass grafting, Circulation **64**(suppl. 2):40, 1981.
17. Many, M., et al.: Effects of depulsation of renal blood flow upon renal function and renin secretion, Surgery **66:**242, 1969.
18. Pappas, G., et al.: Improvement of myocardial and other vital organ functions and metabolism with a simple method of pulsatile flow (IABP) during clinical cardiopulmonary bypass, Surgery **77:**34, 1975.

19. Roberts, A.J., et al.: Systemic hypertension associated with coronary artery bypass surgery: predisposing factors, hemodynamic characteristics, humoral profile, and treatment, J. Thorac. Cardiovasc. Surg. **74**:846, 1977.
20. Salerno, T.A., et al.: Pulsatile perfusion: its effects on blood flow distribution in hypertrophied hearts, Ann. Thorac. Surg. **27**:559, 1979.
21. Salerno, T.A., et al.: Hemolysis during pulsatile perfusion: clinical evaluation of a new device, J. Thorac. Cardiovasc. Surg. **79**:579, 1980.
22. Sarns, E.M.: Engineering department: pulsatile flow: a preview to the Sarns approach, Form 4020, June 1982.
23. Sink, J.D., et al.: Comparison of nonpulsatile and pulsatile extracorporeal circulation on renal cortical blood flow, Ann. Thorac. Surg. **29**:57, 1980.
24. Spiller, P., et al.: Perfusion and assist, J. Cardiovasc. Surg. **22**:422, 1981.
25. Taylor, D.M., et al.: Hypertension and the renin-angiotensin system following open-heart surgery, J. Thorac. Cardiovasc. Surg. **74**:840, 1977.
26. Trinkel, J.K., et al.: Pulsatile cardiopulmonary bypass: clinical evaluation, Surgery **68**:1074, 1970.
27. Zumbro, G.L., et al.: A prospective evaluation of the pulsatile assist device, Ann. Thorac. Surg. **28**:269, 1979.

CHAPTER 30 Pulmonary artery balloon pumping

Much attention has been focused on mechanical assistance to the left ventricle, either by IABP or by the use of a left ventricular assist device (Chapter 32). Comparatively little research and few clinical trials have been pursued in the mechanical assistance of the failing right ventricle. Yet several investigators have recognized the need for right ventricular circulatory assist for patients undergoing certain congenital heart disease corrective procedures,[6] for patients in right-heart failure secondary to right ventricular infarction,[2] and for patients whose conditions are deteriorating from right ventricular failure while being supported by a left ventricular assist device.[1] Eichelter and Schenk[3] established the consequence of right ventricular failure after pulmonary embolism. Therefore the problems of right ventricular failure and its management with pulmonary artery counterpulsation also need to be explored.

Animal trials with pulmonary artery counterpulsation

Researchers at the University of Utah[4] have used pulmonary artery supportive counterpulsation after iatrogenically induced pulmonary embolus in sheep. Animal balloon implantation was achieved through exposure of the right jugular vein and insertion of the 25 cc polyethylene balloon mounted on a curved catheter tip through the jugular vein, right atrium, tricuspid valve, and into the right ventricle. Slight inflation of the balloon facilitated its flotation through the pulmonic valve and out into the pulmonary artery (Fig. 30-1).

During these animal experiments, pulmonary emboli were iatrogenically induced by injection of embolus material (cornstarch or hemologous blood thrombi) into a peripheral vein. The pulmonary artery pressure increased (average of 14 mm Hg), as did the pulmonary vascular resistance (average 680 dynes/sec/cm^{-5}), and cardiac output decreased an average of 0.76 liters/min.

Following a period of balloon pumping from 30 seconds to 10 minutes, the mean pulmonary artery pressure decreased by an average of 13 mm Hg; pulmonary vascular resistance decreased by 432 dynes/sec/cm^{-5} on the average; cardiac output was increased by an average of 0.92 liters/min.

Continuous inflation of the pulmonary artery balloon for 30 seconds increased right ventricular systemic pressure and pulmonary artery resistance and decreased cardiac output. Pulmonary artery diastolic counterpulsation, under normal circulatory conditions, did not net any appreciable hemodynamic effect.

316

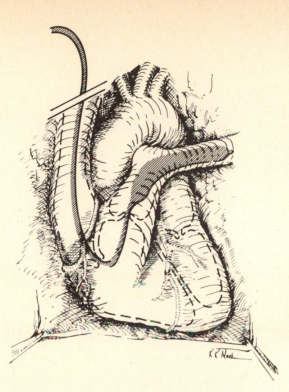

FIG. 30-1 Balloon is inserted through right jugular vein, into right atrium, right ventricle, and through pulmonic valve out to rest in situ in pulmonary artery. By rapid inflation of balloon in diastole and withdrawal of inflating gas just before systole, pulmonary resistance against which right ventricle must eject is lowered. This afterload reduction achieved enables failing right ventricle to empty more easily.

Clinical trials of pulmonary artery counterpulsation in humans

Researchers at Stanford University[5] have adapted the technique of balloon counterpulsation for use in supporting the acutely failing right ventricle. Insertion is undertaken in the operating room with the chest exposed. The patient status necessitating pulmonary artery counterpulsation has been that of profound right ventricular failure and inability to wean from cardiopulmonary bypass. In these trials the patient had previously received conventional IABP to assist left ventricular function and to attempt to facilitate extracorporeal circulation weaning.

Pulmonary artery balloon placement in the open chest is illustrated in Fig. 30-2. The intra-aortic balloon is already in situ. A Dacron woven graft is sutured to the pulmonary artery and a 35 mm single-chambered balloon is implanted into the pulmonary artery through the graft. The fitted balloon catheter is connected to a conventional balloon pump. Fig. 30-3 illustrates the pulmonary artery pressure tracing without and with counterpulsation. It should be noted that 1:1 counterpulsation provides diastolic augmentation and a presystolic afterload reduction.

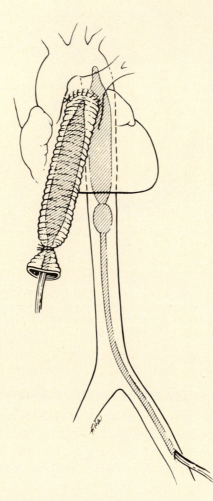

FIG. 30-2 Schematic drawing of balloon inserted into pulmonary artery through Dacron graft. Intra-aortic balloon is also in situ. (Modified from Miller, D.C., et al.: J. Thorac. Cardiovasc. Surg. **80**:760, 1980.)

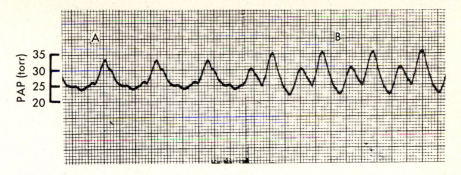

FIG. 30-3 Pulmonary artery pressure without and with diastolic augmentation. **A,** No counterpulsation; **B,** 1:1 counterpulsation, elevating pulmonary artery diastolic pressure and reducing end-diastolic pressure (afterload). (Reproduced from Miller, D.C., et al.: J. Thorac. Cardiovasc. Surg. **80:**760, 1980.)

Pulmonary artery diastolic pressure augmentation may also assist transpulmonary blood flow and thereby improve forward circulation, increasing left atrial and left ventricular blood filling. Thus adaptation of conventional IABP to pulmonary artery counterpulsation affords a life-saving modality for patients with intractable right ventricular failure and/or biventricular failure.[5]

REFERENCES

1. Berger, R.L., et al.: Successful use of a left ventricular assist device in cardiogenic shock from massive postoperative myocardial infarction, J. Thorac. Cardiovasc. Surg. **18:**626, 1979.
2. Cohn, J.N.: Right ventricular infarction revisited, Am. J. Cardiol. **43:**666, 1979.
3. Eichelter, P., et al.: Hemodynamic changes following experimental pulmonary embolism, J. Thorac. Cardiovasc. Surg. **57:**866, 1969.
4. Kralios, A., et al.: Intrapulmonary artery balloon pumping, J. Thorac. Cardiovasc. Surg. **60:**215, 1970.
5. Miller, D.C., et al.: Pulmonary artery balloon counterpulsation for acute right ventricular failure, J. Thorac. Cardiovasc. Surg. **80:**760, 1980.
6. Sade, R.M.: Correcting uncorrectable heart malformations, Contemp. Surg. **12:**16, 1978.

CHAPTER 31 External counterpulsation

Rationale

Intra-aortic balloon counterpulsation requires an invasive procedure for placement. Several investigators have viewed the necessity of an invasive procedure as a limiting factor in balloon pumping and therefore have developed an alternative, noninvasive method, or external counterpulsation.[4,10]

Norton and associates[8] found that aortic diastolic pressure could be raised 40% to 50% by application of a positive pressure pulse during diastole; release of this pressure or application of negative pressure in systole lowered systolic aortic and peak left ventricular pressure. Compression of the legs also increased venous return to the heart and elevated cardiac output. Unfortunately, these pressure waves generated in the lower extremities are propagated throughout the venous system and probably act to impede venous return from the head and splanchnic system.[5]

Clinical application

Clinically, external counterpulsation is activated by encasing the legs from ankle to groin between two halves of a rigid case (Fig. 31-1). The device is completely noninvasive. A water-filled bladder surrounds the legs and totally fills the space between the legs and the outer case. Using the electrocardiogram (ECG) for timing, the bladder and sequentially the legs are pressurized pneumatically during early diastole. Negative pressure or a return to ambient pressure is employed during the remainder of the cardiac cycle to accomplish counterpulsation. The arterial pressure pulse is usually recorded from a finger plethysmograph and is displayed on the console with the ECG. Precise phasing of counterpulsation with the cardiac cycle is established by adjustment of the electronic circuitry through proper delay and duration controls.

Bladder inflation pressures of 150 to 200 mm Hg are required to produce significant elevation of aortic diastolic pressure. Short bursts of high pressures are well tolerated. Less systolic unloading occurs if the bladder is deflated to previous ambient leg pressures, rather than applying negative pressure. Easy applicability allows early initiation as soon as the patient has symptoms of an acute or impending myocardial infarction. Treatments are continued on a symptomatic basis, usually for 50 to 120 minutes four times daily and when necessary.[9]

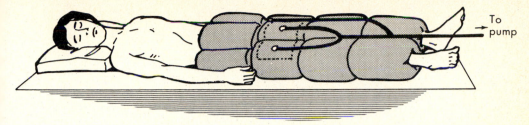

FIG. 31-1 External counterpulsation. Patient's legs are encased from ankle to groin between two halves of rigid case, which is connected to pumping console. Water-filled bladder surrounds legs and outer case. Bladder and sequentially patient's legs are pressurized pneumatically during early diastole. Inflated bladder is released during remainder of cardiac cycle (or negative pressure is applied) to achieve counterpulsation effect.

Use in myocardial infarction without shock

Mueller and co-workers[7] evaluated the effectiveness of external counterpulsation in patients with acute transmural infarction but without evidence of shock. Some patients obtained excellent diastolic augmentation but with little decrease in left ventricular ejection resistance. Significant decreased resistance was obtained in another group of patients but at the expense of less impressive diastolic augmentation. Overall, cardiac index increased, and pulmonary wedge pressures fell.

Amsterdam[1] evaluated the efficacy of application of external pressure circulatory assistance when implemented within 24 hours after infarction. The treatment group consisted of 142 patients, and the control group consisted of 116 patients. There were no significant differences between groups. Compared with control patients, hospital mortality was significantly decreased in the group that received 4 or more hours of external pressure circulatory assistance within the first 24 hours of admission. Circulatory assistance for 3 or more hours also decreased mortality but not as significantly as in those patients who sustained at least 4 hours of pumping. In both groups who underwent pumping for 3 and 4 or more hours of treatment, this modality of circulatory assist demonstrated significant lessening of morbidity as manifested by recurrent chest pain, progression of cardiac failure, occurrence of ventricular fibrillation, change in heart size, and clinical cardiac functional status at discharge.

Use in myocardial infarction following shock

In Soroff's group[12] 45% of the patients survived cardiogenic shock despite a delay of up to 8 hours in instituting external counterpulsation. All patients who responded did so within several hours; the authors found little benefit in extending the treatment beyond that point.

Use with angina pectoris

Banas and co-workers[2] evaluated the effectiveness of 1 hour per day of external counterpulsation pumping for 5 successive days in 21 patients with angina pectoris secondary to angiographically confirmed coronary atherosclerosis. Appreciable diastolic pressure augmentation was produced in 18 patients; 17 patients were free of pain by the fourth day of treatment. Less frequent angina attacks 1 month after pumping were documented in all of the patients studied. Repeat counterpulsation relieved angina attacks, which returned 4 to 6 months after pumping in four of the patients.

Summary of clinical use

In clinical practice the efficacy of external counterpulsation in relieving ischemia and augmenting diastolic perfusion lies in its application in relatively uncomplicated myocardial infarctions. Pollack-Latham's[10] study of clinical usage of external counterpulsation documented that this modality was used most frequently in Killip's Class II patients, exhibiting significant signs of heart failure. Killip's classification[6] of patient cardiac status is outlined in Table 31-1. Anticipated outcomes after external counterpulsation include:

1. Prevention of further ischemia by increasing the aortic pressure during diastole to increase coronary blood flow.
2. Reduction of myocardial oxygen demand and cardiac work by reducing afterload.

TABLE 31-1 Killip's classification of patient cardiac status

Class	Status
I	No heart failure
II	Mild to moderate heart failure (S_3, rales more than halfway up posterior lung fields)
III	Severe heart failure (pulmonary edema by clinical and radiographic confirmation)
IV	Cardiogenic shock (pulmonary edema and hypoperfusion)

Adapted from Killip, T., and Kimball, J.K.: Am. J. Cardiol. **20**:458, 1957.

TABLE 31-2 Comparison of clinical benefits of the IABP and external counterpulsation methods

Parameter	Intra-aortic balloon (n = 10)	External counter-pulsation (n = 10)
Peak systolic aortic pressure (afterload reduced)	Decreased	Unchanged
Right atrial pressure	Unchanged	Unchanged
Coronary blood flow	Increased	Slightly increased
Myocardial oxygen consumption	Decreased	Increased
Lactate use	Improved	Slightly improved
Reversal of shock state	All	

Modified from Singh, J., et al.: Circulation **49**(suppl. 3):108, 1974.

3. Permanent relief of ischemia by accelerating coronary artery collateralization through the use of augmented diastolic pressure.
4. Improved cardiac classification status of the patient before discharge with continued use of conventional medical therapy.[10]

Comparison of IABP and external counterpulsation methods

Ten patients who met the rigorous definition of cardiogenic shock proposed by the Myocardial Infarction Unit of the National Institute of Health were placed in each group to compare the effects of IABP and external counterpulsation. Both methods of augmentation increased diastolic aortic pressure and cardiac index; pulmonary wedge pressure was also decreased. Changes were of greater magnitude, however, with the use of the IABP in all patients.[11] Other comparisons are itemized in Table 31-2.

Patient classification

Specific indications for use of either the IABP or external counterpulsation, when both are available, have been outlined by Pollack-Latham.[10] Killip's patient classification is again used for selection of one of the applications of counterpulsation (Table 31-3).

Nursing management of patients requiring external counterpulsation. A thorough explanation of the procedure that is to ensue is absolutely essential. The patient needs to understand that he will feel pressure in his limbs when the bladder of the leg unit inflates. A simple but precise explanation of how counterpulsation augments coronary circulation should also be included.

The external counterpulsation unit must be stored with the unit plugged in to keep the water storage compartment warm for patient comfort when the unit is activated.

Pollack-Latham[10] outlined essential components of nursing care emphasizing that the patient should void before the procedure begins. If an indwelling Foley catheter is in situ, 50 ml of sterile normal saline solution instilled, and the catheter is clamped during the treatment. Clamping of the catheter prophylactically prevents an oliguric patient from developing a bladder irritation during the pressurized phase of counterpulsation. Other essential comfort measures include padding of the legs and back, keeping the stored water in the console warm, and pressurizing below 200 mm Hg.

Physiological monitoring. Direct ECG leads are attached from the pump to the patient. Pumping is synchronized to allow the pressurized phase of the cycle to be activated during diastole. A plethysmograph is usually applied to the patient's thumb for

TABLE 31-3 Patient selection for use of the IABP or external counterpulsation*

Class	Treatment
I or II	External counterpulsation
III	Initially external counterpulsation; if no improvement in patient status, use IABP
IV	IABP

*Based on Killip's patient classification.

recording a relative arterial pressure. Placement of an arterial line is optional; the unstable patient's care can be facilitated by placement of an arterial line, since auscultation of the blood pressure during the leg pumping action is difficult.

Sequential external counterpulsation pumping

A modification of external counterpulsation in which the legs are compressed sequentially (first distally and then proximally) has been tested. Peak diastolic augmentation was equal in both sequential and nonsequential counterpulsation. Cardiac output was greater when sequenced pumping was employed; this was hypothesized to be the effect of "milking" venous return from the legs.[3]

Summary

External counterpulsation affords a noninvasive, easily and quickly activated method of counterpulsation. Supportive external augmentation appears to be most effective in symptomatic relief for patients in Class I or II of Killip's classification. External compression of the extremities, using rapidly administered high-pressurized hydraulic impulses gated to the cardiac cycle, displaces venous and arterial blood from the extremities. Venous blood propagates antegradely to the central circulation; on release of the inflated bladder apparatus attached to the patient's legs, flow is encouraged in the aorta, providing a potential augmented stroke volume. Continuing evaluation as to the efficacy of external counterpulsation is needed, but in a select patient population its benefits have been demonstrated.

REFERENCES

1. Amsterdam, E.A.: Clinical assessment of external pressure circulatory assistance in acute myocardial infarction, Am. J. Cardiol. **45:**349, 1980.
2. Banas, J.S., et al.: Evaluation of external counterpulsation for the treatment of angina pectoris (abstract), Am. J. Cardiol. **31:**118, 1973.
3. Cohen, L.S., et al.: Hemodynamic studies of sequenced and nonsequenced external counterpulsation, Am. J. Cardiol. **33:**131, 1974.
4. Dennis, C., et al.: Studies on external counterpulsation as a potential measure for acute left heart failure, Trans. Am. Soc. Artif. Intern. Organs **9:**186, 1973.
5. Heck, N.A., and Doty, D.B.: Assisted circulation by external lower body compression, Circulation **64** (suppl. 2): 118, 1981.
6. Killip, T., and Kimball, J.K.: Treatment of myocardial infarction in a coronary care unit, Am. J. Cardiol. **20:**458, 1957.
7. Mueller, H., et al.: Hemodynamic and myocardial metabolic response to external counterpulsation in acute myocardial infarction in man, Am. J. Cardiol. **31:**149, 1973.
8. Norton, R.L., et al.: Effects of change of ambient pressure differential on the effectiveness of peripheral assist, Trans. Am. Soc. Artif. Intern. Organs **17:**169, 1971.
9. Osborn, J., et al.: Circulatory support by leg or airway pulses in experimental mitral insufficiency (abstract), Circulation **28:**781, 1973.
10. Pollock-Latham, C.: Mechanical cardiac assist devices: the efficacy of external counterpulsation. In Pollock-Latham, C., and Canobbio, M., editors: Current concepts in cardiac care, Rockville, Md., 1982, Aspen Systems Corp.
11. Singh, J., et al.: Invasive versus noninvasive cardiac assistance in myocardial infarction shock in man, Circulation **49**(suppl. 3):108, 1974.
12. Soroff, H.S., et al.: Support of the systemic circulation and left ventricular assist leg synchronous pulsation of extramural pressure, Surg. Forum **16:**148, 1965.
13. Soroff, H.S., et al.: External counterpulsation: management of cardiogenic shock after myocardial infarction, JAMA **229:**1441, 1974.

CHAPTER 32 Other ventricular assist devices

Circulatory assist development

Prosthetic arteries, valves, and pacing systems have improved the prognosis for many patients with heart disease. Until recently, however, the only replacement for the pumping action of the heart in patients with severe pump failure was the cardiopulmonary bypass machine used during open-heart surgery. Promising pneumatic, electrical, and nuclear-actuated mechanical assist devices are currently undergoing trials for clinical support of the failing ventricle. Improvements in artificial pump designs and biomaterials and research on blood-synthetic materials have led to development of compact blood pumps with lowered risks of thromboembolism and device failure.

The heart-lung machine is the oldest modality of circulatory assistance and is used to sustain circulation during open-heart surgery procedures. Temporary left heart assist devices have been used successfully in humans when the IABP is insufficient to provide mechanical assistance for the energy demands of pumping blood. All of these devices operate by the simple principle of facilitating decreased work load on the natural myocardium, maintaining systemic pressure, and potentially enhancing coronary artery perfusion.

Cardiopulmonary bypass

Gibbon[15] introduced the technique for cardiopulmonary bypass known as *extracorporeal circulation*. He repaired an atrial septal defect under direct vision with the patient's physiological support maintained exclusive of the heart and lungs. Kirklin of the University of Alabama continued research of Gibbon's principles, developing extracorporeal circulation to the level of physiological support that is appreciated today. Four types of oxygenators are available: sheet or film, bubble, disk, and membrane.[6,11] An example of an extracorporeal circuit is found in Fig. 32-1.

Physiology of membrane and bubble oxygenators

Patient needs dictate the performance requirements of a heart-lung oxygenator. Berger[1] explained that any type of oxygenator should be capable of oxygenating at least 6 liters of blood per minute from a venous oxygen saturation of 40% to 70% to an ''arterialized'' saturation of 100%. The red blood cells must be oxygenated and propelled without breakage.

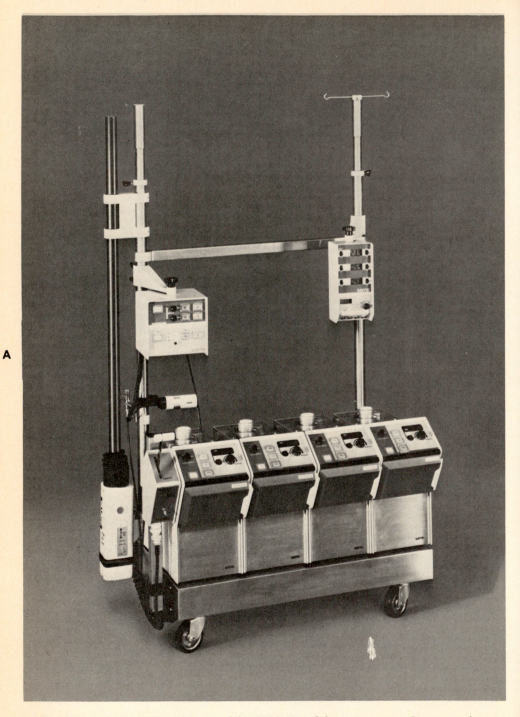

FIG. 32-1 A, Sarns heart-lung machine. Model 7000 MDX modular pump system. Oxygenator hangs on black mast on left. (**A,** courtesy Sarns, Inc., Ann Arbor, Mich.)

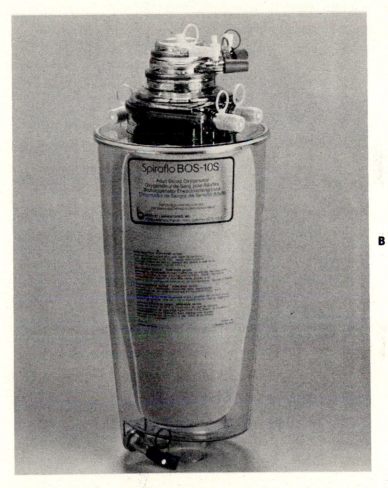

FIG. 32-1, cont'd B, Bentley BOS-10S oxygenator. (Courtesy Bentley Laboratories, Inc., Irvine, Calif.)

Bubble oxygenator.[1,10] An oxygen diffusor that injects gas directly into the incoming venous blood is characteristic of a bubble oxygenator (Fig. 32-2). Fused beads or a simple, perforated plate may serve as the diffusor. Such action produces a column of bubbles, a blood film encasing spheres of gas. Gas exchange takes place between the blood film and the oxygen it envelopes. There is no membranous barrier between the gas and liquid phases in the bubble oxygenator.

Membrane oxygenator.[1,8] Membrane oxygenators impose a thin sheet of permeable material between the blood and gas phases (Fig. 32-3). Oxygen diffuses into the blood through this membrane; hence a barrier exists between the gas and liquid.

Total bypass

Total cardiopulmonary bypass refers to complete circulatory bypass of the heart and lungs.[6] The inferior and superior vena cava are cannulated through the right atrial appendage, and the cannulas are attached to the venous line of the pump oxygenator. Blood flow into the vena cava is diverted out to the oxygenator (Fig. 32-4). Oxygenated blood is pumped back to the circulation via the femoral artery or aortic cannulas. Once the venous blood has been oxygenated, it passes through a heat exchanger that is capable of maintaining the perfusion at a controlled temperature. The roller heads of the pump regulate control of returning blood volume by increasing or decreasing the speed of rotations on the roller heads. Filters and bubble traps are inserted within the arterial side of the circuit for removal of air, fibrin, and platelet aggregates.

Partial bypass

Partial cardiopulmonary bypass has two definitions. Partial bypass is the term used to describe the technique used when perfusing a patient during resection of an aortic aneurysm. Pulmonary circulation is not interrupted. Oxygenated blood is vented through a cannula arising from the left atrium to a roller pump, which in turn pumps the blood back into the common femoral artery (Fig. 32-5). Partial bypass may also be used to describe the weaning phase as the patient is coming off of total bypass. A percentage of the circulatory blood flow is allowed to perfuse through the natural route as flow through the oxygenator is gradually reduced.

Membrane versus bubble oxygenator controversy

Whether or not advantages exist in using the membrane rather than the bubble oxygenator for routine open-heart surgery is controversial. Some studies have suggested improved physiology with the membrane oxygenator,[9,36] and others have failed to show a difference.[10,37]

Physiological benefits of membrane and bubble oxygenators

Theoretically the membrane oxygenator can reduce blood and organ damage by interposing a barrier between blood and gas to which denatured protein can adhere rather than be returned to the bloodstream.[42] Direct contact exists between the blood and gas in the bubble oxygenator; protein denaturation and cell membrane damage may occur when the

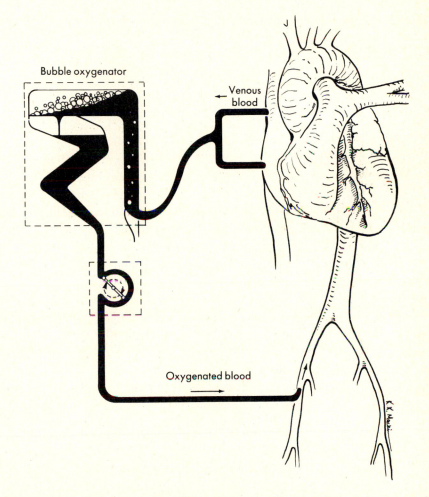

FIG. 32-2 Bubble oxygenator. Oxygen diffusor injects gas directly into incoming venous blood. Such action produces column of bubbles or blood film encasing spheres of gas.

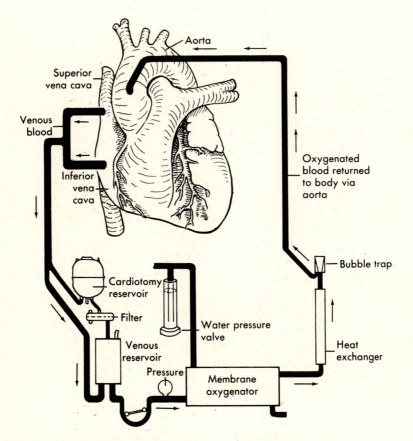

FIG. 32-3 Membrane oxygenator. Oxygen diffuses into blood through thin permeable membrane; barrier exists between gas and liquid.

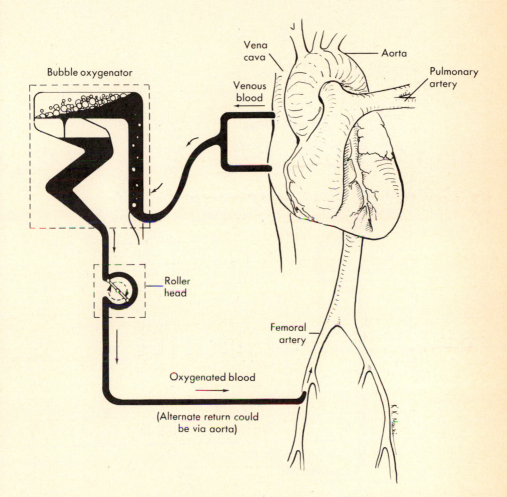

FIG. 32-4 Schematic of total cardiopulmonary bypass. Returning blood is diverted to heart-lung machine through cannulas positioned in inferior and superior vena cava. Oxygenated blood is pumped back to circulation via aorta.

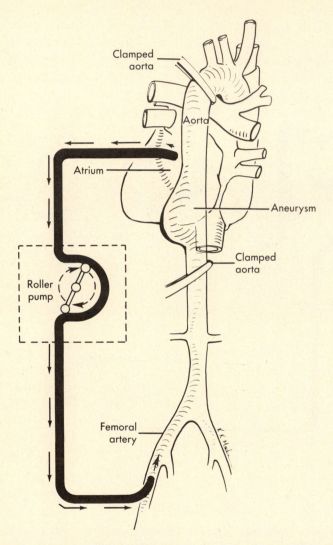

Clamped aorta

Aorta

Atrium

Aneurysm

Roller pump

Clamped aorta

Femoral artery

FIG. 32-5 Schematic of partial cardiopulmonary bypass. Lungs continue to oxygenate blood, which circulates to left atrium. At this point oxygenated blood is diverted to roller pump via left atrium cannula, which reperfuses blood into common femoral artery. Therefore circulation route of natural cardiac system is partially bypassed. This process allows resection of aortic aneurysm.

blood and gas come together.[20] Physiologically problems may be created, such as destruction of clotting factors, hemolysis, and platelet destruction and dysfunction.[39] Intermixing of gas with the bloodstream may increase the likelihood of gas and fibrin microemboli or gas embolization.[36] Microembolization of blood and gas[7] may lodge in the brain and other vital organs. Particle accumulation in the arterial perfusion line has been reported to be of greater magnitude when a bubble oxygenator is used.[9,16] One study reported that the level of trauma from the membrane oxygenator is clinically tolerable for several days, whereas the safe perfusion period with the bubble oxygenator is measured in hours.[10]

Sade and associates[37] at the University of South Carolina studied blood and organ function in children following open-heart surgery during which either a membrane or bubble oxygenator afforded extracorporeal circulation. In this prospective, randomized study no difference was found between the two groups in any variable related to cardiopulmonary bypass (pulmonary, renal, or cerebral function) or in hematological variables, except free hemoglobin. After 5 and 60 minutes of cardiopulmonary bypass and 24 hours postoperatively, plasma hemoglobin was lower in the membrane oxygenator group. The differences were not large, and the author saw them as holding little clinical significance. The lack of dramatic postoperative physiological differences in the two groups may suggest that the oxygenator is not the major source of blood trauma during the open-heart surgery procedure. Contact of extracardiac blood with the pericardium and the use of cardiotomy suction are important sources of blood trauma. Relatively large amounts of cardiotomy suction are required in virtually all open-heart surgery in children. Sade concluded that the physiology of membrane oxygenators is of greater advantage during coronary bypass surgery in which there is less exposure of blood to nonvascular structures as compared to congenital heart surgery; therefore less blood trauma ensues. On the other hand, Pierce[34] editorialized that the tests employed by Sade were predictably too insensitive to or primarily dependent on factors (such as trauma of the surgery or hemodilution) other than the type of oxygenator for their differences after perfusion.

Van den Dungen and associates[41] examined the differences in hemostasis after perfusion with membrane or bubble oxygenators in cardiopulmonary bypass. Significant differences between the two groups were found for postoperative blood loss and transfusions; both were higher in the bubble oxygenator group. Platelet function was better maintained in the membrane oxygenator group until the moment of releasing the aortic cross-clamp, after which it decreased concomitantly with more frequent suctioning. Following protamine administration, an additional drop of platelet function occurred with virtually no platelet function remaining in either group. However, it recovered 90 minutes after bypass, more profoundly in the membrane oxygenator group. In this study hemostasis was better preserved with membrane oxygenator perfusion. Emphasis was placed on the meticulous attention to preventing additional platelet damage by minimal suctioning and administration of a correct protamine dose.

Pierce[34] suggested that meaningful comparisons between the two oxygenators need to be undertaken. Such analysis must be approached with greater attention to moderating cardiotomy suction, appropriate blood filtration, and the development of more sensitive and specific tests for perfusion damage. Pierce concluded that although it is difficult to prove at the present time, there is some significant documentation that leads the clinician to regard the membrane oxygenator as providing superior protection against gas embolization. Further analysis of large numbers of patients needs to be undertaken.

Left heart assist devices

Internal and external counterpulsation, as described in aforementioned chapters, reduces cardiac work. The functionally pumping heart must, however, maintain the circulation. Mechanical flow assistance becomes necessary in the event of circulatory collapse. Several designs of short- and long-term mechanical assist devices have been developed through intensive ongoing animal research at a few major centers, such as the Texas Heart Institute, Cleveland Clinic, Boston Children's Hospital Medical Center in association with Harvard University, Pennsylvania Medical Center at Hershey, University of Utah, Stanford University, and Thoratec Company. A representation of various models of left heart assist devices is presented but is not intended to be all inclusive or to indicate a preference for one device over the other. Rather the reader is merely introduced to a sampling of devices that have been engineered.

Mechanics: flow assistance

Despite variances in design, all mechanical ventricular assist devices support the failing heart by flow assistance. Flow assistance reduces cardiac work by diverting blood from the natural ventricle to an artificial pump that maintains the circulation. Flow assistance is in contrast to the pressure assistance principles of balloon pump augmentation, whereby the resistance to left ventricular ejection is reduced by lowering the aortic end-diastolic pressure before systolic ejection. In comparison with the IABP, which augments existing circulation, left heart assist devices are true blood pumps designed for human compatibility. They can also maintain adequate systemic perfusion during episodes of ventricular fibrillation or asystole.

Analogous to other organs with temporary failure, the heart can potentially regain function if its pumping action can be artificially maintained temporarily, allowing the heart to rest. Myocardial depression, as evidenced by inability to wean from cardiopulmonary bypass intraoperatively, has been successfully treated with employment of a left heart assist device.

Circulation in the left ventricular assist device (LVAD)

Mechanical left heart assist devices divert oxygenated blood from either the left atrium or left ventricle into the artificial pump, which mechanically reinfuses this blood back into the arterial circulation. Ventricular assist devices are attached externally to the patient's chest and connected to the heart by short, large-diameter cannulas to achieve high flow rates. The pumps are pneumatically powered by relatively bulky units similar in size and design to intra-aortic balloon consoles. Pumps can be timed asynchronously, or they can be synchronized with the electrocardiogram (ECG) to eject during any phase of the cardiac cycle. Ventricular assist effectiveness, however, is chiefly the result of its ability to reduce ventricular ejection impedance during biological systole and to eject blood during biolog-

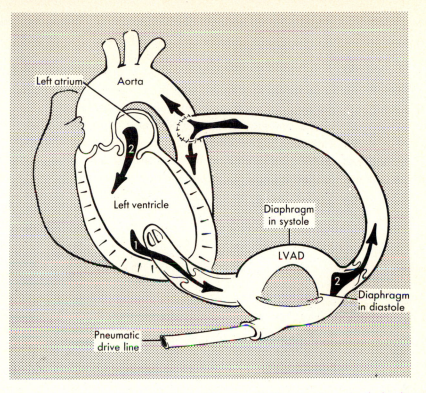

FIG. 32-6 Synchronized blood flow with natural heart and left ventricular assist device (LVAD). In ventricular systole, LVAD is in diastole. *1,* Blood is ejected from left ventricle to LVAD. *2,* During ventricular diastole, LVAD is in systole and pumps blood volume back into aortic cannulas. (Modified from original drawing by Kevin Murray, Salt Lake City.)

ical diastole. Synchronized pumping is instituted to achieve a counterpulsation effect (Fig. 32-6). During ventricular systole blood is diverted out from the natural ventricle into the LVAD. In cardiac diastole the LVAD pumps this blood back into the circulation through a cannula placed in the aorta. Hence counterpulsation circulation occurs; the LVAD is in diastole while the native ventricle contracts and vice versa.

As with balloon pumping, the ECG is used to synchronize triggering of the pump with cardiac action. Left ventricular peak systolic pressure, stroke work index, and oxygen consumption are markedly reduced, thereby reducing the afterload of cardiac work. The biological ventricle is mechanically rested to facilitate any potential reversible ventricular depression.[33]

LVAD and potential clinical physiological effects

The success of IABP counterpulsation has spurred enthusiasm for continued research of mechanical devices that support the circulation. After extensive animal and in vitro testing of device safety and reliability, the National Heart, Lung and Blood Institute's clinical LVAD or partial artificial heart program was initiated in late 1975.[26] This program has demonstrated that in moribund patients with refractory postcardiotomy heart failure, the use of an LVAD is clinically feasible, safe, and often associated with favorable physiological changes that sometimes result in clinical recovery. Other specific findings in the clinical setting have been summarized by Norman[27]:

1. LVADs can provide partial or total support of the circulation.
2. Myocardial function can improve after 48 and 96 hours of LVAD support.
3. Myocardial function can be assessed noninvasively during LVAD support.
4. Mechanical support can be managed with the aid of conventional monitoring of cardiac and systemic blood pressures, cardiac output, and heart rate.
5. LVADs can fully support the circulation throughout episodes of atrial and ventricular dysrhythmias, including fibrillation and asystole.

Direct mechanical left ventricular assist (Skinner)

Skinner and associates[38] have clinically implemented left ventricular assistance by a direct cardiac compression device (Fig. 32-7). The chest is opened when the heart is desperately failing, and the suction cup apparatus is positioned directly over the failing ventricles. Contractile force is mechanically increased through direct compression of the heart, by rhythmic alteration of suction and inflation.

Experimentally this device was used on a fibrillating heart only, never in patients in normal sinus rhythm. The synchronization of this device was found to be extremely difficult. Mechanical trauma inflicted on the heart by the Skinner device and the need for synchronization have greatly limited its use.

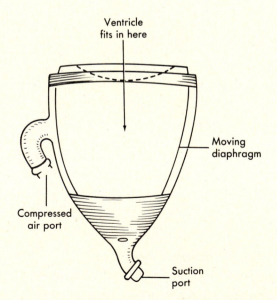

FIG. 32-7 Suction cup apparatus that can be positioned directly over failing heart. Cardiac compression is maintained by alternate suction and inflation.

Atrial-arterial left heart assist (Litwak device)

The Litwak device, developed by Litwak[22] of Mt. Sinai Hospital in New York, consists of atrial and ascending aorta silicone elastomer cannulas with polyester suturing skirts; the first skirt is sutured into the left atrium, and the second is inserted into the lateral aspect of the ascending aorta (Fig. 32-8). One important feature of the Litwak is the technique of cannulation of the left atrium from the right side of the aorta.

The distal ends of both cannulas are positioned subcutaneously in the upper abdominal wall and are connected to a simple extracorporeal circuit, since the blood returning from the left atrium has already been oxygenated. A roller pump is interposed between the left atrium and the ascending aorta, which steadily returns diverted blood into the ascending aorta, maintaining arterial pressure at adequate levels. The maximum flow capacity of the circuit is approximately 5 liters/min. Ventricular preload is reduced as blood volume is diverted from the left atrium into the assist device; left atrial pressure is therefore decreased.

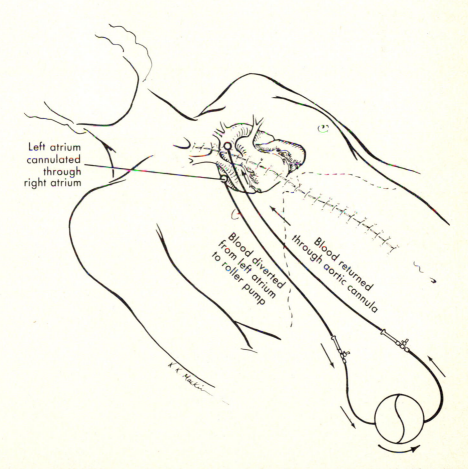

Left atrium
cannulated
through
right atrium

Blood diverted
from left atrium
to roller pump

Blood returned
through aortic cannula

FIG. 32-8 Litwak atrial-arterial left heart assist device. First cannula is sutured with polyester, suturing skirt to left atrium, and second cannula is inserted into ascending aorta. Roller pump is interposed between left atrium and ascending aorta. (Modified from Litwak, R.S., et al.: N. Engl. J. Med. **201**:1341, 1974.)

Avoidance of thoracic reentry to decannulate is an integral part of this device. Circulatory assistance is discontinued simply by exposing the distal cannula tips, disconnecting the mechanical pumping system, and accurately fitting the cannulas with silicone elastomer obturators so that their lumens are totally obliterated. Leaving the cannulas subcutaneously after discontinuation of the LVAD has resulted in serious problems. Infections of these remnants of the LVAD occur frequently and require reoperation for removal.[23]

Abdominal left ventricular assist device (Norman)

The abdominal left ventricular assist device (ALVAD)[28] consists of a single-chambered implantable blood pump, actuated by an external pneumatic drive console that diverts blood directly from the left ventricle into the descending thoracic aorta. The pumping chamber (Fig. 32-9) is symmetrical about a central axis, weighing 470.0 g, measuring 17.0 cm in length, and having a diameter of 6.3 cm. The device houses a polyurethane bladder that collapses in three segments or lobes when pneumatic pressure is applied to the space between the bladder and the titanium housing. The displacement volume is 300 cc with flow rates up to 6 liters/min achieved in humans.

An important difference in Norman's heart is the use of heterograft (porcine) valves. These valves require no systemic anticoagulation, which is a distinct advantage over mechanical valves. However, calcification of heterograft valves remains a problem in calves but is less common in the adult human. Polyester fiber coats all blood-contacting surfaces except the inflow and outflow valves. A neointima develops on the surface of the pump, consisting of fibrin, platelets, erythrocytes, leukocytes, and macrophages.[24,40]

Uniquely the ALVAD is designed for abdominal placement to facilitate implantation without pulmonary compromise and to permit subsequent removal without a thoracotomy.

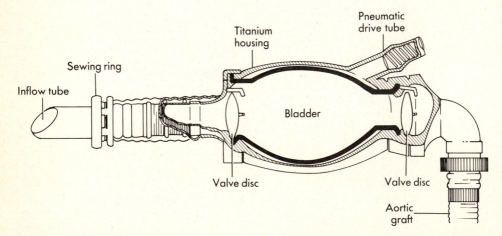

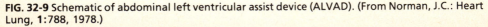

FIG. 32-9 Schematic of abdominal left ventricular assist device (ALVAD). (From Norman, J.C.: Heart Lung, **1**:788, 1978.)

Fig. 32-10 illustrates anatomical placement of the ALVAD in the abdominal cavity. The outflow graft is attached to the infrarenal abdominal aorta. The inflow graft is anastomosed to a cored left ventricular apex to which a Teflon felt sewing ring has been sutured. Exteriorization of the ALVAD pneumatic driveline is achieved through a small left flank incision.

Following priming of the pump with a low-molecular weight Dextran, the clinical drive console can be adjusted to obtain any of the following pumping modes: (1) low-rate asynchronous (35 to 45 beats/min), (2) asynchronous (45 to 140 beats/min), (3) synchronous counterpulsation (20 to 140 beats/min), or (4) intermittent synchronous counterpulsation (1:1 to 1:10).

LVAD (Bernhard)

Similar in design to Norman's LVAD, this device is worn externally rather than internally (Fig. 32-11).[3] The pneumatic pump is tailored with inflow and outflow Dacron conduits, each containing a porcine valve to provide unidirectional flow. The mechanical

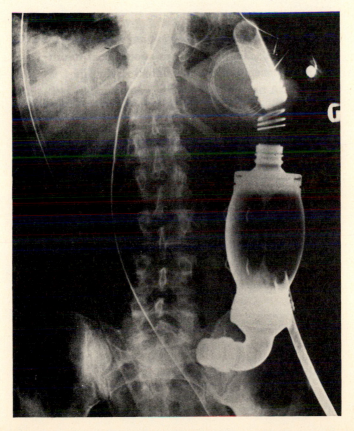

FIG. 32-10 ALVAD in situ in abdominal cavity. (Photo courtesy John Norman, Washington, D.C.)

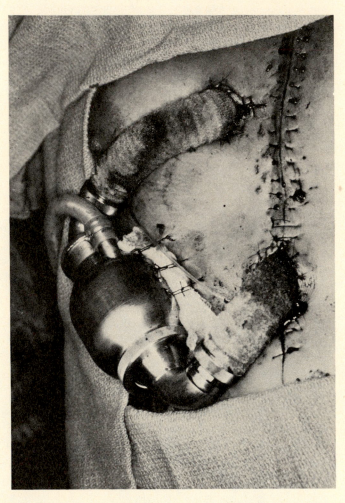

FIG. 32-11 Bernhard's design of LVAD worn externally. (From Berger, R.L., et al.: J. Thorac. Cardiovasc. Surg. **78:**626, 1979.)

ventricle rests on the anterior chest wall, and the afferent and efferent conduits are attached to the left ventricular apex and ascending thoracic aorta, respectively. Fabricated from polyurethane, the pumping bladder is housed in a rigid titanium shell. The blood-contacting surface is flocked with polyester fibrils to facilitate early coating by blood components.

The pumping chamber fills directly from the left ventricle and ejects into the ascending aorta. Ejection may be asynchronous, or it may be synchronized with the electrocardiographic signal to fill during biological systole and empty into the aorta during cardiac diastole. Pumping is accomplished by the introduction of carbon dioxide under pressure into the space between the flexible bladder and rigid housing. Maximal stroke volume is 85 cc, and maximal rate is 100 beats/min.

Transapical left ventricular bypass (Peters)

The transapical LVAD, developed at the University of Utah,[31] withdraws blood via a cannula directly from the left ventricular apex. The blood then passes through a roller pump to an outflow Pall filter and returns to the femoral artery via a Dacron graft (Fig. 32-12). Placement of the apex cannula is achieved by chest entry via a left lateral thoracotomy incision of the fifth or sixth intercostal space under general anesthetic. The ventricular matrix is incised and sequentially dilated. An apical support cuff, withdrawal cannula, and sleeve assembly are sutured into position. A Cooley Dacron graft positioned on the return cannula is anastomosed to the femoral artery. Heparinization is maintained with a continuous intravenous drip. The preprimed pump circuit and outflow Pall filter are connected, and pumping is gradually initiated with removal of any air from the filter. The outflow Pall filter is usually changed prophylactically and cultured every 3 days.

Long-term LVAD (Pierce)

Patients with inoperable coronary lesions, whose left ventricular function precludes separation from the IABP and/or those with myocardial infarction who have little chance of recovering left ventricular function may benefit from a long-term implantable ventricular assist pump.[34,35]

The design of the long-term device developed by Pierce and associates has the added convenience of an implantable energy converter intended for long-term implantable usage. The converter actuates a pusher plate or pressurizes hydraulic fluid that in turn compresses the blood-containing chamber. Of note is Pierce's use of Bjork-Shiley valves, which require long-term anticoagulation.

Ideally such a self-contained implantable device would function much like a pacemaker. Because of the 10 watts of power required to provide energy to drive the pump, an external electrical source is required. Electrical energy may be supplied to the pump via a percutaneous wire (Fig. 32-13). The patient then has the option of obtaining continuous electrical energy from a battery pack or an electrical outlet.

The prospect of an implanted radioisotope power source is not a reality for the near future because of the high cost of development and potential radiation risks. Pierce and associates[34] have used long-term LVADs in animals in which their circulation was sup-

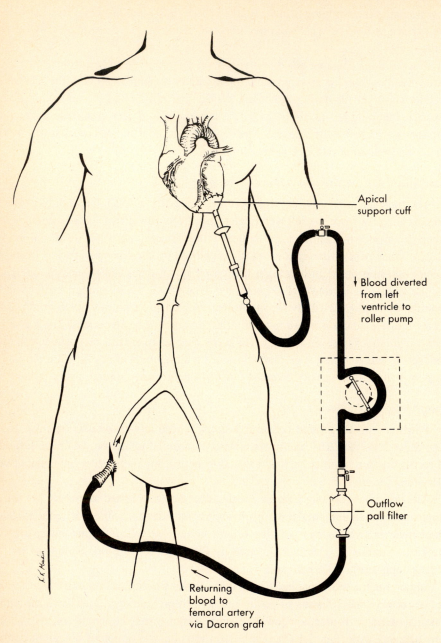

Apical
support cuff

↓ Blood diverted
from left
ventricle to
roller pump

Outflow
pall filter

Returning
blood to
femoral artery
via Dacron graft

FIG. 32-12 Transapical LVAD. (From Peters, J.L., et al.: Artif. Organs **2:**263, 1978.)

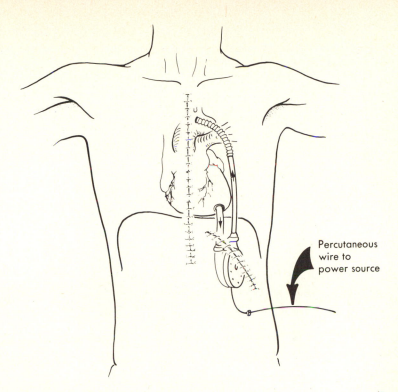

Percutaneous
wire to
power source

FIG. 32-13 Long-term LVAD with percutaneous wire for connection to power source. (From Pierce, W.S., and Myers, J.L.: J. Cardiovasc. Med. **6**:667, 1981.)

ported continuously for more than 100 days. Problems limiting the duration of animal studies include mechanical component failure in the energy converters and calcium phosphate deposits on the high flexion areas where the blood and polyurethane come together. Pierce described the future clinical trials as ones that would involve initial units having functional lives similar to the early pacemakers. When signs of imminent energy converter failure develop, the patient reports to the hospital for replacement. Sudden failures are not catastrophic because the patient's heart is intact and supports life during the few hours required for unit replacement.

Weaning from LVAD

Berger and others[2] reported that in the early phases of LVAD support, the device assumes nearly total left heart output, whereas the biological left ventricle performs little work. Therefore reduction in LVAD flows during this period is poorly tolerated. As the myocardium recovers, usually within 72 hours, the left ventricle resumes a gradually increasing fraction of systemic blood flow, and attempts to wean from the LVAD are undertaken. Temporary reductions in LVAD flow are repeated; if adequate cardiac output and arterial pressures are maintained without marked increase in left atrial pressure, the LVAD is withdrawn. If the circulation deteriorates during attempts at reduced LVAD flow, full mechanical circulatory support is resumed. Berger recommended using the IABP for 24 to 48 hours after LVAD removal as a precautionary measure, but he offered no data to indicate that such support is essential.

LVAD removal

The devices that are worn externally can be removed by dividing the inflow and outflow grafts and burying the stumps subcutaneously. Some surgeons recommend reopening the original sternal-splitting incision and removing all or most of the intrathoracic conduits. Berger and associates[2] emphasized that the risk of retained foreign material is greater than the stress of reopening the surgical wound to remove the device. Usually by the time the patient tolerates separation from the mechanical support, the cardiac reserve is sufficient to withstand re-entry to remove the LVAD.

LVAD and bleeding problems

Excessive bleeding postoperatively has been the major problem with use of the LVAD. The hemorrhagic tendency noted in patients is caused by the extended pump oxygenator time required for repair of the cardiac lesion, repeated trials to wean from the cardiopulmonary bypass, and the period necessary for implantation of the LVAD. This tendency is aggravated by the need for postoperative systemic anticoagulation. Decreased flow through the LVAD in the face of adequate or high filling pressures is strongly suggestive of cardiac tamponade, which may occur as a result of the hemorrhaging.

LVAD and right heart failure

Despite satisfactory left ventricular unloading with use of the LVAD, there is evidence to suggest that the right ventricle simultaneously undergoes an increased work load.[2,28] If the insult that led to left ventricular failure also involves the right ventricle, this chamber will have suffered two insults and will carry a likelihood of concomitant failure. Treatment can be approached either medically with the use of inotropic drugs or surgically with biventricular mechanical assistance. Medical therapy often fails because of the compromised state of the right ventricle.

Anticoagulation and the LVAD

With LVAD flows about 2 liters/min, Bernhard[4] did not recommend anticoagulation, and no thromboembolic complications have been detected. During the final weaning phase, when flow rates are reduced, systemic anticoagulation with heparin is recommended in an attempt to prevent thrombus deposition on the prosthetic surface. The use of porcine valves does not require anticoagulation, whereas the employment of mechanical valves and extracorporeal roller pumps requires continuous anticoagulation.

Balloon pumping versus LVAD circulatory assist

The IABP has been a life-saving technique for tens of thousands of patients who required marginal circulatory assistance. However, it is capable of providing only about 25% of the energy demands of the pumping action of the heart. IABP reduces left ventricular work load and myocardial oxygen consumption by 10% and increases left ventricle output by perhaps 30%. By transferring blood from the left ventricle to the aorta, a left ventricular assist pump reduces ventricular work load by 90% and myocardial oxygen consumption by 40%.[30]

Nursing care of patients requiring the LVAD

Marked myocardial dysfunction has necessitated use of the LVAD. Therefore these patients require continuous one-to-one nursing care and ongoing observations. Postoperative care requires intensive involvement by the nurse, surgeon, and perfusionist or trained cardiovascular technician. Vigilant surveillance to every detail of this critically ill patient affords an immense nursing challenge.

Psychological support. Detailed descriptions are given for the patient's physical care after LVAD insertion, but psychological care for the patient and his family is discussed initially so that the extreme importance of psychological support is not overlooked. The patient and his support systems must be cohesively involved in education and ongoing communications as to developments and procedures of care postoperatively before LVAD insertion. During this time the patient and family need to be assured of adequate meeting time with the surgeon to satisfactorily understand the potential gains and risks associated with the procedure and the anticipated outcomes. If it was not anticipated that the LVAD be used before the operation, the surgeon speaks to the family to obtain consent for insertion at the time that the patient cannot be separated from cardiopulmonary bypass. Often the family members are so stunned by the magnitude of information that is rapidly disseminated that they cannot comprehend or digest the complexity of the procedure that is to ensue.

Once the surgeon has initially explained the procedure to the family (and patient if there is anticipation of the use of the LVAD before surgery), it is imperative that the nurse reinforce the content that has been presented and allow the family to direct the depth of teaching that ensues thereafter. Some families want to have the details of the procedure repeated, and others only want a minimum of information; they cannot cope with the mental stress of trying to comprehend new foreign words. Efforts must be made by the nurse to determine the level suitable for the family.

Social services may be of immense assistance at this point in locating housing for out-of-town families, making phone calls to additional family members, and offering support to the family. During the surgery at least hourly contact must be made with the family to keep them informed of the patient's progress. Families are usually most cooperative of restrictive visiting if they feel that they are a part of the picture and are honestly apprised of the care that the patient is receiving. Preparing the family for the initial visit is an important component of teaching; no matter how detailed the instructions are that have been given the family, the initial visit to the bedside is overwhelming in most circumstances.

The patient is usually kept sedated, but during periods of consciousness, efforts must be made to reassure him that he is not alone, that medical personnel are continuously caring for him, and that basic body function support (i.e., the ventilator breathing for him, the placement of the endotracheal tube preventing his speaking, and a catheter indwelling in his bladder drain his urine) is assured. The patient is questioned as to whether or not he is having pain, and relief measures should be instituted. Despite the fact that the patient must remain relatively immobile, simple comfort measures can be frequently instituted, such as rubbing the patient's shoulders with lotion, offering a cold swab to his mouth, wiping his face, and offering a soothing soaking of his feet in a bath basin of water.

Hemodynamic monitoring. A Swan-Ganz catheter is placed either before or after arrival in the operating room. Ongoing physiological variables that require monitoring include the ECG; systemic arterial, right atrial, left atrial, pulmonary artery, and pulmonary capillary wedge pressures; cardiac output; and temperature. Usually these measurements are monitored via a special data acquisition computer. The extracorporeal component of the LVAD is monitored by the perfusionist or cardiovascular technician trained in its function.

Respiratory care. The patient returns from the operating room intubated, and ventilation is maintained via positive pressure ventilatory support. Assessment of ventilatory and frequent blood gas measurements are essential. Frequent auscultation alerts the clinician pending respiratory complications. Because of the early hemodynamic instability of the patient, vigorous chest physiotherapy and position changes are deferred. However, gentle vibration of the chest may be employed to mobilize secretions along with ongoing pulmonary toilet of secretions. The patient may need to be paralyzed with a drug such as pancuronium to achieve respiratory control with the mechanical ventilator. He can certainly be extubated as is the routine in postoperative cardiac care. A daily chest x-ray film is examined.

Renal function, fluids, and electrolytes. Hourly urine output measurements are made because renal insufficiency is to be anticipated in patients with low cardiac output. Blood urea nitrogen and creatinine are analyzed daily as well as plasma and urine osmolality and serum electrolytes. Patients may have to be dialyzed secondary to decreased cardiac output and impaired renal function. Fluids are administered as necessary to maintain adequate central venous pressure, pulmonary artery wedge pressure, left atrial pressure, and cardiac output. There is no intrinsic need for fluid restriction.

Hematological care. Excessive bleeding is perhaps the most common complication caused by the excessive period the patient was required to be on cardiopulmonary bypass. Daily coagulation profiles, complete blood counts, platelet counts, and reticulocyte counts are performed. These patients sometimes require transfusions of platelets, coagulation factors, and red blood cells. Bilirubin and serum haptoglobin are analyzed to monitor for possible hemolytic end disease states. Ongoing recording of chest tube drainage and examination for bleeding from any other sites are essential. Anticoagulation is adjusted proportionate to the flow rates of the LVAD, since reduced flow rates during weaning require increased anticoagulation to prevent thrombus formation within the LVAD. Additionally the nursing staff must observe the patient for any evidence of septic emboli, such as hematuria and neurological changes.

Infection control. The complexity of the procedure employed and the patient's debilitated state make him a prime candidate for infections. This problem is amplified by the presence of a large foreign body and its associated vascular grafts and mechanical valves. Antibiotics are usually used throughout the time the LVAD is in place. Meticulous hand washing by the staff must be carried out to minimize the risk of spreading iatrogenic infection to the patient. Strict aseptic technique must be maintained for tracheal aspirations, for Foley catheter and intravenous site care, and for dressing changes. The LVAD site is redressed daily, and the incision sites are cleansed with Betadine.

Care of the LVAD pump. Most nurses have limited or no exposure to the LVAD. Cooperative arrangements must be established with the perfusionist or cardiovascular technician for monitoring of the LVAD pump. Nursing responsibility includes preventing kinks and tension on the extracorporeal components of the systems when moving the patient and exposing the junctions of the cannulas and the circuit to observe for any sign of disconnection.

Nursing care of patients requiring the LVAD demands the highest level of competence in the nurse's skills of assessment and understanding of interrelatedness of body systems and the technical aspect of the LVAD. Such expertise is life-saving. The patient and his family usually appreciate the extent of competency required by the nurse, but a reflection on the experience that the patient is undergoing calls for basic nursing skills, such as being kind, keeping the patient and family informed, offering thorough explanations and compassion. It is easy to lose the patient among the maze of tubes and lines if conscious effort is not given to meeting the psychological and emotional needs of the patient and his family, who maintain a vigil and wait unending hours for recovery.

REFERENCES

1. Berger, E.: The physiology of adequate perfusion, St. Louis, 1979, The C.V. Mosby Co.
2. Berger, R.L., et al.: Successful use of a left ventricular assist device in cardiogenic shock from massive post operative myocardial infarction, J. Thorac. Cardiovasc. Surg. **78:**626, 1979.
3. Bernhard, W.F., et al.: A new method for temporary left ventricular bypass, J. Thorac. Cardiovasc. Surg. **70:**880, 1975.
4. Bernhard, W.F., et al.: An appraisal of blood trauma and the blood prosthetic interface during left ventricular bypass in the calf and man, Ann. Thorac. Surg., **26:**427, 1978.
5. Birtwell, W.C., et al.: The evolution of counterpulsation techniques, Med. Instrum. **10:**217, 1976.
6. Bregman, D.: Mechanical support of the failing heart and lungs, New York, 1977, Appleton-Century-Crofts.
7. Brennan, R.W., et al.: Cerebral blood flow and metabolism during cardiopulmonary bypass: evidence of microembolic encephalopathy, Neurology **21:**665, 1971.
8. Byrick, R.J., and Nobec, W.N.: Postoperative lung syndrome: comparison of travenol bubble and membrane oxygenators, J. Thorac. Cardiovasc. Surg. **76:**685, 1978.
9. Carlson, R.G., et al.: The Lande-Edwards membrane oxygenator during heart surgery oxygen transfer, microemboli counts and Bender-Gestalt visual motor test scores, J. Thorac. Cardiovasc. Surg. **66:**894, 1973.
10. Clark, R.E., et al.: A comparison of membrane and bubble oxygenators in short and long perfusions, J. Thorac. Cardiovasc. Surg. **78:**655, 1979.
11. Davids, S., and Engell, H.: Physiology and clinical aspects of oxygenator design, Amsterdam, Elsevier/North Holland, 1976, Biomedics Press.
12. De Bakey, M.D.: Left ventricular bypass sump for cardiac assistance: clinical experience, Am. J. Cardiol. **27:**3, 1971.
13. Dutton, R.C., et al.: Platelet aggregate is emboli produced in patients during cardiopulmonary bypass with membrane and bubble oxygenators and blood filters, J. Thorac. Cardiovasc. Surg. **67:**258, 1974.
14. Galletti, P.M., and Brecker, G.A.: Heart lung bypass: principles and techniques of extracorporeal circulation, New York, 1962, Grune & Stratton, Inc.

15. Gibbon, J.H.: Application of a mechanical heart and lung apparatus to cardiac surgery, Minn. Med. **37:**171, 1954.

16. Hill, J.D., et al.: Neuropathological manifestations of cardiac surgery, Ann. Thorac. Surg. **7:**409, 1969.

17. Ionesu, M.I., and Wool, G.H., editors: Current techniques in extracorporeal circulation, London, 1976, Butterworth & Co.

18. Jarvik, R.K.: Artificial hearts: from engineering ideas to patient care, Report 81-1, Presented at bioengineering seminar, University of California, Berkeley, 1981.

19. Jarvik, R.K.: The total artificial heart, Sci. Am. **244:**74, 1981.

20. Lee, W.N., Jr., and Hairston, P.: Structural effects on blood proteins at the gas-blood interface, Fed. Proc. **30:**1615, 1979.

21. Liddicoat, J.E., et al.: Membrane vs. bubble oxygenators: clinical comparison, Ann. Surg. **181:**747, 1975.

22. Litwak, R.S., et al.: Postcardiotomy low cardiac output, clinical experience with a left heart assist device, Circulation, **54**(suppl. 3):102, 1976.

23. McCormick, J.R.: Infection in remnant of left ventricular device after successful separation from assisted circulation, J. Thorac. Cardiovasc. Surg. **81:**727, 1981.

24. Norman, J.C.: Flecking flocked biomaterial surfaces: initial observations in man during intracorporeal (abdominal) left ventricular assist device (ALVAD) pumping, Topical report to National Heart, Lung and Blood Institute, Bethesda, Md. Oct. 25, 1976.

25. Norman, J.C.: Intracorporeal partial artificial hearts: initial results in ten patients, Artif. Organs **1:**41, 1977.

26. Norman, J.C.: Intracorporeal partial artificial hearts: initial clinical trials, Heart Lung **7:**788, 1978.

27. Norman, J.C.: The role of assist devices in managing low cardiac output. Cardiovascular diseases, Bull. Texas Heart Institute **8:**119, March 1981.

28. Norman, J.C., et al.: An intracorporeal (abdominal) left ventricular assist device, Arch. Surg. **112:**1442, 1977.

29. Parker, J.L., et al.: Membrane versus bubble oxygenators: a clinical comparison of postoperative blood loss, Caridovasc. Dis. **6:**78, 1979.

30. Pennock, J.L., et al.: Reduction of myocardial infarct size: comparison between left atrial and left ventricular bypass, Circulation **59:**275, 1979.

31. Peters, J.L., et al.: Transapical left ventricular bypass: a method for partial or total circulatory support, Artif. Organs **2:**263, 1978.

32. Pierce, E.C., II: Is blood-gas interface of clinical importance? (Editorial), Ann. Thorac. Surg. **17:**526, 1974.

33. Pierce, W.S.: Prolonged mechanical support of the left ventricle, Circulation **58**(suppl. 1):136, 1977.

34. Pierce, W.S., and Myers, J.L.: Frontiers of therapy: left ventricular assist pumps and the artificial heart, J. Cardiovasc. Med. **42:**667, 1981.

35. Poe, W.E., Jr., and Pierce, W.S.: Temporary left ventricular assistance in acute myocardial infarction and cardiogenic shock: rationale and criterion for utilization, Chest **79:**692, 1981.

36. Ratliff, N.B.: Pulmonary injury secondary to extracorporeal circulation: an ultrastructural study, J. Thorac. Cardiovasc. Surg. **65:**425, 1973.

37. Sade, R.M., et al.: A prospective randomized study of membrane versus bubble oxygenators in children, Ann. Thorac. Surg. **29:**502, 1980.

38. Skinner, D.B.: Experimental and clinical evaluations of mechanical ventricular assistance, Am. J. Cardiol. **27:**146, 1971.

39. Solis, R.T., et al.: Cardiopulmonary bypass: microembolization and platelet aggregation, Circulation **52:**103, 1975.

40. Trono, R., et al.: Mechanical properties of neointima formed within experimental and clinical left ventricular assist devices (LVADs), Clin. Res. **24:**523A, 1976.

41. Van den Dungen, J.J., et al.: Clinical study of blood trauma during perfusion with membrane and bubble oxygenators, J. Thorac. Cardiovasc. Surg. **83:**108, 1982.

42. Vroman, L., et al.: Interactions among human blood proteins at interfaces, Fed. Proc. **30:**1494, 1971.

CHAPTER 33 The Utah total artificial heart

Kevin D. Murray and Susan J. Quaal

The history of the total artificial heart (TAH) extends over several decades. Many of the early pioneers in this field were quickly disillusioned about the feasibility of overcoming the numerous complex problems that continually blocked the pathway to success. Yet despite these seemingly insurmountable obstacles, a few dedicated researchers slowly but persistently pieced together the mosaic that has evolved into the artificial heart as we currently know it. Years of study in the animal model have allowed numerous refinements to be made in the construction, function, placement, and regulation of the TAH. The elegance and success of today's artificial heart are credited to the relative simplicity of the device.

We are currently poised on the verge of a potential widespread use of the TAH in humans. This very exciting and challenging prospect will undoubtedly result in new problems and situations that have been heretofore unknown in the clinical setting. Successful use of the TAH in humans therefore requires application of the vast knowledge accumulated in the animal model, along with the expertise and insight of the clinical team who is caring for these patients. Only a handful of researchers and clinical physicians possess the knowledge of how the TAH functions and how to maintain it in animals for many months. As the TAH becomes more widely used in humans, this knowledge needs to be disseminated to physicians, nurses, and auxiliary personnel who are entrusted with the care of the patient who is the recipient of the TAH. Specifically the nurse is a vital member of this team, for he or she is faced with a critically ill patient whose care incorporates extensive measures beyond the familiar intensive care medications and monitoring devices. Standards of care will develop that are unique to these patients.

As experience is gained with patients receiving a TAH, their care will become routine. However, before that state of expertise, the knowledge acquired from years of research in the animal must be made available as a foundation of proven facts regarding the function and management of the TAH. This chapter represents the state of the art of the TAH in the animal model with regard to design, function, regulation, and known problems. The University of Utah received FDA approval for human implantation of the Jarvik-7 (J-7) TAH, and its first clinical application was on December 2, 1982. This historic operation marked the beginning to a new era in cardiac surgery.

History

The first implantation of the TAH inside the chest of an experimental animal took place only a little more than 25 years ago. In 1957 Kolff performed that historic experiment with a TAH that sustained the life of the animal for 90 minutes. Progress was agonizingly slow for the next 12 years with survival time being measured in hours.

Introduction of the diaphragm-type heart in the early 1970s brought a dramatic improvement in performance and furthered the survival of the animal recipients into the 1- to 2-week range, as illustrated in the longevity graph (Fig. 33-1). The problems of design, fabrication, implantation, coagulation, hemolysis, thrombus, mechanical failure, disseminated intravascular coagulaton, respiratory distress syndrome, and many others were slowly, but successfully conquered.

In 1972 an ellipsoidal pneumatically driven diaphragm heart was introduced at the University of Utah. This heart, named the *Jarvik-3* (J-3) after its developer, showed superior design, had compatibility with the blood components, and provided more cardiac output, all of which again lengthened the survival of the experimental animals. Work carried out in many laboratories throughout the United States and around the world continued to advance the success of the TAH. The improvements and innovations that propelled the University of Utah to the forefront of TAH research came under the leadership of Donald B. Olsen, Director of Artificial Heart Research in Salt Lake City, Utah. With further modifications came even longer survival times, ranging into several months. An improved hemodynamic J-3 TAH was designed and fabricated at the University of Utah and was labeled the Jarvik-5 (J-5) TAH. This advanced heart was used by Kolff and Olsen to sustain the life of a calf for 9 months in 1981, which set a world record.

The J-5 TAH was designed to fulfill the stroke volume requirements of experimental animals (165 cc) and has been scaled down to a size that fits the human mediastinum (the Jarvik-7 [J-7]) and yet provides an adequate stroke volume (105 cc). The J-5 and the J-7 TAHs continue to be employed in experimental animals at the University of Utah's Division of Artificial Organs. However, it was the J-7 heart that was implanted in the first human recipient on December 2, 1982, at the University of Utah Medical Center.

J-7 heart

The J-7 TAH has been designed specifically for use in humans. Size and shape are such that it fits the dimensions of the normal adult mediastinum. Long-term testing on an in vitro mock circulation has demonstrated the J-7 artificial heart's durability; testing now exceeds 4 years of continuous pumping. The performance of the J-7 ventricles, when implanted in calf and sheep models, has demonstrated their ability to provide proper cardiac output for several months while causing negligible harm to the recipient's blood components and organs. The J-7 is the culmination in design of a multitude of artificial hearts, and it is the device used by the surgical team at the University of Utah.

Design and function of the J-7

The J-7 TAH consists of several components. They include right and left hemispherical ventricles, two inflow and two outflow quick connects, and four mechanical tilting disk valves (Fig. 33-2).[19]

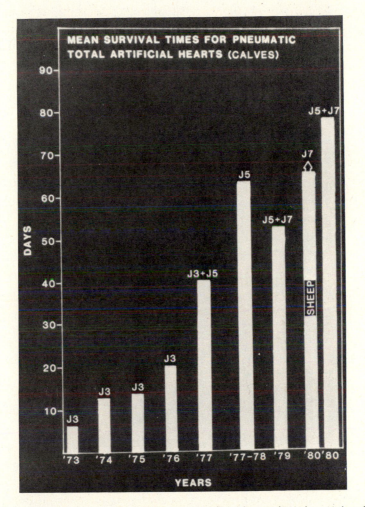

FIG. 33-1 Mean survival times for pneumatic total artificial hearts (TAHs) at University of Utah, indicating improved technology in artificial heart.

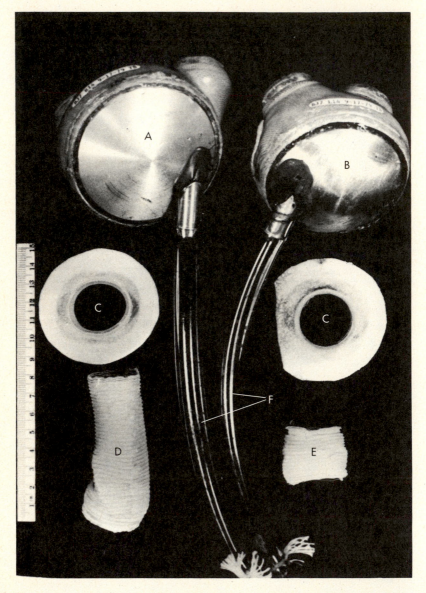

FIG. 33-2 Components of Jarvik-7 (J-7) artificial heart. *A,* Right hemispherical ventricle; *B,* left hemispherical ventricle; *C,* atrial quick connects; *D,* pulmonary artery quick connects; *E,* aortic quick connect; *F,* drivelines. (Photos by Brad Nelson, Division of Medical Illustrations, University of Utah.)

Ventricles. Designing the size and shape of TAH mechanical ventricles was undertaken to meet several important criteria: (1) to fit the space limitations of the adult human mediastinum; (2) to provide the maximum internal volume; (3) to eliminate turbulence, stagnation, and blood trauma. All of these goals have been met in the design of the J-7 hemispherical ventricles. The interior volume capacity is 155 ml with a maximum stroke volume of 105 ml (Fig. 33-3).

The ventricle housing is molded from polyurethane reinforced with Dacron mesh, and the base of the ventricle is fabricated from aluminum or plastic. Both outflow and inflow tracts are angled in such a manner as to provide proper alignment with the native vascular structures and to maintain good hemodynamics (laminar flow without turbulence or stagnation).

The entire interior surface of the J-7 ventricles is formed from segmented polyurethane (Biomer). This substance has been found to be thromboresistant when molded to an ultrasmooth surface. Only when defects, such as cracks or bubbles, appear on the surface of the Biomer does it display tendencies to thrombus formation and calcification. However, with the precision of current molding techniques at the University of Utah, this problem is decreasing in its incidence. Potentially, thrombus formation can also occur in any abnormal flow areas, as well as in seams in the Biomer. A careful study of flow patterns in the J-7 has eliminated stagnation and severe turbulence, and the ventricle's internal lining is molded as one piece, which eliminates seams.

Diaphragm. Four layers of Biomer are used to fabricate the pumping diaphragm (Fig. 33-4). Each layer is 0.006 inches thick. Dry graphite is placed between these layers for lubrication, imparting a black color to the diaphragm. The extreme flexibility of the diaphragm offers a minimal amount of resistance to both inflowing blood in diastole and to the compressed air pumped into the ventricle during systole. Yet these four thin layers of Biomer have proven to be strong and durable.

Constant repetitive flexing in the same area of the diaphragm induces severe stress to these particular points. Excessive stress could cause cracking of the Biomer, which can result in calcification, thrombus formation, and ultimate failure of the ventricle. Therefore design and construction allow the diaphragm to collapse in a random manner with each diastole. This lack of "memory" makes the diaphragm very durable.

When maximally expanded, the J-7 ventricular diaphragm does not touch the housing, thus preventing any hemolysis of red blood cells. Evidence for this success is seen with stable hematocrits, negligible levels of free hemoglobin, and normal lactate dehydrogenase concentrations in animal experiments.

Diaphragm in diastole. The function of the diaphragm is dependent on several factors in each portion of the cardiac cycle. During diastole, the diaphragm collapses in direct proportion to the volume of blood that enters through the inflow port. As more blood enters the artificial heart, the diaphragm collapses in increasing amounts until the maximum volume of the chamber is reached. The rate of collapse is related both to the atrial filling pressures and to the amount of ventricular vacuum. Higher filling pressures and increased vacuum result in more rapid contraction of the diaphragm; however, it only collapses to accommodate that volume of blood delivered via the atria. This behavior is similar to that

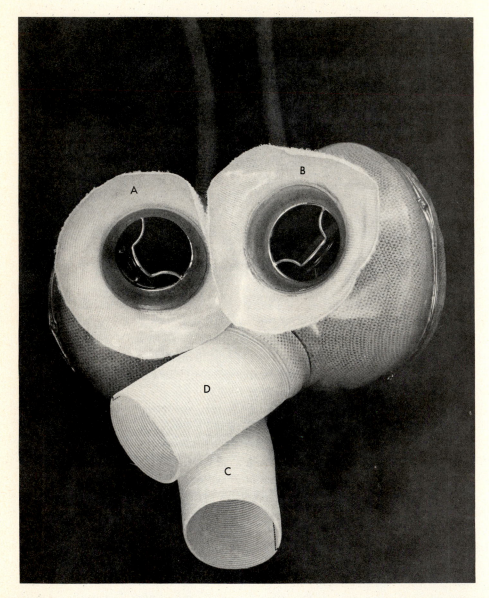

FIG. 33-3 J-7 artificial ventricles with quick connects in place. *A*, Right atrial; *B*, left atrial; *C*, pulmonary artery; *D*, aorta. (Photos by Brad Nelson, Division of Medical Illustrations, University of Utah.)

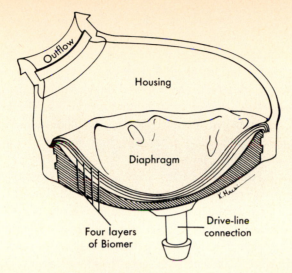

FIG. 33-4 Cross section of J-7 TAH pumping diaphragm. Four layers of segmented polyurethane (Biomer) are used to fabricate this component of artificial ventricle. Each layer is 0.006 inch thick. Dry graphite is placed between layers of Biomer for lubrication.

of the natural heart. Any process that stiffens the diaphragm, such as calcification or rupture of the blood-contacting Biomer, increases its resistance to movement. This increased resistance requires a higher filling pressure and more vacuum to collapse the diaphragm for a given volume.

Diaphragm in systole. During the systolic phase, the diaphragmatic excursion is influenced by the ventricular pneumatic driving pressure, the end-diastolic blood volume, and the resistance to ejection of the blood volume. The optimal situation involves the diaphragm being flexed to its maximum end-systolic position with each heartbeat. This can be accomplished by properly adjusting the pressure generated by the pneumatic heart driver. Driving pressure must be of sufficient force to push the end-diastolic volume of blood through the higher than normal resistance of the artificial valves (aortic and pulmonic). Also, the driving pressure must overcome the afterload pressure of the aorta (aortic end-diastolic pressure plus peripheral vascular resistance) or of the pulmonary artery afterload (pulmonary artery end-diastolic pressure plus pulmonary vascular resistance). Thus with either higher end-diastolic volumes or higher afterloads, the driving pressures must be increased. This explains the difference in driving pressures of the right and left artificial ventricles. The two sides of the TAH may have the same end-diastolic blood volumes and artificial valvular resistance, but their afterloads differ considerably. The right side pumps against an end-diastolic pressure near 5 to 15 mm Hg and the left side from 60 to 90 mm Hg. If the diaphragm becomes stiff for reasons previously discussed or if the outflow resistance increases (valvular malfunction or occluding thrombus), the respective driving pressure needs to be increased to completely empty the ventricle at end systole.

This response serves as a safety factor in case of rupture of the pumping diaphragm. If the internal layer of Biomer (the blood-contacting surface) develops a tear, there is a rapid accumulation of blood between the layers of the diaphragm. A severe degree of stiffness develops in the diaphragm secondary to this trapped blood, and the characteristics just described are noted by the various monitoring devices. Once diagnosed, the ventricle requires immediate replacement before all layers of the diaphragm rupture, and the recipient dies from the massive amount of air introduced into the vascular system.

Artificial valves. The standard surgical procedure for implanting the TAH involves excision of all four native heart valves of the recipient. Replacement of these valves is required to maintain unidirectional flow. Currently the J-7 TAH employs four mechanical tilting disk valves; the inflow valves are larger (29 mm) than the outflow valves (27 mm) (Fig. 33-5). Valve rings are recessed into the inflow and the outflow ports of the artificial ventricles, allowing for less turbulent blood flow and minimizing the chance of thrombus formation at this site. The advantages of these mechanical valves include their durability, their relatively good hemodynamics, and their extensive and successful performance in the animal model. Disadvantages are similar to those found in current clinical practice and include thrombus formation, infection, mechanical failure, and a life-time regime of anti-coagulation.

Porcine xenograft valves have been considered in the TAH design. They would provide improved hemodynamics, diminish the risk of infection and thrombus formation, and require no systemic anticoagulation. However, several problems limit their usefulness in the J-7 heart. The porcine valve support design makes its incorporation into the inflow and outflow ports of the artificial ventricles technically very difficult. Also, a very rapid calcification of the xenograft valve leaflets (<3 weeks) occurs in the calf. This process results in severe valvular malfunction, which can produce potentially fatal hemodynamic alterations.

A technique developed at the University of Utah allows the preservation of the aortic and pulmonic valves in the experimental animal receiving the TAH.[16] Postoperative testing revealed an improvement in the hemodynamics of the TAH in animals with their native aortic and pulmonic valves. Given the same driving measurements, the natural valves improved the cardiac output as compared to TAH animals with four mechanical valves. Also, there was an absence of thrombus, infection, and dysfunction with these native valves. The native valves must be normal in structure and function to be retained and to be compatible with implant of the TAH. The surgical technique is intricate and requires experience to properly isolate these valves without causing them irreparable injury. These limitations preclude the use of this technique in early human TAH implant.

Quick connects. A major consideration in the design of the J-7 TAH was the ease with which the artificial heart could be joined to the remaining portions of the atria, pulmonary artery, and aorta. This emphasis led to the fabrication of the heart in components. It would have been impossible to suture the entire TAH directly to the native vascular structures because the confines of the chest limit exposure. These considerations resulted in the incorporation of quick connects into the design of the TAH.[4] There are two types of quick connects—one for the atria and one for the pulmonary artery and aorta.

Surgical excision of the natural ventricles produces a large defect in the right and left

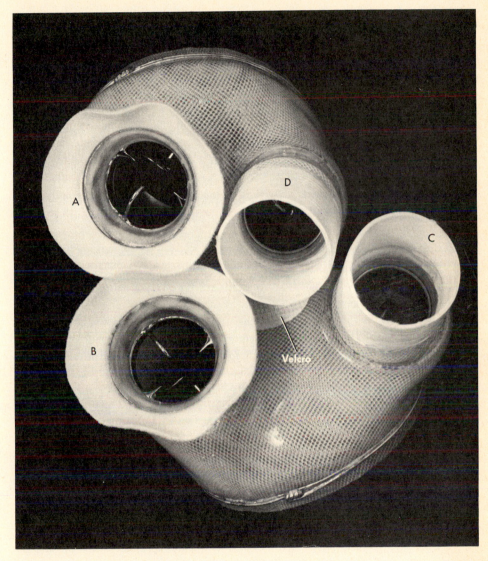

FIG. 33-5 Four mechanical tilting disk valves are used in J-7. Quick connects for atria *(A and B)* incorporate cuff of polyurethane covered felt. Quick connects for pulmonary artery *(C)* and aorta *(D)* consist of short piece of Dacron woven graft rather than cuff. All quick connects are illustrated attached to J-7. During operative procedure, first quick connects are sewn to appropriate remaining remnants of natural heart, and then right and left J-7 ventricles are snapped into quick connects. Positioning of ventricles occurs to align their flat bases adjacent to one another and to form nearly spherical configuration. Small circular patch of Velcro is attached to base of each ventricle to hold two halves in apposition.

atria. The quick connects for these two areas incorporate a cuff of polyurethane covered felt that is anastomosed to the remnant atria (Fig. 33-5). This cuff serves the purpose of anchoring the quick connect and maintaining the volume of the natural atria. Attached to this cuff is the rigid quick connect ring, fabricated of plastic, which has an internal ledge corresponding to a lip on the inflow port of the J-7 ventricle. The quick connects for the aorta and pulmonary artery have the same plastic ring as for the ones just described, but the portion sewn to the native vessels is no longer a cuff but rather a short segment of Dacron woven vascular graft material (Fig. 33-5). The graft portion of these quick connects is only a few centimeters in length and tubular in shape. It must be individually measured for each recipient. Graft material that is too long causes kinks and acute angles, which result in poor hemodynamics. The ability to snap the J-7 ventricle in place after the quick connect is sewn to the aorta or pulmonary artery is the same as that described for the atrial quick connects.

Once the quick connect has been sewn to the appropriate native structure (atria, pulmonary artery, or aorta), the ventricle can be snapped in place. After being locked in position, the lip of the ventricle port is securely resting on the ledge of the corresponding quick connect. This junction is strong, leak proof, and covered internally with the smooth polyurethane (Biomer). The ventricles can be snapped in and out of the quick connects with ease and thus allow inspection of all suture lines for leaks and optimal orientation of the inflow and outflow ports of the TAH (see surgical procedure).

Positioning of the two ventricles allows their flat bases to be aligned adjacent to one another and to form a nearly spherical configuration. A small circular patch of Velcro is attached to the housing of each ventricle to hold the two halves in apposition.

Reaction of the TAH with surrounding tissue

Once the TAH has been implanted in the chest, it becomes enveloped in a fibrous pseudopericardium. This process requires just a few weeks, but when completed, the TAH is isolated from the surrounding structures of the chest. This fibrous tissue acts as a protective barrier. No adjacent tissue damage caused by the TAH has been observed in the longest surviving animals. There is no element of rejection of the TAH once it is implanted. A major potential complication is the establishment of an intrathoracic infection. If such a problem develops, the TAH acts as a foreign body that enhances the infectious process. The only potentially successful treatment is removal of the infected TAH. If the heart is not removed, the recipient will ultimately die of this mediastinal infection.

Extrinsic and intrinsic control of the J-7

The J-7 TAH functions well under a wide variety of physiological conditions. Extrinsic and intrinsic controls are precisely balanced to maintain appropriate cardiac output for the patient. The extrinsic controls (pneumatic heart driver and ventricular vacuum) provide parameters that can be adjusted individually as the hemodynamic requirements of the TAH recipient change. Intrinsic control of the TAH functions on an automatic basis as dictated by the physiological changes in the vascular system and the functional reserve of the TAH.

Pneumatic heart driver: extrinsic control. The pneumatic heart driver processes the extrinsic control mechanisms that are used to regulate the function of the TAH (Fig. 33-6). A backup heart driver is always retained next to the primary heart driver in case of malfunction. The variables that can be adjusted using the heart driver include the heart rate, the individual pneumatic drive pressures for the right and left ventricles, the percent systole, and the delay in the onset of systole as illustrated in Fig. 33-7.

Heart rate. This regulatory mechanism selects the number of beats per minute for both ventricles of the TAH. The rate selected is dependent on cardiac output necessary to meet both the hemodynamic and metabolic demands of the patient. Significance of the heart rate measurement with regard to cardiac output stems from the equation:

$$\text{Cardiac output} = \text{Stroke volume} \times \text{Heart rate}$$

A heart rate of 80 to 90 beats/min is usually selected for a normal 90 to 100 kg calf in the postoperative period. If the animal subsequently develops a need for additional cardiac output, which may occur with exercise, normal growth, infection, pulmonary or systemic venous fluid overload, etc., the heart rate may need to be increased. However, before the heart rate is changed, the function of the ventricles should be evaluated to ensure optimal filling and emptying of these chambers. This establishes that the stroke volume for that particular heart rate is maximal, confirming that the peak cardiac output has been achieved. If the stroke volume were to be less than optimal at the existing heart rate, a further increase in heart rate may then decrease the cardiac output secondary to providing inadequate time for filling and emptying of the ventricle. When the maximum cardiac output is confirmed at the given heart rate, further increases in cardiac output can then be achieved by raising the heart rate. With each increment of change in the rate the cardiac output should be determined, and the filling and ejection of the ventricle should be evaluated to maintain the optimal function of the heart at the newly selected measurements (note COMDU section for cardiac output determinations).

Once very high heart rates are achieved (140 to 150 beats/min), the efficiency of the ventricles reaches a plateau, and eventually a decline in cardiac output is seen. This response of cardiac output results from the progressively shorter time available for filling and emptying of the ventricles. TAH maximal heart rates are considerably less than those seen in the native heart of the normal patient, secondary to the overall inefficiencies of the mechanical components of the TAH.

Percent systole. Approximately 40% of each cardiac cycle in the native myocardium is devoted to systole at a heart rate of 72 beats/min. This percentage continually increases as the heart rate accelerates. As the rate approaches 200 beats/min, the duration of systole exceeds 60% of the cardiac cycle. At this juncture the length of systole erodes a significant portion of the diastolic filling time. Less than optimal ventricular filling eventually ensues, which in turn lowers the resultant cardiac output. Following this same scheme, the TAH requires adjustment of the percent systole as the heart rate increases. The initial setting of a heart rate between 90 and 100 beats/min requires a percent systole of anywhere from 32% to 36%. This range has been found to allow sufficient time for complete emptying of the ventricle and allotting enough time for diastole and optimal filling of the ventricle. The

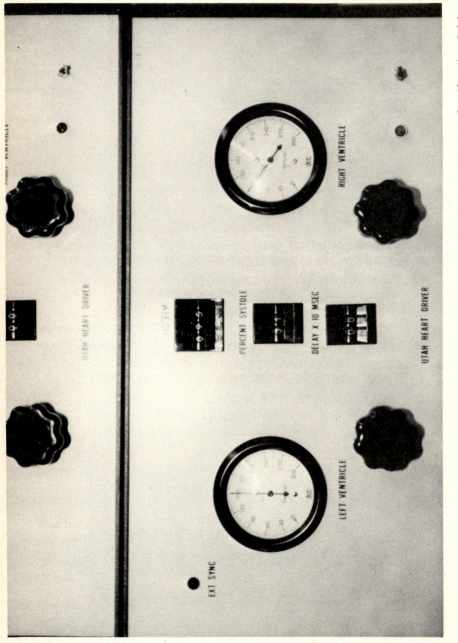

FIG. 33-6 Utah pneumatic heart driver. Backup heart driver is kept in tandem with primary unit in case of malfunction. Driving measurements are preset on second heart driver. Thus in emergency, drivelines need only be changed to new driver and system turned on.

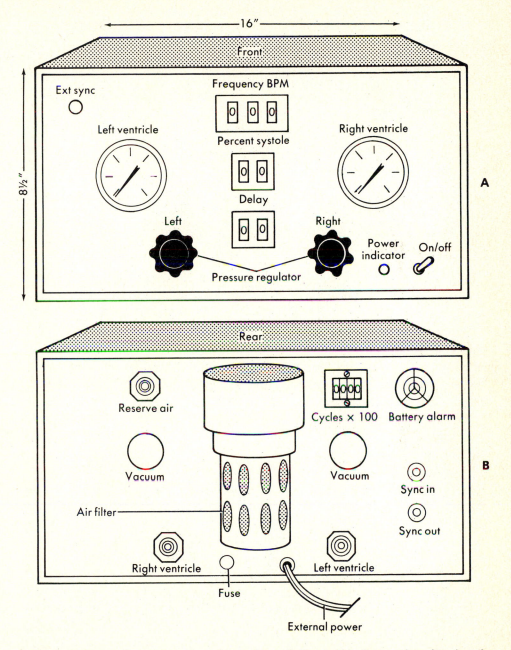

FIG. 33-7 Schematic of Utah pneumatic heart driver. **A**, Front view; **B**, rear view. (See text for discussion.)

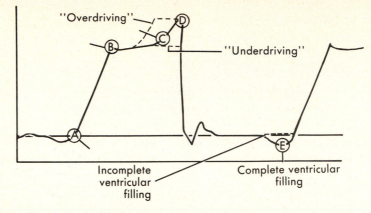

FIG. 33-8 Artificial ventricle driving pressure waveform. Solid line represents ideal pressure waveform. Significant landmarks of pressure waveform are identified. Distortions in pressure waveform that occur with overdriving and underdriving are labeled. *A,* End of diastole; *B,* beginning of aortic flow; *C,* end of effective ejection; *D,* peak driving pressure—full emptying of ventricle; *E,* full filling of ventricle.

complete filling and emptying are dependent on many other factors, such as filling and driving pressures. Given these pressure measurements as being optimal, the percent systole stated previously allows enough time for proper ventricular function.

As the TAH rate is increased (>110 beats/min) in an effort to increase the cardiac output, the percent systole usually needs to be increased. The higher heart rates result in a progressive decline in the duration of each cardiac cycle. Systolic ejection time requires a longer portion of the cycle (increased percentage) to allow full ejection of the end-diastolic blood volume. However, a crucial heart rate is reached with the TAH when increasing percent systole encroaches significantly on the percent diastole and results in suboptimal ventricular filling. This situation causes a reduction of the stroke volume and in turn a decline in cardiac output. In the TAH this becomes evident near 140 to 160 beats/min, or if greater than 50% systole is selected, it shows at lower rates (near 100 beats/min).

The relative inefficiency of the TAH in comparison to the natural heart with regard to the need for increased diastolic and systolic times required at faster heart rates stems from three factors: (1) the TAH lacks the coordinated atrial contraction with the artificial ventricle, which results in a loss of the 20% to 30% of the atrial components of ventricular filling; (2) the decreased orifice size of the prosthetic valves as compared to the natural valves results in a marked increase in resistance to blood flow, which must be compensated for by increased driving pressures to provide full emptying, as well as increased diastolic filling time to ensure complete filling; and (3) a recently recognized problem of intermittent occlusion of the air exhaust port by the flexible pumping diaphragm during diastolic filling. This trapped air in the ventricular housing during diastole diminishes the diastolic blood volume by as much as 30% of its theoretical maximum, which in turn lessens the calculated stroke volume.

Driving pressures. The J-7 ventricle is pulsed by compressed air delivered via Silastic tubing that originates in the pneumatic heart driver (Fig. 33-6). The rhythmic inflow and exhausting of air are responsible for the expansion of the ventricular diaphragm, which in turn expels the blood from the TAH into the aorta or pulmonary artery. Individual selection of the driving pressures (millimeters of mercury) for each ventricle can be made on the Utah heart driver console. Driving pressures can be recorded graphically (Fig. 33-8), and characteristic landmarks can be noted such as the full filling of the ventricle in diastole and peak driving pressure, representing full emptying of the ventricle. Right and left ventricular driving pressures actually recorded in a calf recipient of the J-7 are illustrated in Fig. 33-9.

The amount of pressure that is required to empty the ventricle of its end-diastolic volume of blood is dependent on several factors, which include (1) outflow resistance—mechanical valves, afterload pressures, and vascular resistance; (2) the volume of blood present at end diastole; (3) the flexibility of the pumping diaphragm; and (4) occlusion of the outflow tract by thrombus, endocarditis, pannus, or other pathological processes.

In the immediate postoperative period the ventricular pressure settings are fairly well standardized for the calves and sheep that weigh between 80 and 100 kg. The left driving pressure ranges in the vicinity of 150 to 180 mm Hg and the right driving pressure near 50 to 80 mm Hg. Driving pressures are adjusted to the lowest possible value that completely empties the ventricle. Too low a pressure, underdriving, results in a large end-systolic volume that causes ventricular failure. This failure manifests by inadequate cardiac outputs and abnormally elevated pulmonary or systemic venous pressures. If the driving pressures are too high, the pumping diaphragm will be "overdriven," which can add significant mechanical stress to the components of the TAH and produce unnecessary trauma to the cellular components of the patient's blood.

UNDERDRIVING. When full emptying of the end-diastolic blood does not occur, the ventricle is said to be underdriven. This phenomenon is displayed on the driveline pressure curve as a lack of a peak (meaning the pumping diaphragm is not fully flexed) at end systole (Fig. 33-8). Clinical signs of this situation include those of systemic venous overload and/or pulmonary vascular overload. Underdriving can occur in several circumstances: (1) increased end-diastolic volume, (2) rise in the afterload, (3) development of outflow obstruction (valvular, thrombus, etc.), and (4) stiffening of the diaphragm (calcification, rupture). Correction can be accomplished by increasing the driving pressure or the percent systole for that particular heart rate. Sometimes a combination of adjustments in both these measurements achieves proper function of the TAH's ventricles.

Temporary and random instances of underdriving are results of variations in the physiological changes of the host's body. Events such as exercise, which increase venous return to the TAH, explain a temporary need for increased driving pressures to fully empty the ventricle in systole. However, any rapid, large, or progressive underdriving problems should serve as a warning that some serious and potential catastrophic alteration has possibly occurred. Systematic evaluation of the possible causes is required and should include the problems just listed and discussed in the complication section of this chapter.

OVERDRIVING. If previously satisfactory driving pressures suddenly show an overdriv-

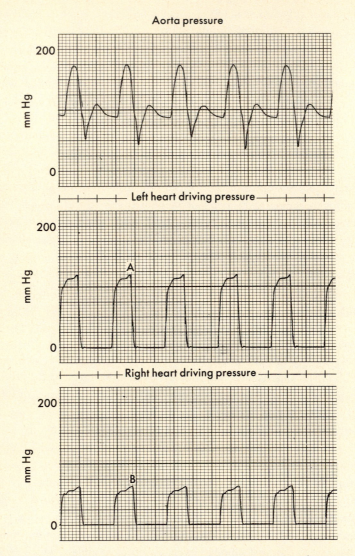

FIG. 33-9 Example of actual right and left ventricular driving pressure waveforms as recorded from calf recipient of J-7 TAH at University of Utah's Division of Artificial Organs. *A* and *B* show end systolic peak that represents full emptying of ventricles. Top aortic pressure tracing, which is indistinguishable from aortic pressure tracing generated from natural myocardium, can be noted.

ing (appears as a spike with a plateau on the end-systolic portion of the drive pressure waveform) of the ventricle, correlation should be made with the stroke volume of the ventricle as well as the central venous pressure or atrial pressure. Overdriving is seen when there is either systemic hypovolemia, inadequate delivery of blood to the affected ventricle, or change in vascular pressure and resistance.

In the hypovolemic setting the stroke volume of the right and left ventricle and the atrial pressures are low. The treatment is volume replacement with intravenous fluids. This should correct the problem with return of normal vascular pressures, stroke volumes, and cessation of the overdriving complication. The other common situation with these changes involves an inadequate delivery of blood from the right to the left ventricle. In this setting the left ventricle shows overdriving while the right ventricular waveform indicates a lack of complete emptying. The stroke volumes of both ventricles are less than optimal, and the central venous or right atrial pressure is elevated. However, these measurements are not monitored on a long-term basis. Therefore the clinical evidence of right heart failure, such as peripheral edema, ascites, and hepatomegaly must be assessed. Correction of this situation requires increased drive pressure of the right ventricle, which in turn results in full emptying and an increased stroke volume. This increased forward flow raises the left atrial pressure and consequently the left ventricular filling pressure. With the left ventricular diastolic volume increased, the left heart driving pressure wave reverts to full emptying without overdriving the diaphragm.

Any decrease in the pulmonary or systemic vascular resistance or mean blood pressure also results in an overdriving of the corresponding ventricle. This situation need not be of any pathological significance but rather a routine variation of the circulatory system. When observed, this overdriving only requires that the driving pressure be decreased until a small spike is seen at end systole on the pneumatic pressure waveform.

Delay in onset of systole. The operative procedure for implantation of the TAH allows the majority of the right and left atria to be left in situ. Study of these remnants has disclosed that they continue to contract in a rhythmic manner and respond to certain drugs for prolonged periods postoperatively. Electrocardiograph monitoring reveals a normal P wave corresponding to these contractions. Ideally synchronization of this atrial rhythm with the artificial ventricles would improve the function of the TAH for two reasons. First it would allow the atrial contraction to contribute to the ventricular diastolic volume. Secondly an additional benefit would perhaps come from regulating the artificial ventricular rate by synchronizing it to the atrial rate: as the body required a change in cardiac output, the atrial rate would also change, thereby automatically adjusting the ventricular rate.

To provide this connection between the atria and ventricle, several electronic modifications were required in the TAH. The P wave had to be continually monitored and then fed into the heart driver; synchronization input and output jacks were placed in the rear of the heart driver console for this purpose (Fig. 33-7, *B*). Activation of the heart driver to begin systole in the TAH needed to be delayed after sensing the P wave; otherwise the mechanical TAH contraction would be superimposed on natural atrial contraction. Thus a variable delay mode was engineered into the heart driver to allow sufficient time between the incoming P wave reaching the heart driver and the initiation of the ventricular systole. With proper adjustment of this delay regulator either the right or left atria could be coordinated with the corresponding ventricle. However, the delay required in each atrium was discovered to be of a different length of time. Since the two artificial ventricles begin systole simultaneously, proper synchronization was impossible with the atria. Also it was found that as the atria's resting rate progressively rose to very high values, improvement in cardiac output of the TAH with P-wave synchronization was insignificant. Because of the aforementioned difficulties, this idea of atrial synchronization has been temporarily abandoned. Therefore the delay adjustment on the front console of the heart driver is not employed with the animal or human recipient.

Intrinsic control: Starling response of the TAH. One of the basic and most significant autoregulatory systems of the human heart is called the Frank-Starling law (Chapter 2). In essence the Frank-Starling law states that the human myocardium responds to increasing diastolic filling volumes (preload) by stretching the myocardial muscle fibers of the ventricle and ejecting a correspondingly larger stroke volume. Autoregulation of the cardiac output as described by Frank and Starling is also found in the functioning of the J-7 TAH.[18]

Given that the TAH is set at a fixed rate and driving pressure, as well as having some diastolic volume reserve, a Frank-Starling-like response is seen as the venous pressure rises. While exercising on a treadmill, the experimental animal's atrial pressures rise as the venous return to the TAH increases. This added volume of venous blood is automatically pumped into the circulation by the artificial ventricle, thereby improving the cardiac output (Fig. 33-10). This intrinsic response of the TAH is limited by the diastolic capacity of the artificial ventricle. Once this value is reached, further improvements of the cardiac output require changes in the external control of the heart.

After this plateau of cardiac output in the exercising animal is achieved, it has been observed that the animal begins to remove more oxygen from the arterial blood. By extracting this additional oxygen, the tissues are able to maintain a stable state during the increased metabolic demands of exercise, an important compensatory maneuver in view of the fact that improved stroke volumes are not possible by the TAH in this setting.

This intrinsic control of the Utah TAH allows for automatic changes of the cardiac output within a certain range in response to the varying needs of the recipient. Therefore during the course of normal activities, such as lying, standing, walking, eating, and mild exercise, the TAH spontaneously adjusts its cardiac output, alleviating the need to frequently change its external controls.

Vacuum. Removal of air from the ventricular housing and the pneumatic drivelines is enhanced with the use of a vacuum. This rapid sucking of air in early diastole helps to decrease the resistance that the pumping diaphragm can provide to the inflow of blood during this filling phase. The effectiveness of the vacuum in this filling period increases as the heart rate becomes more rapid and the time of diastole is shortened.

Two pathological situations exist where the use of vacuum is particularly helpful. (1) If the diaphragm becomes stiff, as in calcification, the use of vacuum can aid the collapse of the diaphragm and thus permit lower atrial pressures to adequately fill the ventricle. (2)

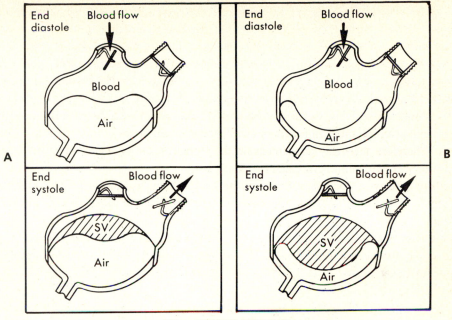

SV = STROKE VOLUME

FIG. 33-10 Frank-Starling response of J-7 TAH. Stroke volume is varied without alteration in heart rate. **A,** With normal venous return, cardiac output is about 6 liters/min. **B,** Increased venous return occurring with activity increases cardiac output to 11 liters/min. (From Jarvik, R.K.: The total artificial heart, Sci. Am. **244:**74, copyright 1981. All rights reserved.)

When ventricular inflow obstruction develops, such as that seen with thrombus or pannus, the application of vacuum increases the pressure gradient across the inflow valve, which provides for more complete filling of the ventricle at a reduced atrial pressure.

Alarms. Appropriate warning mechanisms must be incorporated within the TAH to ensure instant knowledge of any mechanical failures. In conjunction with these alarms, backup mechanical systems must be immediately available to support the TAH should the primary systems malfunction. The Utah TAH employs such alarms and backup systems.

An electric power failure would result in an immediate and automatic assumption of the driving power of the TAH's heart driver by batteries contained within each heart driver. These batteries are in a continuous state of charging as long as outside electricity is being delivered to power the TAH. Once the batteries take over the powering of the heart, an alarm system is activated, which produces a warning every 100 heart beats. This alarm sounds for as long as the batteries are in service. Maximally charged batteries provide sufficient power to drive the heart for 5 hours.

Monitoring of the pneumatic drivelines has a similar scheme of alarms and alternate sources of power. If the air pressure in the drivelines falls below or exceeds the desired level, an alarm system will be activated. Simultaneously a secondary source of compressed air, stored in auxiliary tanks, begin driving the artificial heart. Three backup systems exist to deliver compressed air to maintain proper function of the heart. As in the University of Utah research facility, the homes of human TAH recipients will have a primary air compressor installed along with a bank of compressed air tanks. These tanks are attached to the compressed air system of the TAH so that their activation, via an array of pressure sensitive valves, is automatic and instantaneous.

Cardiac output monitoring and diagnostic unit (COMDU). Measurement of cardiac output is extremely helpful in monitoring the function of the TAH. This information indicates when changes are needed in the driving measurements of the ventricles, provides data about the normal functioning of the TAH, and aids in diagnosing certain pathological processes affecting the performance of the TAH. In the past cardiac output had been determined by implantable electromagnetic flow probes. These devices provided valuable data; however, their lack of durability limited their usefulness.

A recent advancement, the COMDU, has provided continuous and reliable calculations of the stroke volume and cardiac output in the TAH (Fig. 33-11). This innovation is based on an exquisitely simple concept. A pneumotachometer plus a computer are used to calculate the amount and rate of air exhausting from the right and left ventricle of the TAH during the diastolic phase (Fig. 33-12). The volume of air beneath the diaphragm displaced during diastole is directly related to the volume of blood filling the ventricle. These volumes in turn represent the volume of blood ejected in the subsequent systolic phase of the ventricle, which is the stroke volume. If this calculated stroke volume is multiplied by the heart rate, a process performed by the computer, the cardiac output of one ventricle can be determined. The computer calculates the stroke volume and cardiac output for 10 heartbeats and automatically supplies the mean values for these two measurements. Thus continuous monitoring of the heart's function can be determined by this system.

In addition to volume measurement, the configuration of the exhausted air flow curve, displayed on the computer television monitor, can be used to diagnose functional problems with the TAH (Fig. 33-13). Initially, high exhausting air flow rates (Fig. 33-14) can be the result of high pressure filling of the ventricles, which in turn rapidly displaces the measured air. Examples of this problem include pathological aortic or pulmonary valvular regurgitation, high atrial pressures, and elevated pulmonary or central venous pressures. Low flow rates (Fig. 33-15) seen on the computer usually result in less than complete filling of the ventricle. This problem can result from hypovolemia and/or inflow valvular obstruction.

COMDU monitoring is still in its infancy. Research continues to determine proper interpretation of the information displayed by the computer and the most effective clinical contribution rendered by measurement of flow rates in the artificial ventricles. Undoubtedly with further experience, COMDU flow analysis will guide us to more precise adjustment of the TAH function. Also alterations in TAH performance can be more readily diagnosed in earlier states of development, thus allowing for correction before deleterious sequelae develop in the patient. This was evidenced when the prosthetic mitral valve fractured in the first clinical use of the TAH. A COMDU air flow curve was immediately displayed and was diagnostic of a mechanical valve failure. Recognition of the problem was instantaneous, and the patient immediately underwent corrective surgery.

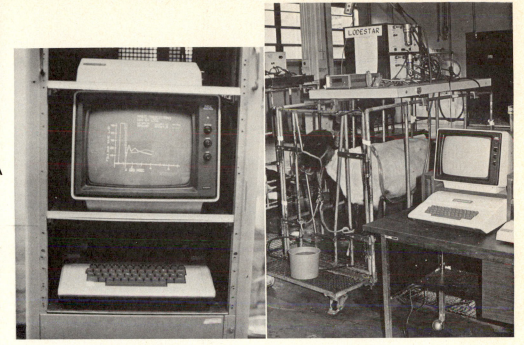

FIG. 33-11 A, Cardiac output monitoring and diagnostic unit (COMDU). (See text for discussion.) **B,** COMDU with animal recipient of TAH.

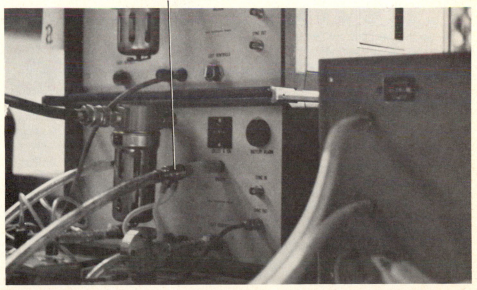

FIG. 33-12 Rear view of Utah pneumatic heart driver, showing insertion of pneumotachometer, which connects to COMDU.

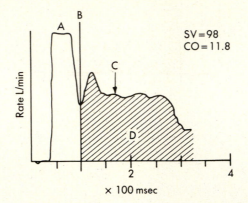

FIG. 33-13 Normal COMDU tracing. *A*, This initial elevation represents earliest portion of diastole, when exhaust valve opens and pressure equilibrates between ventricle and atmosphere. No air has yet left artificial ventricle. *B*, Vertical line displays where computer begins its calculation of stroke volume by measuring area under curve. *C*, Line that represents flow of air from ventricle during diastole. Area beneath this curve, beginning at vertical calibration line, is equal to volume of blood entering ventricle and subsequently ejected (stroke volume). Additionally, configuration of this curve can be used to diagnose several conditions affecting TAH's performance. *D*, Striped region is area representing stroke volume of ventricle being monitored.

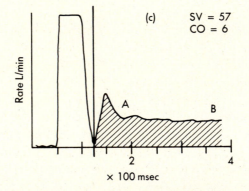

FIG. 33-14 Low-flow COMDU tracing. There is low initial flow *(A)* that continues at slow rate throughout entire diastolic phase, with filling of ventricles never being complete *(B)*. This decreased volume is represented by small calculated stroke volume *(C)*.

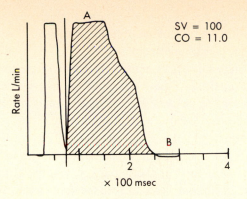

FIG. 33-15 High-flow COMDU tracing. There is rapid initial filling (A) that goes off scale (indicated by plateau of curve) and rapidly falls as ventricle is filled early in diastolic period (B).

Selection of patients

The patients who are eligible for the University of Utah TAH are limited to two categories. Permission for use of the J-7 TAH in these patients has been granted by the FDA.[15] The first group includes any patients who cannot be weaned from the cardiopulmonary bypass machine at the conclusion of a cardiac surgical procedure. This weaning process includes the use of medications and the IABP. The second group embraces all those patients suffering from a severe cardiomyopathy. To quantitate the degree of impairment resulting from the cardiomyopathy, the New York Heart Association's clinical classification scheme has been adopted. Only those patients in Class IV (symptoms at rest that are unrelieved by medications or standard surgical procedures) are considered for the Utah TAH. No specific guidelines regarding age have been formulated. However, with younger patients (<17 years) or women a smaller mediastinum would prohibit the proper fit of the J-7 TAH. Any severe chronic or terminal disease would also preclude a patient from receiving the TAH. Despite these limitations, the number of potential recipients of the artificial heart still numbers in the thousands.

Once selected as suitable candidates for the Utah TAH, the patient and his family undergo a thorough evaluation by a panel of physicians and ancillary personnel to ensure their ability to cope with the great stress that accompanies the implantation of the TAH. The patient must be intelligent, must be motivated, and in general must have a stable personality. Support from the recipient's family is crucial, since they share the burden of stress and assist with the new and at times demanding long-term postoperative care. If this evaluation determines a strong, intelligent, and stable situation, plans can be undertaken to implant the artificial heart.

Surgical procedure

The surgical placement of the TAH has been standardized in the animal model with several hundred successful implantations throughout the world. A few technical differences are necessary in the surgical procedure for humans as compared to the calves and sheep, but these are not of any postoperative clinical significance.[17] The operative procedure is discussed, using the facts obtained from the experimental model, but with alterations that are made for human implantation.

The preoperative preparation is essentially unchanged from the procedures in use for all open-heart surgical candidates. Anesthesia induction is performed with caution to avoid any unnecessary work load on an already compromised myocardium. A median sternotomy incision allows adequate exposure for the removal of the patient's ventricles and replacement with the right and left artificial ventricles. The process of instituting cardiopulmonary bypass is begun after systemic heparinization. The arterial bypass cannula is placed in either the thoracic aorta or femoral artery, and the venous cannulas are introduced into the superior and inferior vena cava via the right atrium. Total body hypothermia is employed to decrease the metabolic rate of all the patient's organs during full cardiac arrest. When adequate flows are achieved with cardiopulmonary bypass, the aorta is cross-clamped, and the vena cavae are occluded, using tourniquets. At this time the native heart is brought into full arrest. Quickly and exactly the right and left ventricles are excised (Fig. 33-16). The two atria are left intact with dissection carefully performed so that all portions of the mitral and tricuspid valves are removed. Additionally the aortic and pulmonic valve leaflets are also excised, and the aorta and pulmonary artery are separated for a short distance (Fig. 33-17).

The four quick connects of the artificial heart are sequentially sewn into place (Fig. 33-18). A permanent suture is used to anastomose each of these connectors independently to the two atria, aorta, and pulmonary artery. Before placement of the TAH's ventricles, the suture lines are tested with specially designed plugs that snap into the quick connects. Through these plugs blood can be injected under physiological pressure to determine any technical errors in the anastomosis. The ventricles of the TAH are then snapped into the quick connects (Figs. 33-19 and 33-20). The pressure drivelines are exited between the ribs and are tunneled for a short distance subcutaneously before exiting the skin (Fig. 33-21). At the exit site from the skin and in the intercostal space, the drivelines are covered with Dacron velour. The patient's tissues can grow into this material, thus providing stability and a barrier to bacterial contamination. This velour covering over the drivelines at the skin level is termed the *skin button* (Fig. 33-22).

Each ventricle is then aspirated via a venting port to evacuate any air that may be trapped in the heart (Fig. 33-20). After all the air is removed, the heart is primed with blood, and the pneumatic drivelines, exiting from the artificial ventricles, are connected to the heart driver console. The clamps and tourniquets on the aorta and vena cavae are released, and the pumping of the TAH is initiated. The rate and driving pressures of the TAH are gradually increased, and the flow of the cardiopulmonary bypass is decreased.

Careful inspection is again made of all suture lines and quick connects to ensure that there is no significant leaking or kinking of the inflow or outflow connections. An additional left atrial monitoring line is brought out through the lateral chest wall. Two mediastinal drainage tubes are placed adjacent to the TAH and exited in the usual manner from the chest. When the TAH is able to sustain full support of the circulation, the cardiopul-

Text continued on p. 378.

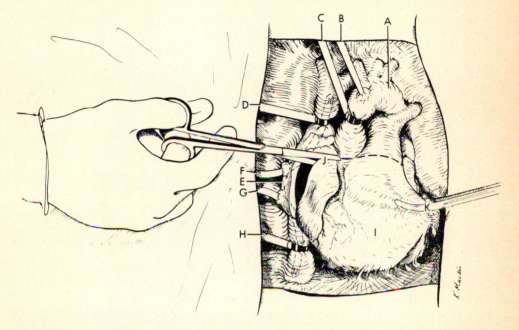

FIG. 33-16 When adequate flows are achieved with cardiopulmonary bypass, aorta is cross-clamped and venae cavae are occluded. Native heart is brought into full arrest. Quickly and exactly right and left ventricles are excised. *A*, Aorta; *B*, aortic cannula; *C*, aortic tourniquet; *D*, superior vena cava tourniquet; *E*, right atrium; *F*, superior vena cava cannula; *G*, inferior vena cava canula; *H*, inferior vena cava tourniquet; *I*, right ventricle; *J*, ventricular incision; *K*, clamp lifting apex of heart.

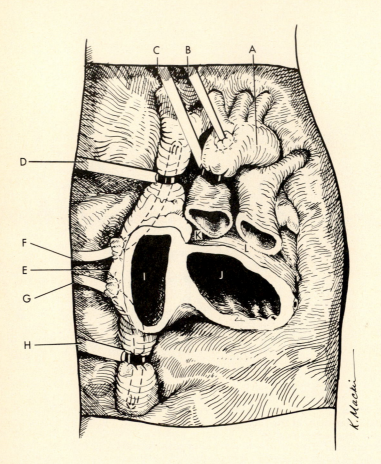

FIG. 33-17 Remnant of natural heart is ready to receive TAH. Two atria are left intact with dissection carefully performed so that all portions of mitral and tricuspid valves are removed. Aortic and pulmonic valve leaflets are excised, and aorta and pulmonary artery are separated short distance. *A*, Aorta; *B*, aortic cannula; *C*, aortic tourniquet; *D*, superior vena cava tourniquet; *E*, right atrium; *F*, superior vena cava cannula; *G*, inferior vena cava cannula; *H*, inferior vena cava tourniquet; *I*, right atrium; *J*, left atrium; *K*, aorta; *L*, pulmonary artery.

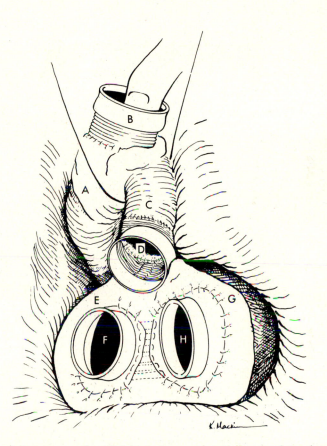

FIG. 33-18 Four quick connects of artificial heart are sequentially sewn into place. *A*, Aorta; *B*, aortic quick connect; *C*, pulmonary artery; *D*, pulmonary artery quick connect; *E*, right atrium; *F*, right atrial cuff and quick connect; *G*, left atrium; *H*, left atrial cuff and quick connect.

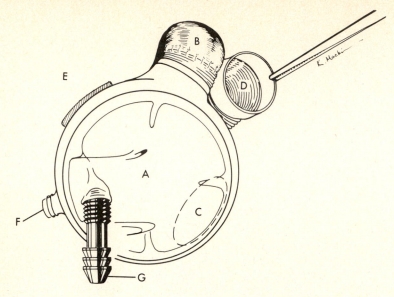

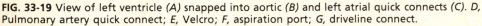

FIG. 33-19 View of left ventricle *(A)* snapped into aortic *(B)* and left atrial quick connects *(C)*. *D*, Pulmonary artery quick connect; *E*, Velcro; *F*, aspiration port; *G*, driveline connect.

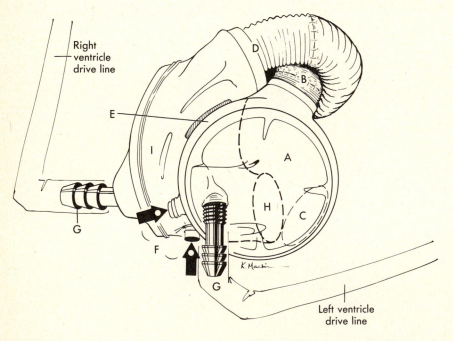

FIG. 33-20 Right and left artificial ventricles snapped into position with quick connects. *A*, Left ventricle; *B*, aortic quick connect; *C*, left atrium quick connect; *D*, pulmonary artery quick connect; *E*, Velcro; *F*, arrows indicating aspiration ports; *G*, driveline connects; *H*, right atrium quick connect; *I*, right ventricle.

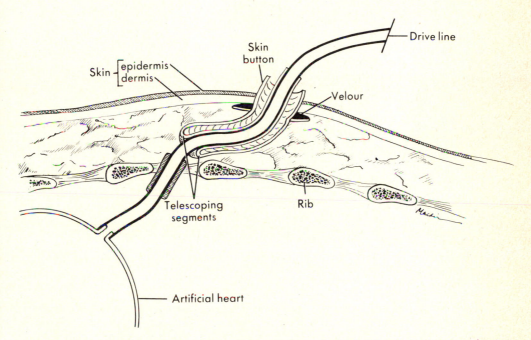

FIG. 33-21 Drive pressure lines are exited between ribs and tunneled for short distance subcutaneously before exiting skin. At exit site from skin and in intercostal space, drivelines are covered with velour. Patient's tissues can grow into this material, thus providing stability and barrier to bacterial contamination.

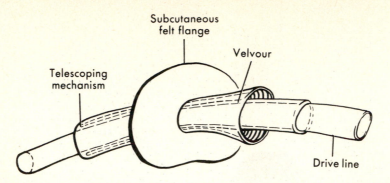

Subcutaneous
felt flange

Velvour

Telescoping
mechanism

Drive line

FIG. 33-22 "Skin button." Dacron velour external surface allows for tissue ingrowth, which diminishes infection and forms secure interface. Telescoping mechanism minimizes tissue trauma imparted by pulsing drivelines and allows movement of driveline without disrupting its connection to artificial ventricle. Felt flange also provides stability to skin button and limits inward extension of any superficial infections. (Modified from Kevin Murray, Salt Lake City.)

monary cannulas are removed. The wounds are closed in the usual manner, and the mediastinal tubes are attached to low suction. As the patient achieves a stable state, he can be safely transferred to the surgical intensive care unit for postoperative care. Fig. 33-23 depicts the postoperative patient following implantation of the TAH. The mediastinal tubes have been removed.

General postoperative care

The surgical implantation of the J-7 TAH in the experimental animal requires between 3 and 4 hours. Postoperative care has been standardized in the calf and sheep in such a way as to facilitate a rapid and successful recovery. In general, however, the postoperative care of human patients with the TAH does not differ drastically from that of currently treated open-heart surgical patients.

A few clinically standard postoperative monitoring techniques and treatment modalities are not applicable to the patient with an artificial heart. Some of these items include (1) monitoring and treatment of cardiac arrhythmias; (2) standard cardiopulmonary resuscitation; (3) use of Swan-Ganz catheters; (4) monitoring and interpreting electrocardiograms; and (5) use of cardiac supportive drugs. A blending of the new and the old is required by the nursing staff to properly and successfully care for these patients. Aspects of postoperative care presented include monitoring, fluid intake, pulmonary care, care of the lines, medications, and psychological care.

Monitoring. Direct monitoring of the J-7 TAH is accomplished by the devices and procedures previously discussed in this chapter (COMDU and driving pressures). Additionally, the more familiar measurements of central venous pressure and left atrial pressure are also available for evaluation. Both these pressure lines are placed for temporary use only.

The two pressure readings do not differ in any significant manner from their use in current clinical practice. Recording of the central venous pressure value serves as a basic

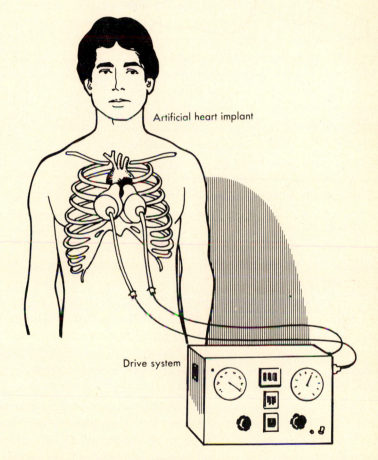

Artificial heart implant

Drive system

FIG. 33-23 Schematic of projected arrangement of TAH in human recipient. Drivelines exit from skin and are attached to pneumatic heart driver.

guide to right atrial pressure and its direct relationship to filling pressures of the right ventricle. This value needs to be maintained in the usual normal range of less than 10 mm Hg. Over several weeks this pressure has been observed to slowly but steadily increase in the animal with a TAH. This often signifies right heart failure with its attendant hepatomegaly, ascites, and peripheral edema; however, it also appears without these signs and symptoms. Whether or not these higher filling pressures are necessary for proper functioning of the TAH or if the venous hypertension represents poor regulation of the TAH remains unsettled. It is known that the total blood volume of the animal with the TAH is increased. The significance of the fact is unknown with regard to atrial pressures.

The left atrial pressure also needs to be maintained at the proper values. The same phenomenon described for the right atrial pressure curve is seen on the left side. The only difference is that the elevated left atrial pressure is manifested by pulmonary hypertension, edema, and insufficiency. Once the patient's condition is stabilized, the central venous pressure and the left atrial line are removed.

Pulmonary care. Postoperatively the patient arrives in the intensive care unit with an endotracheal tube in place and is supported by a mechanical respirator. The usual ventilatory measurements are employed to select the optimal ventilator settings. Standard respiratory care is required for the patient, including endotracheal suctioning, frequent monitoring of the arterial blood gases, and daily chest x-ray films. When the patient's pulmonary mechanics appear adequate to maintain proper respiratory function, he should then be considered a candidate for extubation. After extubation, the use of oxygen by mask, inspiratory exercises, and other standard therapies are employed to prevent atelectasis, hypoxia, and general respiratory insufficiency. The TAH should not interfere with or change this segment of nursing care.

Fluids. Postoperatively the administration of fluids is governed by the hemodynamic requirements of the artificial heart and the peripheral vascular beds. The initial postoperative period is a time when additional volumes of fluids are needed by the patient. Readings from the COMDU, pressure monitors, and driveline pressure waves determine when fluids are necessary and their rate of infusion. The type of fluid selected (colloid, crystalloid, or blood) is at the discretion of the physician in charge. If a low hematocrit is present in conjunction with hypovolemia, the administration of blood is indicated. Once TAH function stabilizes and there is no significant blood loss from the mediastinal drainage tubes, a maintenance volume of IV fluid can be calculated and administered.

When the patient has been extubated and normal gastrointestinal function has returned, he can begin an oral intake of fluids. As his diet is increased, the IV fluids are decreased in volume. If the recipient's medications can also be given orally, the need for the IV is completed, and it can be discontinued.

Fluid overload is also a potential problem in the patient with a TAH. Given normal renal function he should have the capacity for properly regulating his intravascular volume and electrolytes concentrations. However, if there exists excessive body water, the employment of diuretics and fluid restriction should correct this abnormality. A word of caution is necessary regarding presumed fluid overload. The development of signs and symptoms such as peripheral edema, hepatomegaly, ascites, jugular venous distention, dyspnea, and chest x-ray film changes of pulmonary edema could be a result of under-driving of the TAH, as well as distinct fluid overload (refer to driving pressures). Therefore with these clinical findings the physician should determine whether adjustment of the driving measurements of the TAH is necessary in an effort to increase the cardiac output in addition to diuretic therapy.

Care of the lines. In addition to the usual central venous pressure and peripheral arterial lines, the right and left pneumatic drivelines, two mediastinal drainage tubes, and a temporary left atrial catheter are in place when the patient arrives in the intensive care unit from the operating room. The mediastinal chest tubes are positioned adjacent to the artificial ventricle. Blood loss through the chest tubes is monitored as it is with any patient after open-heart surgery. By the third postoperative day, if the chest tubes are draining an insignificant volume of fluid, they can be removed.

The patient is tethered to the heart driver by two 6-foot Silastic pneumatic drivelines. Great care must be taken to avoid any kinking, tension, or puncturing of these tubes. Their insertion site into the patient's chest is protected by the previously described skin button. Frequent inspection of the tissue surrounding the skin button must be done to discover and treat any early skin trauma or infection.

Medications. Cardiovascular medications have a pharmacological activity that stems from the combined response of the myocardium and the peripheral vascular system. Direct cardiac effects of these drugs are null in the TAH recipient. This unusual situation serves to unmask additional and often unexpected vascular and artificial heart responses of several commonly employed medications.

The experience derived from several animal drug studies at the University of Utah's Division of Artificial Organs is summarized in Table 33-1. These results demonstrate the

TABLE 33-1 Drugs given to animals with a TAH

	Dose/kg	RAP	AoP	SVR	CO
Isoproterenol	2 µg	↑	↓	↓	↑ (25%)
Calcium	10 mg	→	→	↓	↑ (16%)
Digoxin	5 µg	↑	→	↓	↑
Glucagon	10 µg	↑	↓	↓	↑
Acetylcholine	20 µg	↑	↓	↓	↑
Nitrous oxide	—	↑	↑	→	↑
Norepinephrine	2 µg	↑	↑	↑	↓
Dopamine	10 µg	↑	↑	↑ (25%)	↓ (11%)
Neo-synephrine	10 µg	↑	↑	↑	↓
Dopamine	50 µg	↑	↑ (45%)	↑	↓ (25%)
Sodium nitroprusside	1 µg/kg/min	↓	↓	↓	↑

RAP, Right atrial pressure
AoP, Aortic pressure
SVR, Systemic vascular resistance
CO, Cardiac output
↑, Increase
↓, Decrease
→, Unchanged
NOTE: All drugs were administered intravenously

effect of various pharmacological agents on the artificial heart and the circulatory system. A general observation from this table implies that when a drug is able to decrease the systemic vascular resistance, the cardiac output can potentially increase. Improving the cardiac output originates from higher stroke volumes, given the fixed nature of the heart rate. To achieve this elevated stroke volume it is necessary to maintain a filling reserve in the TAH, which can accommodate the additional blood used to increase the cardiac output.

At the University of Utah one of the most commonly used cardiovascular drugs has been nitroprusside. During the acute postoperative period there is occasionally a very high peripheral vascular resistance with elevated systemic arterial and pulmonary arterial pressures. These high afterloads require increased driving pressures to ensure full ventricular emptying. Usually a low doseage of nitroprusside (1 to 2 μg/kg/min) improves the pressures, dynamics of the TAH, and blood flow. The duration of use of this medication has been generally less than 48 hours. It appears this regimen is harmless to the animals and improves their recovery from surgery.

As drugs are employed in the care of the human recipients of the TAH, it is extremely important to monitor the function of the artificial heart as well as the pulmonary and peripheral circulation. These accumulated data serve as a guide to judicious use of medications in other patients receiving a TAH.

Psychological care. The psychological response of the recipients of the TAH is an unknown factor. Preoperative psychological screening has been designed to select patients who can tolerate and cope with the wide variety and magnitude of stress to which they are submitted. Implantation of the TAH effects an improvement in the patient's physical status. This amelioration of the signs and symptoms of cardiac disease should provide the basis for a satisfactory adjustment to the mechanical heart. Questioning and teaching before implantation undoubtedly provide some foundation for acceptance of this new device. Yet it can be anticipated postoperatively that the patients and their families will have concerns regarding the reliability, safety, durability, and limitations of the TAH.

Excessive optimism or pessimism must be guarded against when discussing the future of the patient with a TAH until experience with the human implantation has become sufficiently extensive to provide accurate answers to many questions. As with any patient, the policy of honesty coupled with compassion is the most prudent way of dealing with the situations facing these people.

Long-term care

As recovery progresses from the operative procedure, the patient is anticipated to resume a more normal life-style. Activities such as eating, drinking, personal grooming, and general self-care should be assumed by the patient. Intensive teaching must be given regarding care of the pneumatic drivelines, monitoring of the heart driver, and understanding of the general function of the TAH on a day-to-day basis. With the aid of family members, nurses, social workers, and other ancillary personnel, the patient should become relatively self-sufficient.

A major limitation is the lack of mobility. The patient is tethered by the drivelines, heart driver, and compressed air source, although this should dramatically improve with the use of the portable Utah heart driver and compressed air system (see improvement in the pneumatic heart) after recovering from the implantation of the TAH. It is anticipated that the patient will return home, where an intensive and careful follow-up would continue. Frequent evaluations are necessary by the physicians and scientists to determine any changes needed in the driving measurements of the TAH and to assess how the patient's circulatory system and native body organs have adapted to the TAH. These examinations are vital, both providing proper monitoring of the TAH and accumulating data that will assist the future use of the TAH. In time the computer-based COMDU should be able to provide instantaneous information regarding the performance of the artificial heart via messages transmitted through the telephone system between the patient's home and the University of Utah. Experience with long-term experimental animals that have received a TAH indicates that changes necessary in the driving measurements of the Utah Heart Driver occur less than one time per week unless unusual circumstances develop.

Modifications are made in the patient's home to accommodate an air compressor and the air tanks necessary as a backup system. Several outlets for this air are placed in strategic areas in the house, thus allowing the patient to periodically change his immediate environment. Activities such as reading, writing, other tasks that could be performed at a desk, and a multitude of similar diversions would present no problems to the patient (Fig. 33-24). When using the portable driver system, he could be outdoors enjoying light exercise and visiting such attractions as a museum or park. As experience is accumulated, there will be unforeseen problems to be solved. At the same time additional activities will be

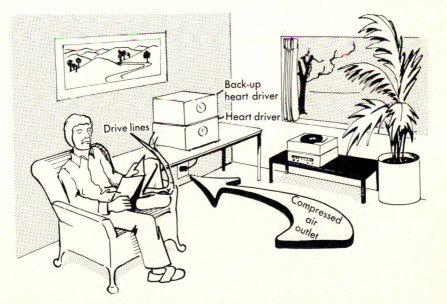

FIG. 33-24 Projected scene of human recipient of TAH in his home. Pneumatic heart driver is connected to wall outlet for compressed air with main compressed air tank being stored in basement of patient's home.

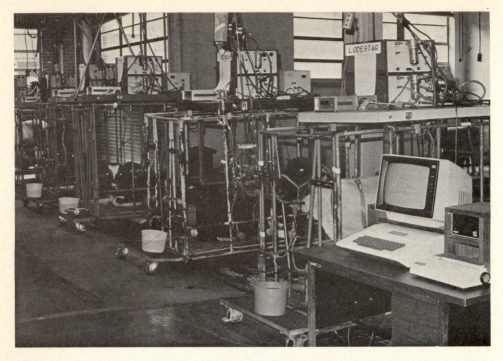

FIG. 33-25 Long-term surviving calf recipients of TAH at University of Utah's Division of Artificial Organs. Survival times after implant range from 30 to 245 days in these recipients.

discovered to allow the patient to enjoy living again. On a long-term basis, the animal recipients are able to eat normally, gain weight, frequently exercise on the treadmill, and essentially lead a normal life (Fig. 33-25).

Complications

Complications that have been observed in the animal recipients of the TAH include infection, thrombus, pannus, embolization, calcification, mechanical failure, and the problem of the animal outgrowing the artificial heart.[13] Each of these is presented in further detail.

Infection. Infection is one of the major complications of long-term surviving animal recipients of the TAH and is often responsible for their deaths. The most lethal site of infection is the interior of the TAH. Additionally, infections can develop along the percutaneous pneumatic drivelines or in the mediastinum. The treatment of established infections at these three sites has met with relatively little success, thus emphasizing the role of preventive care if this problem is to be conquered. The animal with a TAH is very susceptible to infection secondary to a variety of factors, such as exposure to his excretions; this potentiates the risk and clinical course of the established infection process.

Currently more than 50% of long-term surviving animals are found to have bacteria in their blood while alive or at the time of autopsy. The cause of this high incidence of infection appears as a result of a combination of factors, including a large foreign body (the TAH) present in the vascular system with its associated mechanical valves and graft material. The pathogenesis of this problem stems from bacteria lodging in the crevices of the outflow or inflow tracts of the TAH, thus establishing an endocarditis-like picture, or an alternate pathway involves the formation of thrombus, which becomes secondarily infected during an episode of bacteremia. Once present, an infection of the interior of the TAH can cause several problems. This infected thrombus-like material can result in septic emboli to other organ systems, or unimpeded growth can result in hemodynamic compromise of blood flow in the TAH. Most significantly, however, there is a constant bacteremia from this site, which eventually results in sepsis and death. The bacteria most frequently isolated in the TAH animals at the University of Utah include gram negative organisms (45%), *Staphylococcus epidermidis* (25%), and enterococcus (12%).[12] Treatment with intravenous antibiotics alone has met with poor success. These antimicrobial agents are relatively ineffective in this setting of bacteria harbored in a foreign body with a nonvascular environment of red blood cells, platelets, amorphus material, and fibrin. The only potentially successful therapy requires surgical removal of the infected portion of the TAH and replacement, as well as long-term use of synergistic antibiotics. The lethal nature of established intracardiac infections emphasizes the need for a very comprehensive prevention program. This prevention of infections includes the preoperative screening for established infections, an effective prophylactic antibiotic regimen, and meticulous care in the operating room and the postoperative setting. Every episode of bacterial contamination of the bloodstream should be viewed as a potentially lethal event with regard to infection and long-term survival.

Driveline infections have been markedly decreased since the employment of the Dacron velour skin buttons. These buttons promote ingrowth of tissue from the epidermis and dermis, thus forming a secure barrier against bacterial invasion. Additionally, these buttons significantly decrease the tissue damage caused by the pulsatile pressure of the pneumatic drivelines. If an infection does develop, it is usually superficial and requires only debridement and local care, without extension of the process into the thoracic cavity. Fig. 33-26 provides a close-up view of the skin button exiting from a calf.

The preventive antibiotics used at the University of Utah's Division of Artificial Organs include an aminoglycoside and a cephalosporin. They have been found to provide coverage of the most frequently isolated organism, establish good tissue levels before and after surgery, and result in an insignificant complication rate. The administration of these drugs is begun an hour before implantation of the TAH and is continued for 5 days postoperatively or until all temporary monitoring lines and drainage tubes have been removed.

Studies have been carried out at the University of Utah and other institutions, which show a compromise in the defensive ability of animals implanted with a TAH against bacterial invasion.[21] A significant and prolonged decrease in the phagocytic ability of circulating leukocytes has been demonstrated. Additionally, the reticuloendothelial system's capacity to clear bacteria from the bloodstream is impaired.[11] The significance of these dysfunctions is unclear when viewed as separate entities. However, the accumulated

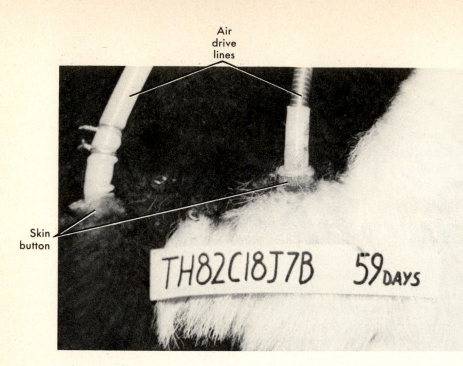

FIG. 33-26 Close-up view of skin button exiting from calf recipient.

evidence stresses the susceptibility of the TAH recipient to severe infections that can ultimately lead to his death.

Thrombus. A thrombus is a conglutinated mass of red blood cells, white blood cells, and platelets covered with a mesh of fibrin. The clinical significance of this pathological process in the TAH is threefold: (1) thrombus is a source of systemic or pulmonary emboli, (2) it is the nidus for the development of infection, and (3) it interferes with the normal function of the TAH (i.e., inflow obstruction and impairment of valvular function). All three of these sequelae to thrombus formation can prove to be lethal to the affected animal.

The J-7 ventricles contain several sites that have a potential for the development of thrombi.[10] The pumping diaphragm has been rendered thromboresistant with the use of Biomer at the blood-material interface. Thrombus formation is initiated only when defects develop in the Biomer blood-contacting surface secondary to fabrication imperfection or stress-related cracks during pumping. The geometry and hemodynamics of the J-7 ventricles have been perfected so that turbulence and stasis of the blood have been corrected, thus eliminating thrombus formation in this area.

The four mechanical valves used in the TAH have the same propensity for thrombus development as those currently in use clinically. Prevention of this serious problem can be achieved by modifying the coagulation system and platelet function with the use of warfarin and dipyridamole or aspirin, respectively.

A significant incidence of thrombus formation has been observed in the experimental animal at the site of anastomosis between the atrial cuffs and the remnant atria. Prevention has not been satisfactorily achieved using anticoagulants and platelet modifiers.

Bacteria are often seen in the thrombus material at autopsy (Fig. 33-27). Whether the

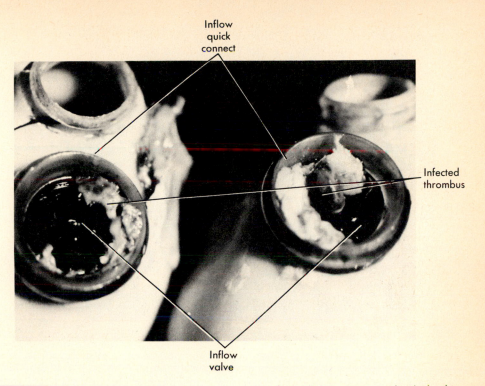

Inflow
quick
connect

Infected
thrombus

Inflow
valve

FIG. 33-27 Infected thrombus at site of quick connects immediately above mechanical valves.

bacteria initiate thrombus formation or secondarily invade established thrombus is unknown. This possibility of thrombus generation by bacteria requires an aggressive posture toward controlling infection (see infection).

Pannus. Pannus is a dense fibrous connective tissue similar to the intimal hyperplasia found in vascular grafts. This proliferative tissue has shown a predilection for growth on the inflow portions of the TAH, specifically at the anastomotic site between the atria and quick connects (Fig. 33-28). Severe blood flow obstruction can develop from enlarged pannus, which impairs filling of both ventricles. This potentially lethal situation has usually been found in long-term animal survivors (of animals surviving longer than 2 months, 78% had pannus at autopsy) and is more severe on the left side of the heart. An additional hazard is the potential for bacterial invasion and the resulting endocarditis-like situation.

The etiology of pannus formation appears multifaceted. The most significant factors include turbulent flow, foreign materials, and platelet damage. This problem has been carefully studied, and specific changes were made in the J-7 TAH's inflow quick connects in an effort to modify the pannus formation.[9] The quick connects were redesigned to eliminate sharp angles and thus provide less turbulent flow (Fig. 33-29). Also the entire blood-contacting surface of the quick connect was lined with ultra-smooth Biomer in place of the previously used polyester felt. These two modifications have resulted in an apparent conquering of the pannus problem. Only 2 of the past 12 long-term surviving animals at

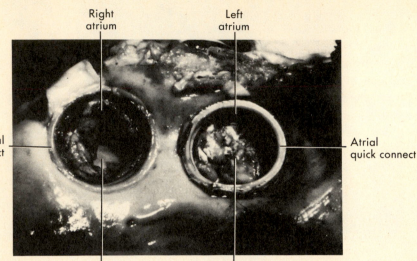

FIG. 33-28 Pannus on right and left side of heart just above inflow valves. Atrial quick connects are in place with ventricles removed. Area seen through quick connects is lumen of right and left atria.

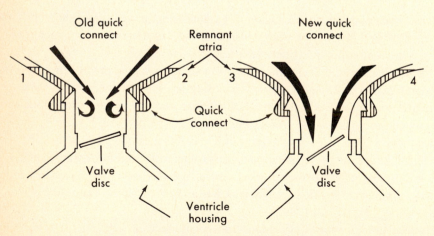

1, 2, 3, 4 = Suture line with quick connect and atria

FIG. 33-29 Cross section of quick connect. **A,** Old design; **B,** new design, eliminating sharp angles and thus providing less turbulent flow.

the University of Utah have developed pannus since the employment of these new quick connects. Both of these cases were hemodynamically insignificant. The contribution of platelet factors remains uncertain. A review of the use of platelet-modifying drugs was inconclusive regarding their role in the prevention of pannus.

Embolization. An *embolus* is defined as a detached intravascular mass that is carried by the blood to a distant site from its point of origin. The vast majority of emboli arise from thrombi. Thus the problem of embolization is intimately related to the previously discussed topic of thrombus in the TAH. The most effective treatment of emboli therefore involves the prevention of thrombus formation. As in the therapy to prevent thrombus, the mainstay of treatment of emboli requires the proper administration of systemic anticoagulants (i.e., heparin or warfarin). Additionally, the prevention of infections within the TAH, which sometimes appear as a nidus for thrombus growth, helps to lower the incidence of embolization.

Once thrombus becomes established within the TAH, whether or not it is infected, the results of embolization are disastrous. Manifestations of emboli can be seen in either the systemic or pulmonary system depending on the side of the artificial heart from which they originate. Some of the signs and symptoms include hematuria, melena, neurological changes, abdominal distress, and pulmonary hypertension or insufficiency. Treatment includes the systemic anticoagulation along with extraction of the emboli (if clinically feasible) and localization of the source of the emboli. Localization is most important, since the risk of further embolization and eventual death is very high. The patient potentially needs to undergo surgery for removal and replacement of the portion of the TAH that harbors the thrombus. Despite the necessity of surgical intervention in the human recipient of the TAH, this approach has never been successfully carried out in the animal model. However, there has been successful reoperations for removal of hemodynamically significant pannus,[5] and the experience gained benefits management of potential thrombus problems in the human recipient.

Calcification. Dystrophic calcification of the blood-contacting surface in the J-7 TAH employed in calves has been a nagging problem. This process is present to some degree in nearly 75% of TAH calves at a median age of 75 days. However, hemodynamically significant calcification usually does not occur until after the TAH calf has survived more than 3 months.

Severe calcification of the blood-pumping diaphragm markedly impedes its mobility, resulting in a nearly rigid device with poor hemodynamic performance. Eventually this complication results in a cracking of the diaphragm that can lead to rupture of the Biomer and the death of the animal (Fig. 33-30).

The cause of this calcification has been difficult to determine. It is well known that the growing, immature calf rapidly calcifies artificial surfaces ranging from polyurethane to porcine xenograft heart valves. This parallels the experience in children who also calcify the flexion points of xenograft cardiac valves in a relatively short period of time.[6] Adult sheep are being used in TAH experiments at the University of Utah; it is hypothesized that their calcium metabolism will be less dynamic and destructive than that of adolescent calves. Preliminary results appear encouraging with less significant calcium deposits

Calcium

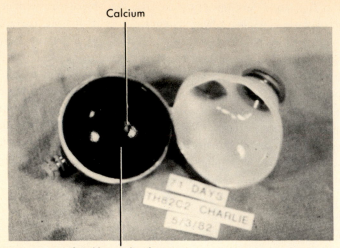

Artificial heart diaphragm

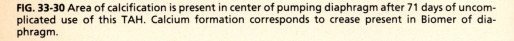

FIG. 33-30 Area of calcification is present in center of pumping diaphragm after 71 days of uncomplicated use of this TAH. Calcium formation corresponds to crease present in Biomer of diaphragm.

found on the pumping diaphragm in long-term sheep survivors as compared to calves. Ideally this improvement will also be seen in the adult human recipients of the TAH; however, this remains unknown. Additional biochemical investigations are underway in an effort to further delineate this problem.

Defects in the segmented polyurethane blood-pumping surface, such as cracks, microbubbles, and foreign substances, also serve as a nidus for calcification.[3] These imperfections can be minimized by the precise fabrication techniques and by elimination of any stress points on the diaphragm.

Some recent experimental results demonstrated inhibition of calcium deposition in xenograft cardiac valves in calves. In this work the xenograft material was washed with an organic-type soap consisting of a chemical called C-12 acyl-sulfate. This process inhibited calcium from destroying these biological valves during a 14-month period of use in calves. These remarkable results are currently undergoing further investigation in an effort to elucidate the mechanism of protection. Understanding this protective process and the pathogenesis of the abnormal calcium formation could lead to a process that would protect the Biomer of the TAH.

Mechanical failure. A criterion of the J-7 TAH that is extremely important with regard to its use in humans is its durability and reliability. Both of these areas have been evaluated in vitro and in vivo.

While constantly pumping water at physiological pressures on a mock circulation, the J-7 ventricle has successfully functioned for an equivalent of more than 4 years. Simultaneously the J-7 TAH continues to be used in animal experiments in which survival extends for several months. Mechanical failure of the J-7 heart is infrequently a cause of death in these animals. Yet occasionally a vital component malfunctions or breaks. The areas most susceptible to these problems include the mechanical valves, the pumping diaphragm, and the pneumatic drivelines. The tragedy of these failures stems from their lethal consequences in an otherwise healthy animal. Great care is taken to ensure against these problems during design and construction of the J-7 TAH. However, unpredictable and incorrectable malfunctions can develop and ultimately jeopardize the life of the recipient. Mechanical valve failure stems from the significantly higher dp/dt (change in pressure during changes in time, usually millimeters or mercury per second) of the J-7 ventricles as compared to the natural myocardium. The artificial ventricle dp/dt exceeds the native heart by several thousand millimeters of mercury per second. This added stress is a known factor in mechanical valve failure.

Heart transplantation

The idea that the patient receiving a TAH eventually undergoes a heart transplantation is a possibility but is not mandatory. In an effort to study this potential clinical situation, experiments involving twin calves have been conducted at the University of Utah.[20] One of the twins would have a J-7 TAH implanted as previously described in this chapter. After recovering from the operative procedure, the animal would be maintained with the TAH for a period of 30 to 70 days. With the calf in good health and acclimated to the TAH, it would undergo removal of the artificial heart. During this same operation the heart of its twin would then be implanted. Because of their genetic likeness, these transplant animals did not require any immunosuppression. Although some technical difficulties were encountered with the transplantation procedure initially, three long-term survivors have been produced in this experiment (Fig. 33-31). Following transplantation, no serious sequelae have been found in the recipient animals, and they continue to grow and be physiologically normal. This experience demonstrates the feasibility of using the TAH as an intermediate step in heart transplantation. It would offer several advantages: provide an increased pool of potential heart recipients; stabilize the clinical condition of the patient before the heart transplant, making the implantation of a cadaver myocardium safer; and allow more time for immunological and genetic testing.

The human recipients of the TAH at the University of Utah receive no guarantee regarding a future heart transplant. Postoperatively they would have the option to seek an evaluation from a transplant center. If they would be determined to be a good candidate and a donor heart was available, a heart transplant could be undertaken.

An example of a major difference in candidates for a TAH and a transplant is pulmonary hypertension. This disorder of elevated pulmonary vascular pressures, so commonly seen in heart disease, would not impair the function of the TAH. The artificial ventricle is able to generate enough force to overcome this abnormally increased pulmonary afterload. However, a transplanted heart would be severely stressed by such vascular resistance, and all too commonly it would result in right ventricular failure. Thus patients with this disorder are usually not considered as potential recipients of a heart transplant and yet remain candidates for a TAH.

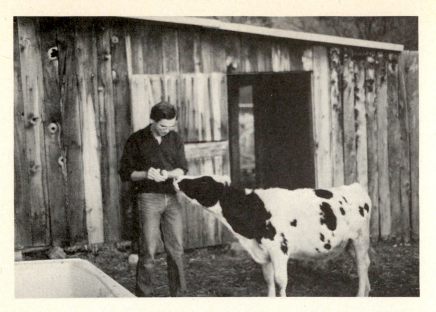

FIG. 33-31 Charlie, 198 days after his heart transplant. He was recipient of artificial heart for 71 days before transplant. At time of transplant, he weighed 96.5 kg, and at time of photo his weight was 182.5 kg.

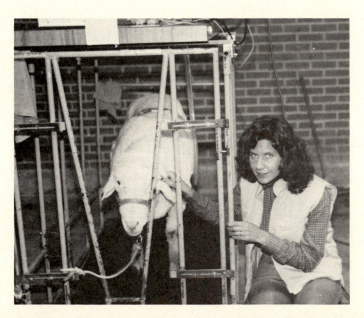

FIG. 33-32 Ted E. Bear. Longest surviving sheep recipient of TAH—297 days.

Animal outgrowing the TAH. The great majority of the implantations of the TAH have been performed using young calves as the recipients. These animals have been an excellent research model in several respects. Over the years a vast amount of information has been acquired regarding the physiological response of calves in the preoperative state as well as after TAH implantation. Simultaneously the details of the technique for implanting the TAH, the use of the cardiopulmonary bypass, and the immediate postoperative care have been studied and reported. This information has contributed to the ability to maintain calves with a TAH for up to 9 months.

Longer periods of survival are limited in calves because of rapid growth. The calves used for implantation of a TAH are 3 to 4 months old. At this age their size suits the requirements for proper fit of the TAH; their weight, however, is already 85 to 100 kg. They continue to grow after surgery at a rate of nearly 0.3 kg per day, reaching a weight that is 100 to 200 kg more than their operative weight. These full-grown animals require a cardiac output of about 60 ml/kg/min, which is far in excess of what the J-7 TAH can deliver. This in turn limits the long-term survival of the animal.

To circumvent this problem, TAHs have been implanted in sheep. They are of a size to accommodate the TAH (about 100 kg) as well as being nongrowing adults. Disadvantages recognized with sheep models include limited intensive study in their preoperative preparation, TAH implantation, and postoperative care. Experience, however, has already refined the techniques in the care of this animal. At the University of Utah a sheep received a TAH implant on June 2, 1982, and lived 297 days, a record for survival with a TAH (Fig. 33-32). Another sheep had survived for 169 days before succumbing to a mechanical failure. It is anticipated that in the future these animals will provide long-term survivors (>1 year) that can be studied to elucidate problems that may develop in this advanced time frame.

Improvements in the pneumatic heart

The basic design and function of the J-7 TAH have been found to be excellent in the experimental animal. Yet improvements are being continually made in the design, production, implantation, and postoperative care of the University of Utah TAH. In conjunction with these advancements, new problem areas are discovered that require investigation and correction. Many of these areas have already been addressed under various headings in the previous sections of this chapter.

One of the most significant recent innovations deals with the heart driver and compressed air source. Air used to operate the pneumatic TAH has routinely been supplied via large air compressors or pressurized air tanks. Both of these sources are too large and bulky to permit any freedom to the TAH recipient. Additionally, the standard Utah heart driver limits the mobility of the TAH patient. However, these obstacles have been overcome by engineers at the University of Utah's Division of Artificial Organs. They have designed and built a portable heart driver and compressed air source that fit into a standard camera case. The compressed air is produced from a small piston and the power from batteries that last for more than 3 hours. The system has been successfully employed with the experimental animal, permitting the animal to walk outside free of encumbering

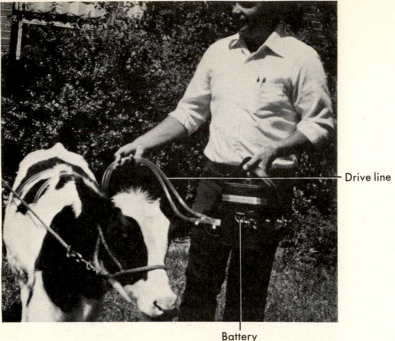

Drive line

Battery
and compressed
air source

FIG. 33-33 Calf recipient of TAH, walking with portable heart driver and compressed air source contained in camera case.

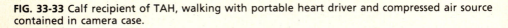

devices (Fig. 33-33). Although this breakthrough does not eliminate the air drivelines exiting from the chest, it does permit the human recipient the luxury of increased mobility and the joys derived from this freedom.

Electrohydraulic heart

Despite the success of the pneumatic TAH in the experimental setting, its application in humans exposes some less than optimal characteristics. Using air as the driving force permits the TAH to be reliable, efficient, and versatile in its response to the ever changing needs of the recipient. However, the use of a pneumatic system dictates the need for two large drivelines exiting the chest, as well as a relatively large power source and heart driver (see improvements of the pneumatic heart).

In an effort to improve on the TAH's power source, experiments have been ongoing at the University of Utah, employing an electrohydraulic system (Fig. 33-34).[8] A brushless DC motor, the size of a flashlight battery, powers a turbine-like impeller that pumps silicon fluid back and forth between the right and left ventricles. This turbine and motor are capable of producing a speed of 10,000 revolutions per minute in one direction, and in less than 25 msec they can reverse direction and achieve the same speed in the opposite direction. This rapid shifting of hydraulic fluid results in an asynchronous pumping of the

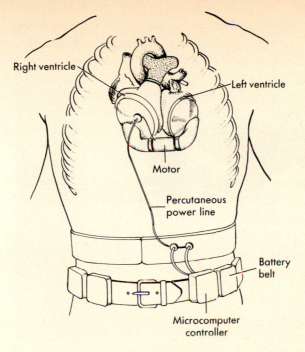

FIG. 33-34 Electrohydraulic heart. Prospective arrangement of system with human implant. Power source is from batteries worn on belt and transmitted through transcutaneous cable. (Modified from Jarvik, R.K.: Am. **244**:74, 1981.)

ventricular diaphragm; that is, when the right heart is in systole, the left heart is in diastole and vice versa. In essence the hydraulic fluid replaces the air used to eject blood in the pneumatic TAH. A controlling system has been designed to maintain proper balance of both sides of the heart, thus providing proper cardiac outputs for the pulmonary and systemic circulation.

Advantages of this system include (1) complete implantability of the heart and motor in the mediastinum, (2) a single exiting cable that attaches to a belt of batteries or an electrical outlet and a pacemaker-sized controller, (3) elimination of pneumatic drivelines and compressed air requirements, and (4) the use of two J-7 ventricles that employ the successful and reliable technology demonstrated in the pneumatic TAH.

Extensive testing of the electrohydraulic heart in vitro and in vivo is necessary before it can be considered for human use. Most importantly, an automatic control system is imperative to reliably adjust the motor speed and the duration of systole and diastole in each ventricle. This system must sense and respond to the recipient's circulatory needs on a beat-to-beat basis to be successful.

New devices

Despite the success and continued improvement in the University of Utah's TAH, new devices are continually sought that might provide a better replacement for the diseased human heart.

The concept of leaving the native myocardium in situ and providing mechanical circulatory support is not new. However, in the past these devices were usually a singular artificial ventricle placed extrathoracically and used temporarily until the natural heart could sustain the circulation (Chapter 32). Recently a design has been proposed at the University of Utah by Kolff that incorporates two flattened J-7-like ventricles. These ventricles would be placed on either side of the native heart permanently. Air would be employed to drive the ventricular diaphragms, and the same Utah heart driver could be used to regulate function. The advantage of this design is the retaining of the patient's heart.

A revolutionary innovation is the design, construction, and preliminary evaluation of a magnetically suspended rotary blood pump.[2] Simplistically this system consists of a rotor placed in the bloodstream and suspended by a magnetic field. As the magnetic field is sequentially altered electronically, the rotor can be made to spin and thus pump blood. This system provides continuous nonpulsatile blood flow that appears to be well tolerated by animals for long periods of time. Major advantages include (1) no moving parts that undergo wear; (2) only the rotor in contact with blood; (3) no need for valves, pumping diaphragms, or bulky ventricles; and (4) a single, small cord exiting the chest for electrical power and appropriate control mechanisms.

Human implantation of the J-7 TAH

Human implantation of the J-7 TAH took place on December 2, 1982, at the University of Utah Medical Center. The artificial heart was implanted in a patient with cardiomyopathy. The cause of this pathological situation can be diverse, but the manifestations are the same—a failing myocardium. This failure is usually a slow but progressive deterioration of the heart's pumping ability.

With great deliberation and extensive education about the J-7 TAH, including a visit to the artificial heart laboratories at the University of Utah, the patient decided to have the J-7 artificial heart implanted when his own myocardium became ineffective in supporting life. A heart transplant was another potential treatment for this end-stage heart disease. However, the patient's age of 61 years excluded him from this procedure.

The surgery, as described earlier in this chapter, was performed by a team of surgeons at the University of Utah. Although the implantation was tedious, its success can be attributed to the vast experience derived from many animal experimental implants of the TAH, performed by Drs. Olsen, DeVries, and Joyce. The most significant technical difference in the human implantation of the artificial heart, as compared to research animals, stems from the chronically debilitated state of the recipient's other organs and tissues.

All experimental calves and sheep are healthy when undergoing the TAH operation, whereas the human patient had suffered years of deteriorating heart function that affected other organs. Also his need for steroids resulted in tissues becoming very delicate and friable, thus making suturing during the surgical procedure more difficult.

The postoperative recovery was slow with various problems arising, which necessitated three additional operations. However, all of these difficulties, including a pneumothorax, fractured mitral valve, seizures, and prolonged epistaxis, were corrected before any irreparable harm was suffered by the patient. Only the tremendous experience and knowledge of the TAH possessed by the physicians and scientists caring for this patient allowed for such serious and life-threatening problems to be successfully corrected.

The TAH performed well during its 112 days of pumping. Sepsis, secondary to pseudo membranous colitis, was the ultimate cause of death. Postmortem examination of the TAH revealed no infection, thrombus calcification, or pannus or mechanical failures.

The wealth of information gained from this initial human experience provides unique data concerning the manner in which the human body operates when cardiac function remains optimal at all times. Also, new areas of animal research have been instituted to further explore mechanisms of how certain problems developed in this patient.

In addition to the mechanical aspects of the TAH, concerns have been voiced regarding economical and ethical issues. These areas will require more in depth investigations and future policy decisions. However, with this initial success, the future of the Utah TAH appears optimistic.

Conclusion

The TAH is not meant to be a substitute for the normal myocardium. The magnificence of the natural heart has been underscored by the difficulty that has been encountered in mechanically duplicating its performance. Rather the TAH is science's effort to replace a diseased and failing organ with a device that will improve the recipient's quality of life.

As a research tool, the TAH has been invaluable in a wide variety of disciplines ranging from polymer chemistry to circulatory physiology. This time consuming, demanding, and at times frustrating research has been responsible for making the University of Utah's TAH suitable for human implantation. However, the use of this mechanical heart in humans does not indicate that this device is perfect or that research can no longer be useful. On the contrary, the basic scientific investigations must continue in an effort to further improve the TAH as well as deal with difficulties that will undoubtedly continue to arise in the clinical setting.

The information detailed in this chapter has been derived primarily from the investigative group at the University of Utah's Division of Artificial Organs, in addition to various scientific publications. These researcher's talents and efforts have set the stage for human application of the TAH. As the clinical team that implants the TAH receives the accolades of the patients and the public, this handful of unpublicized researchers take quiet satisfaction that their labors have resulted in a device that will help others.

REFERENCES

1. Akutsu, T., et al.: Permanent substitutes for valves and hearts, ASAIO **4**:230, 1958.
2. Bramm, P., et al.: A free-floating body as the rotor of a centrifugal blood pump for LVAD or TAH, Int. J. Artif. Organs **6**:161, 1982.
3. Coleman, D.E., et al.: Calcification of nontextured implantable blood pumps, Trans. Am. Soc. Artif. Intern. Organs **27**:97, 1981.
4. Foote, J., et al.: Quick-change connections for the artificial heart (abstract), Am. Soc. Artif. Intern. Organs **5**:26, 1976.
5. Fukumasu, H., et al.: Re-operative surgery in calves with a total artificial heart, Int. J. Artif. Organs **3**:24, 1980.

6. Geha, A.S., et al.: Late failure of procine valve heterografts in children, J. Thorac. Cardiovasc. Surg. **78:**351, 1979.
7. Iwaya, F., et al.: Studies of the remnant atria of the total artificial heart: P-wave response to surgery, treadmill exercise and drugs, J. Artif. Organs Suppl. **3:**324, 1979.
8. Jarvik, R.K.: The total artificial heart, Sci. Am. **244:**74, 1981.
9. Jarvik, R.K., et al.: Determinants of pannus formation in long-term surviving artificial heart calves, and its prevention, Trans. Am. Soc. Artif. Intern. Organs **27:**901, 1981.
10. Kessler, T.R., et al.: Elimination of predilection sites for thrombus formation in the total artificial heart—before and after, Trans. Am. Soc. Artif. Intern. Organs **24:**532, 1978.
11. Kusserow, B.K., et al.: Decreased reticuloendothelial phagocytic function following prolonged *in vivo* blood pumping—preliminary observations, Trans. Am. Soc. Artif. Intern. Organs **21:**388, 1975.
12. Murray, K.D.: Infection in total artifical heart recipients, Trans. Am. Soc. Artif. Organs **29:**(In press), 1983.
13. Murshita, J., et al.: Current major problems in long-survival animals with pneumatic total artificial hearts, ASAIO, 1983. (In press.)
14. Olsen, D.B.: The total artificial heart—a research tool for potential clinical reality. In Unger, F., editor: Assisted circulation, New York, 1979, Springer-Verlag.
15. Olsen, D.B., and DeVries, W.D.: The experimental total artificial heart in transition to the clinical arena, Proc. Int. Soc. Artif. Organs **5:**40, 1981.
16. Olsen, D.B., et al.: Saving the aortic and pulmonary artery valves with the total artificial heart replacement, Trans. Am. Soc. Artif. Intern. Organs **22:**468, 1976.
17. Olsen, D.B., et al.: Implantation of the total artificial heart by lateral thoracotomy, Artif. Organs **1:**92, 1977.
18. Olsen, D.B., et al.: The noncardiac intrinsic autoregulation of tissue perfusion in calves with total artificial hearts, Trans. Europ. Soc. Artif. Organs **4:**263, 1977.
19. Olsen, D.B., et al.: Fabrication, implantation and pathophysiology of the total artificial heart in calves for six months. In Pierce, W.S., editor: Circulatory assistance and the artificial heart, USA-USSR joint symposium, Tbilisi, USSR, Pub. No. 80-2032, Washington, D.C., 1980, National Institute of Health—Department of Health and Human Services.
20. Olsen, D.B., et al.: Artificial heart implantation, later cardiac transplantation in the calf, Trans. Am. Soc. Artif. Intern. Organs **27:**132, 1981.
21. Paping, R., et al.: White blood cell phagocytosis after artificial heart implantation, Trans. Am. Soc. Artif. Intern. Organs **24:**578, 1978.

Glossary

Actin filament Thin, protein, oval-shaped filament of the myocardial cell that communicates with another filament, myosin, during cardiac muscle contraction.

Action potential Electrical changes across the cell membrane.

Adrenergic receptors Tissue-receptor sites responding to catecholamine-mediated stimuli.

Afterload Resistance against which the left ventricle must eject its volume of blood during systole.

Allen test Test for patency of the radial artery that contains an indwelling catheter.

Alpha receptor Tissue receptor, when stimulated, causes arteriolar vasoconstriction, gastrointestinal and genitourinary sphincter constriction, glycogenolysis, and sweat gland activity.

Augmented diastolic pressure Increase in diastolic pressure that occurs with inflation of the intra-aortic balloon.

Beta receptor Tissue receptor that, when stimulated, causes increased cardiac impulse generation and conduction in the sinoatrial and atrioventricular nodes, enhanced myocardial contractility, dilation of arteriolar and bronchial smooth muscles, promotion of insulin and renin secretion, and stimulation of lipolysis and lactate production.

Biomer Registered patented name for a specific type of segmented polyurethane; it is a medical grade of the elastic material Lycra.

Bubble oxygenator Heart-lung bypass device that oxygenates the blood that is diverted outside the body into this machine.

Calibration Applying a known amount of mercury pressure to a transducer to assess transducer accuracy.

Cardiac index Cardiac output per square meter of body surface area.

$$\text{Cardiac index} = \frac{\text{Cardiac output}}{\text{Body surface area}} = 2.4 \text{ to } 4.0 \text{ liters/min/m}^2$$

Cardiac output Amount of blood pumped by a ventricle during 1 minute. It is determined by stroke volume and heart rate.

COMDU Cardiac output monitor and diagnostic unit. Using the pneumotachometer plus a computer, the air exhausted from the artificial ventricle can be used to determine the stroke volume of each heart beat as well as disclose functional data regarding the total artificial heart's performance.

Coronary autoregulation Process of coronary artery vasodilation in response to myocardial ischemia.

Counterpulsation Raising of the intra-aortic pressure in diastole by inflation of an intra-aortic balloon and deflation of the balloon with rapid withdrawal of the inflating gas, just before the next systole. Balloon inflation and deflation occur in opposition with systole and diastole.

Damping Property of an oscillatory system that diminishes and eventually arrests the fluctuations recorded from closure of a flush device.

Depolarization Reduction of a membrane potential to a less negative value.

Dopaminergic Stimulates the dopamine receptors in the kidney, which causes renal vasculature to dilate.

dp/dt Rate of pressure rise with respect to time. d, Change; p, pressure; and t, time.

Driving pressure Amount of compressed air (millimeters of mercury) used to eject blood from the artificial heart's ventricles during systole.

dv/dt Rate of change of voltage with respect to time. d, Change; v, voltage; t, time.

Dynamic cardiac work Energy transfer that occurs during the process of ventricular ejection.

Dynamic response Fidelity with which the physiological monitoring system will simulate the hemo-dynamic event recorded; it is determined by driving the system with a known input signal and observing the oscillatory ringing response.

Ejection fraction Index of left ventricular function; the percentage of total ventricular volume that is ejected during each ventricular contraction. Normal, 65%.

Electrohydraulic heart Jarvik-7 artificial heart that is modified so that no longer is air used to drive the artificial ventricles but rather the alternate pumping of hydraulic fluid by a compact electrical motor. This entire device is implantable with only one cord exiting the chest for electrical power and control of the heart's performance.

External counterpulsation Noninvasive method for providing counterpulsation consisting of encasement of the legs in a rigid case housing a water-filled bladder. Using the electrocardiogram for timing, the bladder and sequentially the legs are pressurized pneumatically during diastole.

Extracorporeal circulation Heart-lung bypass circulation, whereby venous blood is diverted outside the body to a mechanical oxygenator and is returned to the body through a cannula in the aorta or femoral artery.

Extrinsic control of the total artificial heart Measurements that can be adjusted on the Utah heart driver, which control the function of the total artificial heart.

Fick method of cardiac output determination Uptake of oxygen by the body is the product of the body's blood flow rate and its arterial mixed venous oxygen difference. The formula for cardiac output determination by Fick is:

$$CO \text{ (liters/min)} = \frac{\text{Oxygen consumption in ml/min}}{\text{Arterial-venous oxygen content difference}}$$

Frank-Starling law of the heart The greater the stretch on the myocardial fibers before contraction, the greater the force of contraction up to a certain physiological point.

Frequency Number of cycles of a particular wave that is generated per second.

Hydrostatic pressure Weight exerted by any object resting on a surface.

In situ To be in the natural or original position.

In vitro Performed outside the body of a living animal and in an experimental setting.

In vivo Performed inside the body of a living animal.

Inotropic Increasing the force of myocardial contraction.

Intercalated disk Boundary that separates each cardiac cell.

Intramural Within the walls of a hollow organ or cavity.

Intrinsic control of the total artificial heart Physiological changes that influence the function of the total artificial heart.

Isovolumic contraction Early phase of systole whereby the left ventricle is generating enough tension to overcome the resistance of the aortic end-diastolic pressure.

Jarvik-7 Pneumatic, ellipsoidal artificial heart designed by R.K. Jarvik for use in humans.

Laminar flow Airflow concentrated into a narrow pathway.

Laplace's law Law of physics that states that the tension on the wall of a chamber is the product of the pressure in the chamber times the radius of the chamber.

Left ventricular assist device (LVAD) Mechanical pump that temporarily and artificially rests the pumping action of the left ventricle.

Mediastinum Central portion of the chest cavity bounded by the right and left pleura and the diaphragm. The middle of this space is occupied by the heart.

Mitochondria Cylindrical bodies found arranged systematically between and in close approximation to the parallel rows of contractile units in the cell. Oxidative phosphorylation, the process by which adenosine triphosphate is produced with the energy contained in carbohydrates, lipids, and proteins, occurs within the mitochondria.

Morbidity Number of cases of a specific disease in a calendar year per 100,000 population.

Mortality Death rate.

Myofibril Small group of branching longitudinal, striated strands found in muscular tissue, running parallel to the cellular long axis, from one cell to another.

Myosin Protein present in muscle fibrils that is in the shape of a rod with a globular enlargement at one end. These proteins come together with another protein, actin, in a sliding mechanism during cardiac contraction.

Overdriving Providing excess compressed air to the artificial heart's ventricle during systole, given the corresponding end-diastolic blood volume.

Pannus Abnormal growth of dense fibrous tissue found at the remnant atria suture lines, which interfere with diastolic filling of earlier total artificial hearts.

Pattern logic Feature of the Kontron intra-aortic balloon pump in which the QRS complex is recognized on a width basis.

Peak logic Feature of the Kontron pump in which any positive waveform is recognized to trigger the pump.

Percent systole Amount of time of each heartbeat devoted to the ejection of blood from the ventricle. This measurement is adjusted using the heart driver.

Phlebostatic axis Approximate location of the right atrium, found by drawing an imaginary line from the fourth intercostal space to the right of the sternum, crossed with the midaxillary line.

Pinocytotic Vessels that are capable of absorbing liquids by phagocytosis and are presumably involved in cellular metabolism.

Pneumatic heart driver Mechanical device that regulates compressed air delivery to the artificial heart and controls heart rate, percent systole, and delay in systole.

Pneumotachometer Small cylindrical device that measures the change in pressure from the exhausting air of the artificial ventricle. The pressure gradient is directly related to flow, thus allowing the computer to derive an exhaust flow curve (liters/min) for use by the COMDU.

Preload Ventricular end-diastolic volume.

Pulmonary vascular resistance (PVR) Resistance in the pulmonary vascular bed against which the right ventricle must eject.

$$PVR = \frac{\text{Mean pulmonary artery pressure} - \text{Pulmonary artery wedge pressure}}{\text{Cardiac output}}$$

Normal, 0.5 to 1.0 unit

Pulsatile assist device (PAD) Flexible valveless balloon conduit contained within a rigid plastic cylinder that is inserted into the arterial line close to the aortic root of an extracorporeal circuit to provide pulsatile cardiopulmonary bypass perfusion.

Pulsus alternans Alteration in the peripheral arterial pulse (strong alternating with a weak pulse), despite a regular rhythm, observed in patients with myocardial dysfunction.

Quick connect Plastic push-fit connector is first sewn to the native structures of the recipient (atria, aorta, and pulmonary artery). A plastic lip found on the artificial ventricle is securely snapped onto a plastic ledge of the quick connect, thus forming a strong, watertight bond.

Renin Protein formed in an ischemic kidney, which acts as an enzyme in a chain of events that finally produces a potent vasoconstrictor, angiotensin.

Resistance Opposition to force. In the vascular system the retardation of blood flow caused by constriction of peripheral vessels.

Sarcolemma Cell membrane.

Sarcomere Portion of a striated muscle fibril lying between two adjacent dark lines considered to be the contractile unit.

Sarcoplasmic reticulum Intracellular system of tubules, which forms a membrane-limited network around each fibril in muscular tissue. Calcium is bound within the sarcoplasmic reticulum. When a wave of depolarization spreads throughout the sarcoplasmic reticulum, calcium is released.

Skin button Inverted piece of Silastic tubing covered externally with Teflon and a felt collar attached perpendicularly at the midpoint of the tubing. This device covers the drivelines of the total artificial heart at their exit point from the skin and eliminates pressure transmission to the surrounding tissues.

Static cardiac work Energy transfer that occurs during the development and maintenance of ventricular pressure before the opening of the aortic valve.

Stroke volume Volume of blood ejected with each heartbeat and governed by afterload, preload, and contractility. Stroke volume equals cardiac output divided by heart rate.

Stroke volume index Stroke volume divided by body surface area.

Sympathetic amine drug Produces effects resembling those manifested from stimulation of the sympathetic nervous system.

Syncytium Group of cells in which the protoplasm of one cell is continuous with that of adjoining cells.

Systemic vascular resistance (SVR) Resistance against which the left ventricle must eject to force out its stroke volume with each beat. As the peripheral vessels constrict, the SVR increases.

$$SVR = \frac{\text{Mean arterial pressure} - \text{Right atrial pressure}}{\text{Cardiac output}} = 12 \text{ to } 18 \text{ units}$$

Or above formula $\times$ 80 = 900 to 1500 dynes/sec/cm^{-5}

T-tubule system Originates from invaginations along the surface of the myocardial cell membrane and provides an extension of the cell membrane into the cell. It is a storehouse for calcium and may be involved with the movement of substrates into the cell and the removal of metabolic end products from the cell.

Thermal dilution Method of cardiac output determination. A bolus of a solution (volume and temperature are known) is added to the bloodstream. The resultant cooling of blood temperature is sensed by the thermister, located at the tip of a catheter placed in the pulmonary artery.

Transducer Instrument that converts a patient's physiological pressure into an electrical signal.

Troponin Protein in the myocardial cell ultrastructure that modulates the interaction between actin and myosin by binding with calcium.

Underdamping Transmission of all frequency components without a reduction in amplitude.

Underdriving Providing insufficient compressed air during systole to eject the entire end-diastolic volume of the artificial heart's ventricle.

Ventriculography Opacification of the ventricular cavity with contrast medium during heart catheterization.

Windkessel effect During systole the aorta stretches to accommodate the stroke volume ejected. Energy that was stored propels this volume out into the peripheral arterial tree during diastole.

Index

Pump failure—cont'd
  methoxamine in treatment of, 67
  nitrates in treatment of, 74-75
  phentolamine in treatment of, 75
  prazosin in treatment of, 75
  sodium nitroprusside in treatment of, 74
  Tridil in treatment of, 74-75
  vasodilator agents in treatment of, 74-75
  vasopressors
    combined use of vasodilator drugs and, in treat-
        ment of, 75
    and intra-aortic balloon pumping, comparison of
        treatment of, with, 88
Pump function, effects of
  arteriolar vasodilation on, 72, 73-75
  venodilation on, 73-76
Pyruvate, 39

Q

Quick connects in Jarvik-7 total artificial heart, 356-
    358

R

RA pressure waveform, 192-193, 198, 199
Reflex vasoconstriction in cardiogenic shock, 60, 61
Removal
  of balloon; *see* Balloon in intra-aortic balloon
      pumping, removal of
  of left ventricular device, 344
Renal function
  adjustments in, in heart failure, 56-59
  effect of intra-aortic balloon pumping on, 107-
      108
  of patient with left ventricular assist device, 346
Renal perfusion, effect of pulsatile flow versus non-
    pulsatile flow on, 312
Renin-angiotensin mechanism in heart failure, 57,
    59
Repolarization, 8-9
Respiratory care of patient with left ventricular assist
    device, 346
Retrograde insertion of balloon in intra-aortic balloon
    pumping; *see* Balloon in intra-aortic balloon
    pumping, insertion of, retrograde
Right atrium, 6, 7
Right coronary artery; *see* Coronary artery, right
Right heart failure and left ventricular assist device,
    344
Right ventricle, 6, 7
Right ventricular failure, 44-47
Right-sided failure, 44, 49
  as reflected on pressures in series circuit, 47, 48
RV pressure waveform, 194

S

Safe timing in intra-aortic balloon pumping, function-
    al range of, 132-133
Sarcolemma, 28, 29
Sarcomere, 30
Sarcoplasmic reticulum, 32
Sarcotubular system, 32
Sarns heart-lung machine, 326
Sarns pulsatile flow pump, 309, 311
Sensory deprivation, potential for, nursing care of
    patient with intra-aortic balloon pump and,
    239
Sequential external counterpulsation pumping, 324
Shock
  cardiogenic; *see* Cardiogenic shock
  myocardial infarction following, use of external
      counterpulsation in, 321
  myocardial infarction without, use of external coun-
      terpulsation in, 321
Sinuses of Valsalva, 17-21
Skin button, 372, 378
Skinner device, 336
SMEC Model 1300, 275-279
  abbreviated operator's manual for, 277-278
  improper timing for, 150
  pacemaker signal for, 179-180, 181-182
  specifications for, 275-277
  timing of intra-aortic balloon pump for, 136-139,
      143-144
Sodium nitroprusside (Nipride)
  and dopamine in combination with intra-aortic bal-
      loon pumping, 92-93
  in treatment of pump failure, 74
Sodium-potassium adenosine-triphosphate (ATPase),
    75-76
Staircase effect, 14
Staple graft closure after removal of balloon, 300,
    301
Starling response of Jarvik-7 total artificial heart, 366,
    367
Starling's curve of heart, 14, 209
Static external dynamic work, 39-41
Stenosis, coronary artery, effect of intra-aortic balloon
    pumping on myocardial blood flow distal to,
    99
Strain-gauge transducer in hemodynamic monitoring,
    219
Stroke volume, 11, 206
Stroke volume index, 206
Stroke work index, 208
Subclavian artery approach for insertion of balloon in
    intra-aortic balloon pumping, 120
Surgery
  cardiac; *see* Cardiac surgery